D1488570

The Powerful Placebo

The Powerful Placebo

From Ancient Priest to Modern Physician

ARTHUR K. SHAPIRO, M.D.

and

ELAINE SHAPIRO, PH.D.

The Johns Hopkins University Press

Baltimore and London

06 05 04 03 02 01 00 99 98 97   5 4 3 2 1

The Johns Hopkins University Press
2715 North Charles Street
Baltimore, Maryland 21218-4319
The Johns Hopkins Press Ltd., London

A previous version of Chapter 2 was published in A. K. Shapiro,
"Semantics of the Placebo," *Psychiatric Quarterly* 42:653–95.
Portions of chapter 11 also appear in *The Placebo Effect,* edited
by Anne Harrington (Cambridge: Harvard University Press, 1997).

Library of Congress Cataloging-in-Publication Data will be
found at the end of this book.
A catalog record for this book is available from the British Library.

ISBN 0-8018-5569-1

To our children, Peter, Moira, and Kaethe,
and their children, Laura, Elisa, and Paige

Contents

Preface and Acknowledgments

In 1953, while a second-year medical student with time on my hands because of a hospitalization for infectious mononucleosis, I began to study the psychiatric literature. I became intrigued by the frequency with which new treatments were announced with enthusiasm and fanfare, followed by several supporting papers, only to disappear from the literature and eventually reappear in a new guise. I saw the same phenomenon in the frequent announcements of crucial discoveries in the treatment of psychiatric and other disorders.

My readings revealed numerous references to the work of Henry Beecher, Stewart Wolf, and Harry Gold. My pursuit of their writings opened up for me a whole new area of interest and amazement, the powerful placebo effect. This phenomenon also stimulated my interest in the importance of controlled methodology, especially the double-blind procedure, a method to control the placebo effect of treatment. The double-blind procedure was used in many studies of antipsychotic, antidepressant, and antianxiety agents and drugs introduced in the 1950s, and eventually in studies of psychotherapy. The development of reliable and valid methods of evaluating such studies became major areas of research in the 1950s, 1960s, and 1970s.

I continued my interest in the placebo effect during my residency at the Boston Psychopathic Hospital (now the Massachusetts Mental Health Center), notably with the excellent guidance and support of Harry C. Solomon, M.D., chair of the Mental Health Center, and Milton Greenblatt, M.D., director of research. Dr. Daniel Levinson (also of the department), and Dr. Greenblatt published an article on the placebo effect with which I assisted, and I was very gratified to find they had included my name as one of the authors. Dr. Greenblatt encouraged my research by providing facilities, including a separate research office and patient volunteers to assist in typing the very large reference file that I had by then collected about the placebo effect.

I wrote a paper about the history of the placebo in medical treatment, which was accepted by the *American Journal of Psychiatry* before I completed my residency. Other papers were accepted by various journals. Most gratifying to me was the publication of a long scholarly article, "A Contribution to the History of the Placebo Effect," published by the *Behavioral Science Journal* at the University of Michigan. It has been printed twice in the *Congressional Record* and re-published once in the monthly journal *Classic of the Month*.

Of great importance to my pursuit of understanding of the placebo effect was the support I received from Dr. William Lhamon, chair of the Department of Psychiatry at Cornell University Medical College. Dr. Lhamon proposed that my wife and I join the department in the 1960s. At last I had an affiliation that provided encouragement, research space, and some financial support, as well as an intellectually gifted and curious chair's interest in our research. Within a short time the Placebo Studies Laboratory (later renamed the Special Studies Laboratory) was officially established at the Payne Whitney Psychiatric Clinic, at the New York Hospital–Cornell University Medical Center. Its main purpose was to study the placebo effect of treatment and the methodology necessary to control for this effect.

My studies on the placebo effect were initially supported by a grant from the National Institute of Mental Health. A large sustaining grant from Hoffman-LaRoche supported studies contributing to the improvement of methodology for the evaluation of new drugs, as well as well-controlled studies of drugs of interest to Hoffman-LaRoche. Many other grants were obtained throughout the years. This was an especially fruitful and productive period.

I continued some of the placebo research at the Division of Epidemiology at Columbia University, with the collaboration of Elmer Struening, Ph.D. Somewhat later, I also relied on the advice of Dr. James Schmeidler, a statistician in the Mount Sinai Department of Psychiatry. Dr. Struening's participation, which had extended over many years, came to an end as funding decreased and his other interests became paramount. I am greatly indebted to Dr. Struening, who was instrumental in the original design and data analysis of my placebo research.

In the 1990s I again began to plan the present volume on the placebo. My work on the book took longer than had been anticipated. During 1994 I became ill with cancer, which limited my ability to work, and by 1995 it had become impossible to continue working. In addition, the historical research, the statistical analysis of the data, and the need to review and integrate voluminous documentation and references was time consuming. The more thoroughly each detail was checked, the more details became available for checking. Over time I came to the conclusion that it would be impossible to satisfy my obsessive desire to confirm every detail. I hope that any remaining errors are outweighed by otherwise correct conclusions about the data.

I would also like to thank the following individuals who consented to be interviewed about the development of the double-blind method and controlled clinical trials: Dr. Harry Gold, Dr. Nathaniel Kwit, Dr. McKeen Cattell, Dr. Walter Modell, Dr. Stewart Wolf, Dr. Ted Greiner, Dr. Oskar Diethelm, Dr. Harry Marks, Dr. Muriel Gold Morris, Dr. Walter Riker, Dr. John Bull, Sir A. Bradford Hill, Dr. P. Pichot, and Dr. D. Lawrence. Adele A. Lerner, archivist at Cornell, steered us through that institution's labyrinthine medical archives. I am indebted to all of them for their gracious and unstinted help. I am also indebted to Dr. Ted Greiner, Dr. Stewart Wolf, and Dr. Muriel Morris for their helpful criticisms of selected chapters of this book.

In addition to those mentioned above, I wish to express my gratitude to the following individuals who contributed to these studies: Gail Brody, M.A., Louis Morris, Ph.D., Gerald Raabe, M.S., and Drs. Kurt Rawitt, Theodore Finkle, Jerome Haber, and Jack Chassan.

ARTHUR K. SHAPIRO
Clinical Professor
Department of Psychiatry
Mount Sinai School of Medicine
New York, New York

I began my collaboration with my husband in 1966 at Cornell University Medical College. In the 1990s, we began our voluminous research, the analysis of the data, and the writing of the present volume. It is my deepest sorrow that my husband's untimely death in 1995 prevented him from completing the manuscript and seeing it in published form. In the light of his abiding, almost forty-year-long interest in unraveling the mystery of the placebo effect, I can think of no greater testimony to his dedication than my completion of this volume as a legacy to him. I hope I have done so in a worthy manner.

ELAINE SHAPIRO
Associate Clinical Professor
Department of Psychiatry
Mount Sinai School of Medicine
New York, New York

The Powerful Placebo

chapter one

The Placebo Effect in Medical History

I t is a mystery how a ubiquitous treatment used since antiquity was unknown, unnamed, and unidentified until recently. It is even more remarkable because this is the only treatment common to all societies and cultures. When we examine the long history of medicine, it is the only common denominator between the Egyptian physician who prescribed crocodile dung and the modern physician who prescribes penicillin. Moreover, its effectiveness has been attested to, without exception, for more than two millennia.

One of the many secrets enshrouding this remarkable treatment is that when its effectiveness wanes, it metamorphoses into a new, seemingly different, and culturally more appropriate form of effective treatment—somewhat as bacteria develop a resistance to antibiotics. Trousseau (1833) discerned this covert mischievousness in the middle of the nineteenth century, and he urged healers to hurry and use new drugs while they still worked.

The treatment, however, is not limited to drugs. It can take the form not only of oral, parenteral, and topical drugs but also of magic; religious rituals (such as prayer and exorcism); incantation; intubation or incubation; purgation (in the form of clysterization, phlebotomy, catharsis, vomachics, diaphoretics, and other forms of dehydration or reduction of guilt by ridding the body of the bad or evil); and cleansing the mind by talking out the evil (as in psychoanalysis and psychotherapy). The medium for these myriad treatments, of course, is the placebo, and the underlying matrix for its effectiveness is the powerful placebo effect.

What is a placebo? Briefly defined, a placebo is any treatment (including drugs, surgery, psychotherapy, and quack therapy) that is used for its ameliorative effect on a symptom or disease but that actually is ineffective or is not specifically effective for the condition being treated. The placebo effect, then, is primarily the nonspecific psychological or psychophysiological therapeutic effect produced by a placebo, but may be the effect of spontaneous improvement attributed to the placebo. A placebo therapy may be used with or without knowledge that it is a placebo. Included among placebos are treatments that are given in the belief that they are effective but that actually are placebos by objective evaluation. A placebo may be inert (such as a sugar pill) or active (such as an in-effective drug or a drug used at an ineffective dosage), and placebos may include, therefore, any treatments, no matter how potentially specific and no matter who administers them.

Increased recognition of the power of the placebo came in the 1930s. Two seminal papers highlighted the importance of the placebo and the placebo effect: Gold et al.'s initial study (1937) describing the "blind test" as a control for the placebo effect of treatment and Houston's proposal (1938, 1416–18) that the his-tory of medicine was largely the history of the placebo effect:

> A recognition of the importance of the relationship between doctor and patient, even though belated . . . has a long history. In the early history of medicine, it comprised all that the doctor had to offer the patient. It is only very recently that medicine has had more to give. A survey of medical his-tory acquaints us with many illustrious names . . . but . . . they had very lit-tle to give by which the patient could profit. Historians sentimentalize the practical values of ancient medicine. One scans the pages of Hippocrates in vain for any treatments of specific value. The pages of medical history read like the log of an old-fashioned ocean voyage, in which it noted that on such a day a whale spouted, on such a day a flying fish was sighted, or a bit of driftwood, but in which no mention is made of the huge prevailing fact that what was constantly seen day by day, almost to the exclusion of other sights, was the unending green waste of water. And this inevitable circumambient ocean is, by analogy, in medical history the "personal relationship between doctor and patient." In a word, the medicines used were placebos. . . . The great lesson, then, of medical history is that the placebo has always been the norm of medical practice, that it was only occasionally and at great inter-vals that anything really serviceable, such as the cure of scurvy by fresh fruits, was introduced into medical practice. . . . The medical historian is apt to mislead us when he speaks of the learned and skillful doctors of the past. . . . Their skill was a skill in dealing with the emotions of men. They themselves were the therapeutic agents by which cures were effected. Their therapeu-tic procedures, whether they were inert or whether they were dangerous, were placebos, symbols by which their patients' faith and their own was sus-tained. The history of medicine is a history of the dynamic power of the relationship between doctor and patient.

This chapter traces the history of the placebo effect in prescientific medicine. That history provides ample evidence for the hypothesis that until recently the history of medical treatment was essentially the history of the placebo effect.

The history of the placebo effect affords lessons and insights about how to evaluate the effectiveness of treatment and how to detect and study placebo effects. Let us consider the details of this history, because those who forget the past are condemned to repeat it—although even those who do know the past may be destined to repeat it.

The Placebo Effect in Prehistoric Times

According to Sir William Osler (1932), the desire to take medicine is one feature that distinguishes hominids from their fellow creatures. A reasonable assumption from the study of primitive societies and early medical records is that placebos were the dominant treatment in preliterate cultures. It is probable that whatever beneficial effects accrued to early treatment could only have been due to the placebo effect. Although nothing is known about the earliest medications or about the first physician, historians date the earliest portrait of a physician to Cro-Magnon times, 20,000 B.C. (Haggard 1934; Bromberg 1954). This horned, tailed, hirsute, and animal-like apparition had great psychological effect, and it is likely that the treatment used was simply a vehicle for the psychological or placebo effect and was without any intrinsic merit (Modell 1955).

Babylonia and Assyria

The recorded history of medical treatment, although concordant with medical progress, is at the same time incredible. The fifteen remedies described in the oldest Sumerian medical tablet, dating to 2100 B.C.—the treatments of the *ashipu* (sorcerer) and the *asu* (physician)—were, as were all the remedies of the ancient cultures, placebos. Most of the current knowledge regarding the medicine of the ancient Babylonians and Assyrians is derived from baked clay tablets covered with cuneiform writing. The earliest medical records from Babylonia and Assyria mentioned 250 drugs of vegetable origin and a smaller number of animal and mineral origin. As in past cultures, animal and human excrement was used for myriad conditions. Modes of administration included medicated wines, draughts, plasters, lotions, infusions, decoctions, and fumigations (Kremers and Urdang 1940). The treatment for a person's head full of sores was boiled dung, the head having been shaved until blood oozed (Majno 1975). Gastric complaints were treated by pouring burning juice of cassia or cold water over a kneeling person; or, with the person's head down and feet up, the cheek was forcibly struck, the person rubbed violently, and the stomach admonished, "Be good" (Rapport and Wright 1952).

Egypt

The Ebers Papyrus, estimated to have been written about 1500 B.C. (Ghalioun-gui 1963), is one of the most important medical papyri and is a compilation of recipes for various illnesses. It contains 842 prescriptions and mentions more than 700 drugs of mineral, vegetable, and animal origin—all, with a few possible exceptions, worthless (Kremers and Urdang 1940; Estes 1989). Patients were treated with dirt and flyspecks scraped off walls. Other treatments included blood of lizard, cats, and other animals; fat of goose, ox, cat, snake, hippopotamus, mouse, and eunuch; grated human skull; ram's hair; beetles; tortoise shell; teeth of swine; hoof of ass; laundry sops; molds covering bread or wood long soaked in water; and the urine of children, adults, and menstruating women, which were credited with different medicinal effects.

The ancient Egyptian healers were fond of dung, recommending excrement from humans and eighteen other creatures, such as the crocodile, the cat, the ass, the pig, the dog, the sheep, the gazelle, the pelican, and the fly. Hog and donkey dung were considered noxious, but animal and human dung and urine were used to repel bad spirits. Breasted, a pharmacologist before becoming a famed Egyptologist, praised dung because it is "ammoniacal" (Majno 1975, 109). The treatment for various disorders of the rectum included suppositories containing dung. A better explanation than referring to dung as ammoniacal is that the suppository was a male *deconcupiscent,* but there has been no controlled study to determine its worth. To restore a husband's potency, the head of a baby crocodile and oil were rubbed on his phallus.

The extensive use of medication is suggested by the many different modes of administration: decoctions, infusions, clysters, pills, tablets, troches, capsules, powders, potions, inhalations, lotions, ointments, plasters, fumigations, packs, and suppositories, which were eaten, drunk, masticated, swallowed, inserted into bodily orifices, and spread over all parts of the body (Kremers and Urdang 1940). Bloodletting began in Egypt in 1000 B.C. Disease was viewed as a curse cast on an individual by an evil spirit, and bloodletting was used to purify the body of evil spirits (Seigworth 1980).

The ancient Egyptians were obsessed with the anus, conceiving it as a secondary source of the circulation that could distribute *ukmedy* (a rotten stuff in feces) to other parts of the body. The anus is referred to in eighty-two prescriptions from ancient Egypt; it was soothed, refreshed, smoked, and kept from slipping or twisting. Enemas were sanctified by a legend about Thoth, the Egyptian god of medicine and science, who landed on the waters in the form of a sacred ibis, filled his beak with water, and injected it into his anus; this was later

called the Divine Clyster. Enemas and diuretic drenches were used for three consecutive days each month for hygienic purposes and for many ailments (Majno
1975).

Egyptian medicine had a far-reaching effect on Greek, Roman, and Western
medicine, and probably contributed to the humoral concept in Greek medicine.
The Egyptians were the first to write medical texts; to use a medical vocabulary;
to make observations about human anatomy; systematically to describe facts
about medical illness; to use splints, bandages, and surgical and drug therapies; and
to make more rational diagnostic, prognostic, and therapeutic decisions (Majno
1975; Estes 1989). It has been suggested that the symbol used on prescriptions, the
Rx, represents one of the restored eyes, Rx xR, of Horus (Ohashi 1995).

Greece

Asclepius

The history of Greek medicine goes back to the centaur Chiron, the teacher of
pharmacy, who was half human and half horse. Chiron taught Apollo, who
handed down his knowledge about healing to his son, Asclepius (Edelstein and
Edelstein 1945; Phillips 1987). Asclepius (referred to as Aesculapius by the Romans) surpassed all other healers and later became a god. At the more than three
hundred sanctuaries for healing referred to in literary sources (Edelstein and
Edelstein 1945; Veith 1972), his daughters Hygieia, who represented health,
and Panacea, who represented healing, were the personification of all earthly
remedies.

The only indication that a patient was about to enter a sanctuary of Asclepius in Pergamon were two pillars that flanked an inviting but portentous-
appearing dirt road that disappeared in the distance. Inscribed on one of the
pillars were the words "Death Cannot Enter Here." The temples of Asclepius
were built in healthful pastoral settings, usually with mineral springs, bathing
pools, gymnasia, gardens, exercise grounds, a racetrack, and in Epidaurus a the-
ater seating twelve thousand persons. Admission to the healing sanctum was preceded by elaborate ritual. First the patients were bathed, then they underwent
purification by rigorous fasting, sea baths, and fumigations. Each day, at the
temple's entrance, they read votive tablets describing medical cures, and in the
inner court of the temple offerings were made before the gold and ivory images
of the god. After a sacrifice, priests, acolytes, masseurs, and bath attendants prepared them for the special rite of incubation, or temple sleep. They slept on pal-
lets made of the skins of animals sacrificed to the deity and were dressed in white
to induce healing dreams.

Incubation, sleep in the temple as a means of obtaining a cure of disease, involved an elaborate ritual. Patients dreamed that Asclepius walked among them, followed by his daughters Hygieia and Panacea, and his ever-present serpent and sacred dog. The sleeper, in the state between sleep and waking, saw a priest dressed as a god who spoke with a harmonious voice. According to Jayne (1962), the priests came to the patient's room during the night to anoint the diseased parts with salves and medicinal herbs and directed the serpents or dogs to creep over the sleeper, lick the diseased area, and whisper remedies in the sleeper's ear. The gods asked the patient about the illness, touched the patient or laid on hands, and gave advice and directions for future treatment. Priests were paid in money, supplications, or songs, according to the patient's means. Votive offerings were frequently of silver and gold. Since Asclepius was reported to give advice that was not medical, Phillips (1987) called him the forerunner of confessors or psychotherapists. No subsequent retreat, hospital, institute, spa, or academic treatment center can rival the impressiveness of an Asclepian sanctuary; the extensive support and tender loving care of the Asclepiads, attendants, and staff; the power of the healing rituals; the comprehensive, multimodal treatment; and the impressive cures. The recorded cures included the delivery of a woman pregnant for five years; the cure of a bald man, who was endowed with hair overnight; and the cure of a Spartan girl suffering from dropsy, whose head Asclepius cut off, held upside down to drain the fluid, and finally replaced on her neck.

Various explanations have been offered for the cures: miracles and divine healing, the application of natural remedies, animal magnetism and somnambulism, interpretation of dreams, hypnosis, suggestion, and autosuggestion. The most powerful element underlying these therapeutic procedures was the placebo effect, possibly enhanced by the emotionally charged and elaborate ritual.

The Four Humors

The all-encompassing and compelling theory of humors, first taught in Greek medicine by the Pythagoreans, became the fundamental concept in Hippocratic medicine and was further emphasized by Galen and most other subsequent physicians (Phillips 1987). It was based on the idea that the basic elements of matter were earth, air, fire, and water. Similar constituents in humans are the four humors: blood (secreted by the liver), phlegm (secreted by the lungs), yellow bile (secreted by the gallbladder), and black bile (secreted by the spleen), with the brain secreting only mucus. Corresponding qualities are moist and warm, moist and cold, dry and warm, and dry and cold, each different from the others in color, temperature, and humidity.

Dominant humors were also associated with constitution or temperament (from *temperamentum,* blending of humors): the sanguine person, with excessive hot and moist blood, was prone to obesity and laughter; the phlegmatic person, dulled by cold phlegm, was inclined to sloth and rest; the choleric person, driven by hot yellow bile, was inclined to great anger; and the melancholic person was depressed by cold, dry black bile, which made him or her pensive, peevish, and solitary (Bettmann 1956). The mixture of the humors, affected by diet, weather, and climate, determines the basic condition, temperament, health, and disease. A person is healthy when the humors are properly balanced and ill when they are improperly mixed. Treatment followed the theory and involved propitious adjustment of the humors by drugs and other procedures, such as bloodletting to adjust the humors to a proper balance.

A fortuitous element of the theory was that nature itself can heal by adjusting the relationship among the humors. This idea led to the aphorism that nature is a great healer and that the physician's role is to aid nature and not hinder it by interfering with the natural course of an illness. Thus, relying on the possibility of spontaneous improvement was less harmful to the patient than was treatment with many of the ineffective drugs available at the time.

Hippocrates

Although Hippocratic medicine coexisted alongside Asclepieia apparently without conflict, medicine as practiced by Hippocrates (called the Father of Medicine), described in about seventy essays making up the Hippocratic Corpus, replaced the religious, mystical, magical, and fanciful theories that formerly dominated treatment by the temple priests with a commonsense approach of careful clinical observation (Hippocrates 1964). From 195 to 400 drugs, mainly of vegetable origin, are mentioned in the corpus (Kremers and Urdang 1940). The modes of administration included fomentations, poultices, gargles, pessaries, pills, ointments, oils, cerates, collyria, looches, troches, and inhalations. Medicine became more practical and humanistic. Treatment was usually confined to fresh air, good diet, tisanes of barley gruel, hydromel (honey and water), oxymel (honey and vinegar), massage, and hydrotherapy, but also included purgatives with more than sixty cathartic drugs, and bloodletting (Garrison 1929; Phillips 1987). Hippocrates strongly emphasized diet but discouraged vegetables and fruits, a practice that probably resulted in vitamin deficiencies, especially among the rich (Majno 1975). Frequent references are made to purgatives, sudorifics, emetics, and enemas, consistent with Hippocratic theory requiring the purification of the body from disease-producing humors.

According to Guido Majno, the direct treatment of wounds did little harm and some good. Subsequent treatment, however, is characterized as "bad to hair-raising. Imagine cutting the veins of a patient who has already half bled to death through his wound, plus the combined effects of enemas, purges, and vomiting, plus the side effects of poisoning with hellebore, and all of this on a starvation diet" (1975, 188). They also used sarcotics to make flesh grow, epispastics to attract cathartics to excite the tissues, mundifiers to clean ulcers, emollients to produce supple scars, and so on. At the same time, demonstrating the Hippocratic respect for nature's healing, and reflecting the insight of almost all healers that something else beside their ministrations goes into healing, there was the observation that "Nature, without instruction or knowledge, does what is necessary. Natures are the physicians of disease" (*Epidemics*, quoted by Majno 1975, 200).

Although Hippocratic medicine freed medicine from superstitions and philosophic constraints, eventually laying the foundation for more rational treatment, and the ancient Greeks' theory of disease was developed by the best minds of the time, it was wholly imaginary, and treatment was largely impotent and often the opposite of what we now know should have been done. Despite this, Hippocratic precepts guided medicine for more than two thousand years.

China

Chinese medicine, built on ancient humoral theories (Huard and Wong 1968), flowered in the fourth or fifth century B.C. with the appearance of Lao Tzu, Confucius, the *I Ching (Book of Changes)*, the *Chou Li (Institutions of the Chou)*, and the medical compilation known as the *Huang Ti Nei Ching Su Wen (The Yellow Emperor's Classic of Internal Medicine)*. This book dominated the medical canon in China without major changes for centuries (Veith 1972; Majno 1975). Like the Greeks, the Chinese were enamored of numbers and symmetries. They developed a complicated system that held that everything was made of five elements: water, fire, wood, metal, and earth; as well as the legendary sixty-four combinations of yin and yang; number lore, with numerous intercorrelations among these elements; and especially, acupuncture and moxibustion. Simple diseases were treated with five tastes (vinegar, wine, honey, ginger, and salt), five kinds of grain, five kinds of drugs (herbs, trees, insects, stones, and grains), and five flavors (pungent, sour, sweet, bitter, and salty). Pungent food was used to dispel disintegration of the liver and sour food to drain it; salty food was used for a weakened heart, and sweet food to drain the heart. People living in eastern China who were prone to ulcers were treated with acupuncture with flint needles; people in the west prone to internal disease were treated with poison medicine (from five creatures: viper, scorpion, centipede, toad, and lizard). Northern people exposed to cold were treated with moxa; southern people suffering from contracted muscles and numbness required acupuncture with fine needles; people living in the center of the country who were predisposed to chills, fevers, and paralysis were treated with massage, breathing, and exercise of the extremities. Chinese medicine used almost every known substance (Morse 1934; Hume 1940), the pharmacy totaling over eighteen thousand drugs and prescriptions.

Acupuncture was the most extensively used treatment in China for twenty-five hundred years; it is still in use today. Although acupuncture is used in many countries and is believed by laypeople and by some physicians to be an effective treatment for many conditions, and despite the licensing of acupuncturists in many states in the United States, adequately controlled studies have failed to confirm its effectiveness. Moreover, it is likely that acupuncture in the past killed many more people than it helped, since the use of unsterilized needles probably was responsible for homologous serum jaundice, which was endemic in China for centuries.

India

The major Indian medical writings appeared in the Atharvaveda, the Choraka, and the Sushruta. The dates are uncertain and may be anywhere between 1500 B.C. and 1000 A.D., later than the earliest such writings of other ancient civilizations, in part because of reluctance to commit ideas to writing. Treatment of wounds that could be seen with the naked eye—which resulted from perennial warfare, as in most ancient societies—was more advanced than other medical treatment. Indians developed military hospitals, techniques of rhinoplasty, couching for cataract, amputation of limbs, repair of torn or stretched earlobes, the use of hot oil to stop bleeding, and the use of ant heads to suture and clamp wounds.

The cornerstone of ancient Indian treatment was the use of mantras, dieting, drugs, and withdrawal of the mind from injurious or harmful thoughts. Other treatments included abstinence from sex, meat, and emotions; fasting; vomiting; purging; venesection; and enemas. Enemas were also given to elephants: Indians are credited with developing the most massive clyster in medical history to treat recalcitrant boils on the buttocks of an elephant driver, in the belief that poisons in the elephant could be transferred to humans.

Medicine was less advanced in India than in Greece, and there is no record that the use of the six hundred or so drugs known in early India was effective, as is true for most other cultures at the time.

Alexandria

Little information about Alexandrian medicine, except for some scattered references by Celsus, Pliny, and others, survived the destruction of the library in Alexandria. The major known Alexandrian contributions to medicine were the introduction of ligatures for bleeding blood vessels and the development of the syringe.

Rome

The ancient Romans were suspicious of and had derogatory attitudes toward physicians. Although Greek and later Roman physicians such as the Asclepiads, Celsus, Galen, and others speckled Roman medical history, Romans relied primarily on folk medicine for six hundred years. This may have left them just as well off as, or even better than, they would have been if they had used physicians. These attitudes are reflected in the first century A.D. by the rational observations of Celsus (after whom Paracelsus named himself). Celsus held that surgical treatment was more effective than medical treatment (as it seems to have been throughout much of medical history before the twentieth century): "The third part of the Art of Medicine is that which cures by the hand. . . . It does not omit medicaments and regulated diets, but does most by hand. The effects of this treatment are more obvious than any other kind; inasmuch as in diseases since luck helps much, and the same things are often salutary, often of no use at all, it may be doubted whether recovery has been due to medicine, or a sound body, or good luck. . . . But in that part of medicine which cures by hand, it is obvious that all improvement comes chiefly from this, even if it be assisted somewhat in other ways" (Majno 1975, 355).

Almost a half-century later, Pliny, who willy-nilly assembled twenty thousand facts from two thousand volumes by a hundred authors, commented: "Physicians acquire their knowledge from our dangers, making experiments at the cost of our lives. . . . Physicians acquire enormous amounts of money, up to 600,000 sesterces a year [roughly 100 times the minimum living wage]. . . . Heaven knows, the medical profession is the only one in which anybody professing to be a physician is at once trusted [there being no recognized medical diplomas], although nowhere else is an untruth more dangerous. We pay however no attention to the danger, so great for each of us is the seductive sweetness of wishful thinking" (Majno 1975, 348).

Galen is acknowledged as a creative, imaginative, and productive luminary in the history of medicine, having written more than thirty volumes on all aspects of medicine. He also was dogmatic and pompous, proclaiming, "Never as yet have I gone astray, whether in treatment or in prognosis, as have so many other physicians of great reputation. If anyone wishes to gain fame . . . all that he needs is to accept what I have been able to establish" (Haggard 1934, 98). His therapy was based on the principle of opposites: if a drug causes or is thought to cause fever, it can be used to treat chills; if a drug causes emesis, it can be used to treat constipation. He wrote a whole book on the use of dove dung as a dressing for wounds, and another about theriac. Galen's pharmacopoeia of 540 vegetable, 180 animal, and 100 mineral substances—a total of 820 placebo substances—dominated treatment for fifteen hundred years. Galen's answer for every question and explanation for every phenomenon, authoritatively and dogmatically proclaimed, may have contributed to the tenacious hold his theories had on medical practice, although their preeminence slowly eroded and they were finally put to rest with the development of bacteriology and the work of Bernard, Pasteur, Koch, and others in the nineteenth century. Galen said that pus was a necessary part of healing. Because of this belief, many thousands died of infection. Yet he was able to observe insightfully: "He cures most in whom most are confident" (Osler 1892, 117).

Majno commented: "The Hippocratic books had spelled out the theory, the Alexandrians had reinforced it, Galen, who gave it the final touches, thereby became responsible for rivers of blood—and for cemeteries prematurely full" (1975, 419). The physicians who followed Galen forgot about experimentation. Thus, from Asclepius through Hippocrates to Galen, and until very recently, the history of medical treatment was largely the history of the placebo effect, because all medical treatments, with rare exceptions, were at best placebos, at worst unknowingly deadly.

Classic Placebos during the Reign of Galenic Medicine

Medicine's Universal Remedy: Theriac

Theriac, one of medicine's oldest and most expensive drugs, contained between thirty-three and more than one hundred substances and took six months to concoct (Watson 1966; Majno 1975). Viper's flesh, medicine's magical restorative, was the main ingredient, and opium was often added for good measure. Theriac, originally an antidote to poisons and venoms, was developed during the reign of Mithridates VI (king of Pontus, in Asia Minor, from 114 to 63 B.C.), who was concerned about being poisoned. Galen wrote a whole book on theriac, originally called mithridatum, and claimed that it drew out poisons like a cupping glass and divided the overlying tissue of an abscess more quickly than a scalpel.

He increased the number of ingredients and the time required for the concoction to mature, and enlarged its indications.[1] Nero's physician, Andromachus, further increased the number of ingredients to sixty-four, added chunks of viper flesh, and increased the opium content considerably, the mixture taking several months or years to achieve maturity. Theriac later was embossed on beautiful porcelain jars as *theriac Andromachus,* or less frequently as *theriac galene* (the name *theriac galene* was given by Andromachus and means tranquillity). Theriac eventually was used less as an antidote to poisons and venoms than as a remedy for "almost every human ailment—chronic headache, hardness of hearing, dimness of sight, blackout and giddiness, epilepsy, shortness of breath, spitting of blood, indigestion, nausea, liver trouble, the stone; it strengthens the tongue, soothes delirium, is an excellent soporific, calms the worries and stresses of the mind, is the only cure for tetanus" (Watson 1966, 46).[2] It was included in the 1872 German and 1874 French pharmacopoeias, and was even bought as Venice treacle in Vienna shortly after World War II.

Theriac could have been useful for pain, as well as anxiety, depression, and other psychological symptoms, if its preparation contained an adequate amount of opium and the administered dosage was adequate, which is doubtful. However, an adequate dosage could result unknowingly in addiction and severe symptoms of withdrawal. Because of theriac's large number of ingredients, the time required for its preparation, its innumerable ineffective ingredients, its expense, and the fact that it contained only one remotely and unpredictably effec-

1. The ingredients for Galen's electuarium theriacale magnum, given in Greek verse so that they could be remembered, included "Root of Florentine iris, licorice, 12 ounces each; of Arabian costus, Pontic rhubarb, cinquefoil, 6 ounces each; of Ligusticum meum, rhubarb, gentian, 4 ounces each; of birthwort, 2 ounces; herb of scordium, 12 ounces; of lemon grass, horehound, dittany of Crete, calamint, 6 ounces each; of pennyroyal, ground pine, gemander, 4 ounces each; leaves of laurus cassia, 4 ounces; flowers of red roses, 12 ounces; of lavender, 6 ounces; saffron, 2 ounces; fruit of amyris, opobalsamum 4 ounces; cinnamon, 12 ounces; cassia lignea and spikenard, 6 ounces each; Celtic nard, 4 ounces; long pepper 24 ounces; black pepper and ginger, 6 ounces each; cardamoms, 4 ounces; rape seeds, agaric, 12 ounces each; seeds of Macedonian parsley, 6 ounces; of anise, fennel, cress, seseli, thlaspi, amomum, sandwort, 4 ounces each; of carrot, 2 ounces; opium 24 ounces, opobalsamum 12 ounces; myrrh, olibanum, turpentine, 6 ounces each; storax, gum arabic, sagapenum, 4 ounces each; asphaltum, opoponax, galbanum, 2 ounces each; juice of acacia and of hyocist, 4 ounces each; castor, 2 ounces, Lemnian bole, calcined vitriol, 4 ounces each; trochiscs of squill 48 ounces; of vipers, of sweet flag 24 ounces each" (Macht 1915, 479).

2. The use of theriac as an antidote to poisons and venoms suffered a severe blow in 1745 with the publication of a monograph by the physician William Heberden denying theriac's antidotal abilities (Paulshock 1982).

tive substance, psychotherapy was later referred to by Pierre Janet (1924) as a psychological theriac.

Bizarre Placebos

In the sixth century, the Byzantine compiler Alexander of Tralles recommended, as a treatment for gout, myrrh mixed with the nipplelike projection from the cecum of a young pig, wrapped in the skin of a wolf or dog, and worn by the patient as an amulet during the waning of the moon. In the seventh century, Paul of Aegina outlined the use of blood in treatment: hot pigeon and turtle blood for black eyes and during trephination; owl blood for dyspnea; bat blood for preserving the breasts of virgins; bat, frog, chameleon, and dog-tick blood to prevent breast hirsuteness; goat blood for dropsy and kidney stones; domestic fowl blood for cerebral hemorrhages; lamb blood for epilepsy; kid blood for hemoptysis; bear, wild goat, buck goat, and bull blood for apostemes; land crocodile blood for visual acuity; and duck, stag, and goose blood for deadly poisons (Rapport and Wright 1952). Galen rejected these remedies but recommended others equally bizarre.

Clysterization (the purification, purging, or removal of evil bowel contents), currently called enema, is another famed method of catharsis that was used in most periods of history. Medical history is replete with testimonials by physicians about the virtues of enemas, and they were commonly used by the laity. Voltaire advised every young man to secure a wife who could give an enema pleasantly and quickly to keep the passages open. Despite their extensive use, enemas cause dehydration, the exact opposite of the hydration required by many illnesses, making them potentially lethal. Commonly used in the United States and other countries through the 1940s, they are used today only for diagnostic procedures, to instill some medications, and to clear fecal impactions.

Bleeding, first used by the Egyptians, spread to Greece and Rome and continued to be used until the end of the nineteenth century as a common remedy for a multitude of conditions. Leeches were only one of many methods used to bleed. In 1827 alone, France imported 33 million leeches because domestic supplies had been exhausted (Sigerist 1958).

A bizarre remedy for gout which was recommended in the thirteenth century was made up of oil of skinned puppy, vulture, goose, bear, fox, wax, and seven other substances (Jastrow 1913). The seventeenth-century edition of the *London Pharmacopeia* (Rapport and Wright 1952) recorded the use of worms, lozenges of dried vipers, powders of precious stones, oil of bricks, ants, wolves, spiders, earthworms, fur, feathers, hair, human perspiration, saliva of a fasting man, spiderwebs, wood lice, moss scraped from the skull of a victim of violent death, crabs' eyes and claws, and human urine. Most human, animal, and insect excretions and matter were used in most cultures throughout history: "hotte horse dung" for ague, goose dung for baldness, sheep dung for gallstones (Castiglioni 1947), bulls' balls, macerated vulva, and usnea (the moss scraped from the skull of a hanged criminal)—an official drug in the pharmacopeia until the nineteenth century for the relief of nervous or wasting diseases (Haggard 1929). Many of these medications were so expensive that only the wealthy could afford them.

Mattioli, an Italian physician in the sixteenth century, concocted an antidote to poison and the plague. It contained as many as 230 ingredients, including mithridatum and theriac Andromachus. It is highly improbable that any of the ingredients cured disease; all were placebos, except perhaps for the variable amount of opium, which could be effective for pain.

Legends about the unicorn existed in ancient China and India, appeared in the Bible, emerged in the literature of the Western world in the fourth century B.C., and became important in materia medica in the sixteenth century (Shepard 1930). Medicinally, the horn of the unicorn was taken as ground horn, as scrapings for fevers, and as jellies to restore failing strength, and was thought to detect and protect against poisons in wines and foods. It was seen as a cure for poisons, fevers, bites of mad dogs and scorpions, worms, fluxes, the plague, the falling sickness, memory loss, and all other complaints; and was believed to assist the memory, fortify the animal spirits, and prolong youth. Although the horn was believed to come from a unicorn, it was in fact the left upper incisor tooth, spiraled counterclockwise, of a male whale called a narwhal. An article of commerce for more than eight centuries, unicorn horn is the most expensive placebo in the history of medicine, selling for ten times its weight in gold at the height of its popularity in the sixteenth century. At that price, based on the cost of gold in 1995, a mature nine-pound unicorn horn would cost about $55,000. For a penny, poor people were able to buy a "unicorn drink," a glass of water run through a hollow horn or taken from a beaker in which a unicorn horn had been dipped. Disputations about how to distinguish a real horn from a fabricated one, or about whether, in fact, real ones existed, began in the twelfth century and continued over the next five centuries as the price escalated.

The most important event in unicorn lore occurred in the seventeenth century. Merchants in Copenhagen, concerned about the true nature and origin of the substance they were selling as unicorn's horn, and wondering whether investment in unicorn was worthwhile, appealed to Ole Wurm, a zoologist and antiquarian of high attainment, to decide the question. Wurm delivered a learned dissertation in Latin in 1638, concluding that "the alicorns of Europe are the teeth of narwhals" (Shepard 1930, 261). Although the price of unicorn horn declined, exposure of the true nature of alicorns had little effect on the remedy's vogue. It remained in the *London Pharmacopoeia* for more than a century. Though it has not been in general use since the eighteenth century, ground unicorn horn is still being dispensed in Japanese herbal shops.[3]

Bezoar stone came from Arabic medicine to Europe and was used as a treatment for poisons and melancholia and as a universal antidote. According to legend, a bezoar stone was the crystallized tear from the eye of a deer bitten by a snake. In reality, it was a gallstone, or a concretion found in the stomach or intestine of animals such as the goat. Bezoar stones were often counterfeited, pebbles being used instead. There are records of individuals being tried and punished for the offense, and international conferences were held to curb the counterfeiting. Ambroise Paré remarked at one of these conferences that it didn't make any difference whose counterfeits were used, as all were equally ineffective.

Babylonians, Hebrews, Greeks, and Nero used mandrake *(Mandragora officinarum)* as a sedative, purgative, emetic, aphrodisiac, and hallucinogen; for the treatment of ulcers; and in magical rites and orgiastic rituals. According to popular superstition, the mandrake, which resembled a man, would shriek when pulled from the earth. Because a person hearing the shriek was thought to go insane or die, a horn was blown to drown out the shriek when the plant was collected. For further protection, a dog was tied to the plant with a rope and food was left nearby. When the dog attempted to escape or reach the food, it would pull out the root (and presumably go mad and die).

Shakespeare referred to many of the drugs, therapies, and diseases known in his day in his thirty-seven plays. Possibly part of his extensive medical knowledge was provided by his son-in-law, who was a physician. He mentioned mandrake more frequently than all other drugs, and there is an exceedingly descriptive reference to it in *Romeo and Juliet* (4.3.47): "And shrieks like mandrakes torn out of the earth / That living mortals hearing them, run mad."

Mandrake, henbane, and belladonna were constituents of the fabled witches' brew. Mandrake was the first drug referred to as an aphrodisiac and was described in the Bible as having been successfully used by Jacob and Leah; it was

3. We have two five-foot unicorn horns, which would have cost $1,360,000 in the sixteenth century but were obtained at the bargain price of $1,500. One is in each of our offices, behind the patient's chair—they help in our therapy too! History always in the background contributes to our psychotherapeutic interpretations a sense of humility, an attribute of which psychiatrists can never have too much.

valued in ancient Greece and Rome, was discussed by Dioscorides and Pliny, was used extensively throughout the centuries, and is still esteemed in Asian countries. Hundreds of other substances were extolled as aphrodisiacs throughout recorded history; all were placebos (Walton 1958). A bizarre but typical example of the desperate, primarily male lust for aphrodisiacs came to our attention while browsing Alan H. Walton's book on aphrodisiacs: "Macerate an ass's verge with oil, and use the fluid thus obtained . . . for anointing . . . and drinking of it" (the ass was known for its considerable amorous propensities). Curious about the meaning of *verge,* we found it defined as a noun referring to the male organ of copulation in certain invertebrates. Other aphrodisiacs included gander's foot, jackal's gall, placenta of a newly foaled mare, menstrual blood, mixture of mother's and daughter's milk, bull's balls, macerated vulva, powdered skink flesh from the genital area drunk with wine for erection of the virile member and miraculously exciting sexual desire and ability, and innumerable bizarre recipes that were said to give one the strength of ten men and enable one man to satisfy ten women, to enable a man to enjoy a hundred women, to enable the organ to attain the largeness of the member of a horse, or to enable a bald man to have sex twice during the day and twice in the evening. Owl flesh was said to excite desire but at the same time turn a man into a fool. Hardly any substance was not used. Despite the persistent quest for aphrodisiacs, it is doubtful that any are truly effective. The traffic in aphrodisiacs has not diminished, however, as indicated by the many sex shops, advertised herbal remedies, and classified notices in magazines and papers. The quest for aphrodisiacs probably lags only slightly behind the pursuit of drugs for dissipating pain, curing illness, and prolonging life.

Powdered Egyptian mummy, resembling and tasting like rosin, was believed to heal wounds and to be an almost universal remedy. Several official conferences were convened to discuss the adulteration and counterfeiting of the powdered mummy from Egypt (and the impurity of the unicorn horn and bezoar stone as well), possibly when they were no longer effective. Paré, who was also skeptical of Egyptian mummy, said that the mummy was sometimes made in "our France" from bodies stolen from the gallows. "Nevertheless I believe they are just as good as those brought from Egypt, because they are none of them of any value" (Haggard 1929, 324). It is unlikely that patients were treated with authentic powdered Egyptian mummy. If they were, it would be a dramatic example of how a placebo remedy believed to be helpful could harm, since the main ingredient in the embalming process would have caused arsenic poisoning when ingested.

Despite the long use of these remedies, some physicians doubted their efficacy. Pliny, for one, criticized the use of some remedies, calling them compounds specifically devised for the luxurious and opulent (Watson 1966). And despite the extensive use of these and many other distasteful, useless, and often harmful drugs, and the continued prescription of the flesh of vipers, the spermatic fluid of frogs, horns of deer, animal excretions, holy oil (Leslie 1954), and other bizarre substances, the physician continued to be a respected and honored member of society. Fortunately, humans managed to survive not only the diseases but also the remedies (King 1966).

The Laying On of Hands

The laying on of hands is one of the oldest and most persistent treatments, still used today. The Bible describes Christ's touch as curing blindness, dropsy, leprosy, stroke, and insanity. Paintings portray Christ as exorcising evil by touching insane persons; the evil is symbolized as expelled monsters, distorted animals, and evil-appearing humans. The number of lesser clerics and inspired laypeople—recorded and unrecorded, in all religions throughout the world—who healed by touching and other faith procedures is so large that the technique appears to be a major constant in history. Psychiatrists today do not expel evil by exorcism or touching (in fact, touching a patient often is proscribed), but they encourage patients to externalize or speak out the evil. Thus, possibly in the same way, patients cathartically verbalize aggression, forbidden libidinal impulses, nefarious evil, and guilt.

The royal touch, by which a royal personage was thought to cure by touching, stroking, or making the sign of the cross over a patient with the King's Evil (usually scrofula or skin disorder, but at times, any type of illness), first appeared in 300 B.C.: the Greek king Pyrrhus of Epirus is reputed to have cured colic by touching (with his toes). Touching was used by the Roman emperor Vespasian in the first century B.C., the Norse king Olaf in the tenth century A.D., and many English, French, and Spanish monarchs. Thomas Aquinas, by testifying to the cure of a page by King Clovis of France in the fifth century, helped sanctify the practice. King Edward the Confessor was reported to have restored sight to several blind men, as well as to have effected other cures (Rubin 1974). Samuel Johnson was not cured when touched for scrofula by Queen Anne when he was two years old.

Many quarrels occurred over lineage and the right and ability to cure by touching. Patients were carefully screened, and only one treatment was allowed for each person, thus decreasing the possibility of failure. King Charles II, who treated more people than anyone else, touched almost one hundred thousand patients during twenty-five years of his reign in the seventeenth century. Richard Wiseman, the surgeon to Charles II, in his treatise on scrofula, bore witness to the many hundreds of cures performed by the touch of his king (Bloch 1973). It is noteworthy that more people died of scrofula in the time of Charles II than in any other period of English history (Haggard 1929). Shakespeare described touching by the king for the King's Evil in *Macbeth* (4.3.140–59): "'Tis called the evil; a most miraculous work in this good king; / Which often . . . I have seen him do. How he solicits heaven, / Himself best knows; but strangely-visited people, / All swoln and ulcerous, pitiful to the eye, / The mere despair of surgery, he cures, / Hanging a golden stamp about their necks, / Put on with holy prayers; and 'tis spoken, / To the succeeding royalty he leaves / The healing benediction."

Early attempts by Italian philosophers to explain these cures attributed them to the effect of imagination. However, it is more likely that when there were cures, the diagnosis of scrofula had been invalid. There was little differentiation between scrofula and other swellings; or epilepsy and muscular spasms, or other possible seizures or neurotic manifestations. Spontaneous remission of the symptoms no doubt accounted for many of the cures. Documents indicate that the royal touch rarely healed, and that individuals returned to be touched again and again. Most of those who recovered their health did so only incompletely or temporarily, often a long time after being touched. The practice of royal touch disappeared in England in the eighteenth century and in France in the nineteenth century. Its demise was attributed to political revolutions, which caused a shattering of faith in the supernatural character of royalty and in the idea of absolute monarchy (Bloch 1973).

The ability to heal by touching was soon claimed by commoners who believed that their powers were given by divine revelation. The first prominent commoner to do so was Valentine Greatrakes, a Puritan, a soldier, and a respected merchant, who in seventeenth-century England claimed to effect cures by stroking, for patients with the King's Evil, ague, pain, falling sickness or convulsions, and hysterical passion (Haggard 1929); he rarely accepted payment. Others followed in the eighteenth century, some of the more famous being the seventy-year-old English housekeeper Bridget Bostock, called the "healer of Coppenhall," who treated up to seven hundred people daily suffering from hysteria, dyspnea, palsy, and almost everything else, never accepting remuneration for her ministrations. She is reputed to have fasted during treatment hours and to have stroked and anointed the sick with her saliva, praying at the same time. The Austrian priest Joseph Gassner treated with a combination of prayer, exorcism, commands, and a form of trance that was a precursor of hypnosis.

In the nineteenth century, the priest-prince Von Hohenlohe used prayer, stroking, laying on of hands, and direct commands for healing, seeing up to eight thousand sufferers yearly; he later used "absent healing" and "synchronized prayer" as far away as the United States. Zouave Jacob, formerly a trombonist in the Zouaves military band, and a Jew not professing belief in a personal God, was a healing celebrity in nineteenth-century France. He did not charge for his ministrations or claim supernatural powers, and did not know the source of his power. Jacob treated many different diseases and was positive that his powers could work only when he was in the room with one supplicant or groups of supplicants. He did not ask patients about their complaints but simply looked at the sufferer and uttered commands such as "Be well" or "Arise and walk."

These are only a sample of the thousands of religious, royal, and common healers that trafficked in healing throughout the world, and continue to do so in our time.[4] Medical practice in the seventeenth century continued to be characterized by beliefs in folk medicine. The materia medica was composed largely of remedies that were simples, animal and vegetable, such as worms, lozenges of dried vipers, oil of ants, and other insects and animals. In this period, the status of the physician and of the quack was at its zenith (Garrison 1929).

Animal Magnetism

Franz Mesmer, a physician with four doctorates, including one in astrology, has a special place in the history of faith healing and psychological healing. The controversial story of Mesmer and animal magnetism is well known. He is extolled as a saint by some, romantically described as rediscovering and developing psychological healing by some (Zweig 1932), and called a faith-healing charlatan by others (Podmore 1963). Although his methods changed over time, one of his healing procedures took place in a sumptuous room with mirrors, flowers, stained glass, incense, and soft music. An oaken tub in the center of the room contained "magnetized" bottles of water resting on layers of powdered glass and iron filings. Slender iron rods, jointed and movable, were inserted through holes in the tub; they could be applied to a person's body. Patients were seated around the tub holding hands, or a cord was attached at one end to the tub and passed around the body of each patient, thus binding the patients into a chain. Another group of patients stood in a second circle, connected by holding hands. Mesmer (in a silk lilac robe) or an associate would stare into the eyes of each patient, touching or pointing his finger or a rod at the affected parts (Podmore 1963).

These methods were adopted by many mystics but were viewed skeptically

---

4. Touching is still extensively used in many primitive and religious healing rituals. Therapeutic touch is one of the techniques used today by alternative medicine practitioners.

by others, who believed the methods to be charlatanism and quackery. A committee appointed by the Royal Academy of Medicine in Paris, which included Benjamin Franklin, investigated some of the practices used by proponents of animal magnetism. The committee's report, published in 1784, concluded that it had been "finally shown by conclusive experiments that the imagination without the aid of Magnetism can produce convulsions, and that Magnetism without the imagination can produce nothing"; that "there is no proof of the existence of the Animal Magnetic fluid; that this fluid having no existence, has in consequence no utility"; and that the effects were caused by "touches of the operators, the excited imagination of the patient, and . . . the involuntary instinct of imitation" (Podmore 1963, 59). A change in the zeitgeist is indicated by the official appointment of a distinguished panel of physicians and scientists to study therapeutic claims (it was the first to do so), by the thoroughness of the committee's evaluation, and by its conclusions. Moreover, more rational study of the therapeutic effects of trancelike phenomena and suggestibility began with the Marquis de Puységur, James Braid (who gave hypnotism its name), Hippolyte-Marie Bernheim, and others, providing a link to the next phase in psychological healing, namely, psychotherapy.

Thus, the evolution of psychological healing began with primitive supernaturalism, magic, incantation, fetishes, amulets, and religion administered by shamans, witch doctors, and priests. The Greeks and Hippocratic physicians added rationality to physical and mental illness by considering them natural phenomena. Religious mysticism returned with Christian faith healing and exorcism, practiced by clerics who treated by invoking redemption by the Almighty; this was followed by divine treatment by royalty (referred to as the royal touch). The ability to heal by touching was soon claimed by the commoner Greatrakes, who paved the way for many other mortals to touch and participate in venerated healing pursuits, their powers believed to be based on divine revelation or diverse mystical concepts. The subsequent healing lineage included notables such as Mesmer, Elisha Perkins, James Graham, Phineas Quimby, Mary Baker Eddy, and the hypnotists; it was extended to other kinds of lay therapists, and finally to psychotherapists belonging to well over 250 different schools.

Placebo and Nonplacebo Drugs during the Decline of Galenical Medicine

The First Nonplacebo Drug: Cinchona

Cinchona bark, introduced into Europe in the seventeenth century, both reflected and contributed to the end of Galenism (Garrison 1929; Bruce-Chwatt

1988; Jarcho 1993). According to legend, the countess of Chinchon was cured of an ague (the name for fever at the time) by a bark long known to Peruvian Indians. It was introduced to Europe by Jesuits in about 1638 and became known as Peruvian, or Jesuits', bark, later referred to as pulvis cardinalis and pulvis patrum, and finally given its generic name, *cinchona,* by Linnaeus, who erroneously omitted the first *h* in the countess's name.

Thomas Sydenham and Thomas Morton introduced cinchona (later known to contain quinine) into English medicine and were the first to differentiate its effect on malaria (then known as intermittent and tertian fever, and ague) from its ineffectiveness in other fevers. The demonstration that cinchona bark was specific only for fevers of malarial origin and not for all febrile infections was an important advance in medical treatment, because previously there had been no way to distinguish between placebo and nonplacebo. Robert Talbor, an apprentice apothecary, took up its use and in 1672 cured Charles II of a tertian fever, a deed for which he was later knighted. Charles sent Talbor to France to cure Louis XIV, which he promptly did, after which Louis XIV made him a chevalier with an annual pension, granted him a monopoly on the sale of the remedy for ten years, and later purchased the secret remedy, which turned out to be cinchona bark in claret wine.

Reliance on authority, particularly Galenical theory, was so unyielding that most physicians at the time rejected the use of cinchona bark. Another factor contributing to the rejection of the bark was the raging contention about its worth which resulted from anticlerical attitudes toward Spanish Jesuits, who first introduced, strongly recommended, and proselytized the use of the bark for the malarial scourge that had been endemic in Europe for centuries. Leonard J. Bruce-Chwatt (1988), however, proposed instead that the rejection was related to the use of adulterated or substitute products, which made it difficult to determine the bark's effectiveness.

According to Fielding H. Garrison, "No other event . . . did so much to upset the current school systems of medicine as the discovery of Jesuits' bark. Bernardino Ramazzini said that cinchona did for medicine what gunpowder had done for war. The fact that it rapidly cured a protracted intermittent fever, for which the older remedies had been employed for months at a time to void the 'corrupted humors', was the end of Galenism in medical practice" (Garrison 1929, 290).

Cinchona can be considered the first drug that was not a placebo (Houston 1938; Findley 1953) because it was specific for the treatment of malarial fevers and not useful for other fevers. The empirical basis for its discovery and use did not adhere to authoritative Galenical principles for determining when a drug was useful. The history of cinchona illustrates the way in which powerful a priori beliefs prevented intelligent and highly trained physicians from recognizing an effective treatment and led them to reject one of the most useful drugs in the history of medicine. Also contributing to this recurrent theme in the history of medicine is the placebo effect, which causes ineffective remedies to appear effective and thus obscures the recognition of new effective drugs.

The Treatment of Charles II in 1680

Medical reasoning about treatment languished during the seventeenth century in a primitive state: the lungs of a fox, a long-winded animal, were given to consumptives; the fat of a bear, a hirsute animal, was prescribed for baldness. Despite the massive ineffectiveness of their treatments, physicians must have benefited their patients in some way, because they continued to be held in high esteem. Consider the treatment of Charles II by fourteen of his celebrated physicians:

The King was bled . . . to the extent of a pint from his right arm. Next [the physician] drew eight ounces of blood from the left shoulder; . . . gave an emetic to make the King vomit, two physics, and an enema containing antimony, rock salt, marsh-mallow leaves, violets, beet root, camomile flowers, fennel seed, linseed, cardamom seed, cinnamon, saffron, cochineal, and aloes. The King's head was then shaved and a blister raised on his scalp. A sneezing powder of hellebore root was given to purge his brain, and a powder of cowslip administered to strengthen it, for it was the belief in those days that the nasal secretion came from the brain. The emetics were continued at frequent intervals and meanwhile a soothing drink given, composed of barley water, licorice, and sweet almonds, light wine, oil of wormwood, anise, thistle leaves, mint, rose, and angelica. A plaster of pitch and pigeon dung was put on the King's feet. Next there was more bleeding followed by the administration of melon seeds, manna, slippery elm, black cherry water, extract of lily of the valley, peony, lavender, pearls dissolved in vinegar, gentian root, nutmeg, and cloves. To this mixture were added 40 drops of the extract of human skull. Finally in desperation a bezoar stone was tried. The King died. (Haggard 1934, 267–68)

Cures for the Falling Sickness

Mistletoe was thought by the ancient druids to have curative virtues against St. Anthony's fire (erysipelas), corns, frostbite, muscular atrophy, apoplexy, infertility, chorea, and bubonic plague. It was Galen's drug of choice, and since he believed it to be a plant that grows on the oak and hence cannot fall, he reasoned that it should be a specific for the falling sickness (Lennox 1957). Colbatch, however, reported in 1719 that mistletoe was just as effective when grown on a lime tree. The reputed powers of mistletoe increased, and by the seventeenth century it was thought to be effective for edema, impotence, leprosy, syphilis, epilepsy, and other diseases. It was used by Sir Charles Locoock, who thought that epilepsy might be caused by crowded teeth, and hysteria associated with menses and onanism (Lennox 1957).

The revival of learning during the Renaissance marked the transition to modern civilization. Disciplines flourished, and progress in science and medicine, although inconstant and haphazard, accelerated in the seventeenth and eighteenth centuries, resulting in the end of Galenism.

The Seventeenth Century

Although medicine made rapid progress during the seventeenth century, treatment was still primitive. For example, the first edition of the *London Pharmacopoeia,* published in 1618, included remedies such as the celebrated antidote of Mattioli, mithridate, theriac Andromachus, Vigo's plaster (viper's flesh with live frogs and worms), worms, lozenges of dried vipers, fox lungs (for asthma), powders of precious stones, and oil of bricks, ants, and wolves. "The very witches' caldron was brewed in the pharmacopoeia of the seventeenth century" (Haggard 1934, 269). The 1650 *London Pharmacopoeia* contained moss from the skull of victims of violent death; and Gascoyne's powder made of bezoar, amber, pearls, crabs' eyes, coral, and black tops of crabs' claws. The 1677 *London Pharmacopoeia* included many new medications, such as cinchona bark, but also human urine. Other weird remedies contained in the three pharmacopoeias were "blood, fat, bile, viscera, bones, bone marrow, claws, teeth, hoofs, horns, sexual organs, eggs, and excreta of all sorts; bee-glue, cock's comb, cuttlefish fur, feathers, hair, isinglass, human perspiration, saliva of a fasting man, human placenta, raw silk, spider-webs, sponge, seashell, cast-off snake's skin, scorpions, swallows' nests, wood lice, and triangular Wormian bone from the juncture of the sagittal and lambdoid sutures of the skull of an executed criminal" (Garrison 1929, 289).

The ineptitude of physicians in the seventeenth century is reflected in the derisive comments by characters in Molière's plays: a medical candidate asked about his treatment for a string of ailments responds, "Clysterium donare, Postea seignare, En Suita purgare," thus advocating the incontestable merits of clyster, lancet, and purge for every disease, to which the august medical faculty responds,

"Bene, bene" (Garrison 1929). Guy Patin, dean of the faculty of the University
of Paris, bled his wife twelve times for a fluxion (excessive flow of fluid or blood)
in the chest, his son twenty times for fever, himself seven times for a head cold,
a friend thirty-six times for fever, and another sixty-four times for rheumatism
(Garrison 1929). Robert Boyle, a contemporary of Molière and the founder of
modern chemistry, after expunging many questionable remedies from the re-
vised pharmacopoeia, included the sole of an old shoe "worn by some man that
walked much," which was to be ground into a powder and taken for stomach
ache, true mistletoe of the oak for falling sickness, and album Graecum and goose
grease for hemorrhoidal pain (Haggard 1929). Sick patients continued to submit to purging, puking, poisoning, cutting, cupping, blistering, bleeding, freezing, heating, sweating, leeching, and shocking. The vast number of proprietary
preparations was another curious feature of seventeenth-century therapy.

The Eighteenth Century

The eighteenth century is variously characterized as "laying the foundations for
modern or scientific medicine" (Veith in King 1958, vii) and as "the adolescence
of modern medicine" (King 1958, viii), and is described by Garrison as "the age
of theories and systems" (King 1958, viii). Several important well-known therapeutic advances occurred in this century. William Withering learned about the
use of foxglove (digitalis) for dropsy (edema), a primary disease at the time, from
an old grande dame in 1776. He used it for heart disease but was unaware of the
distinction between cardiac and many other causes of edema. Although included in the Edinburgh Pharmacopoeia in 1783, digitalis was not included in the
London Pharmacopoeia until 1809. The story of Edward Jenner's use of vaccination for smallpox is well known. So too is James Lind's simple and straightfor-
ward study of the efficacy of lemons and oranges in prevention of scurvy, a result not accepted by physicians for another 160 years and not fully appreciated
by Lind himself.

   The value of a well-designed therapeutic trial was not appreciated in the eighteenth century (Gaddum 1954). Although pharmacopoeias continued to drop
questionable remedies, the 1746 London Pharmacopoeia retained mithridate, theriac, bezoars, crabs' eyes, and wood lice and included many new drugs that were
no more effective than the older drugs. Physicians compounded, dispensed, and
sold their own secret remedies, writing long-winded prescriptions, and English
clerics such as Bishop Berkeley and John Wesley dabbled in therapeutics. A fashionable theory in the eighteenth century, together with the vogue for clysters,

was the "doctrine of infarctus," which held that fecal impaction was the *causa causans* of most human ills (Garrison 1929).

The treatment of George Washington, who developed a cold and then quinsy (tonsillar abscess) at the age of fifty-seven, epitomizes treatment at the end of the eighteenth century. Within twelve hours, he was bled 2.5 to 2.8 quarts, followed by a moderate dose of American calomel, an injection, 5 grains of calomel, 5 to 6 grains of emetic tartar, frequent inhalations of vapors of vinegar water, blisters applied to the extremities, and a cataplasm of bran and vinegar applied to his throat, on which a blister had already been raised. The amount of bloodletting, especially with the likely dehydration from fever, a calomel purge, and the absence of hydration, was enough to have killed him, or at least to have hastened his death. Thus, once again an ineffective placebo treatment was capable of harming—even the "father of our country"—without being detected for many centuries.

The Nineteenth Century

The nineteenth century was marked by Claude Bernard's 1865 classic exposition of the scientific method, "founded on observation and proved by experience" (Modell 1976, 10). Bernard's ideas about experimental medicine, although conditioned by the time in which he lived, nevertheless strongly influenced the direction of experimentation in this century and are as relevant today as they were when they were written. Important developments included the study of morbid anatomy early in the century, physiology in midcentury, and the science of bacteriology and the beginning of pharmacology in the latter part of the century (Modell 1976).[5]

Therapeutics, however, without scientific knowledge of physiology, pathology, or chemistry, was primitive and irrelevant. Attempts to develop systems of therapy based on theory alone were totally unsuccessful (Modell 1976). Allopathy, which spread throughout the world, selected drugs to produce effects opposite to the symptoms of a disease. Massive dosages of drugs were used to sup-

---

5. For example, in 1864 Pasteur demonstrated that spontaneous generation did not exist and that the cause of fermentation and putrefaction was an as-yet-invisible microorganism. Lister followed in 1865 with antiseptic methods, paving the way for modern surgery. Koch isolated the anthrax bacillus in 1876, the tubercle bacillus in 1882, and the cholera vibrio in 1884; the streptococcus bacillus was identified in 1882; Pasteur developed the preventive vaccination for rabies in 1885, and Behring developed an inoculation against diphtheria in Koch's laboratory in 1894.

press the dominant symptoms of a disease and often resulted in death. For example, treatment for malaria and dysentery included purging with colonics until collapse.

Homeopathy is based on the principle of *similia similibus curantur*, or "like cures like" (the belief that the healing power of medicines depends on the resemblance of the symptoms they produce to the symptoms of the disease) and the principle of signatures of drugs, also used by Paracelsus (Holmes 1891). The latter principle is based on the astrological conception that stars impress the "signatures of disease" on drugs, and that the signatures are manifested by the form and color of the plant from which a drug is obtained. Thus, the similarity in shape of the root of the orchid to a testicle was the rationale behind its use to treat diseases of the testicle; and nutmeg, resembling the brain, was used to treat diseases of the brain. Another future development in the medical reasoning of homeopathy was the belief that the smaller the dose, the greater the effect, and the belief that drug action is potentiated by dilution. "From 1829 onward, [Hahnemann] recommended the administration of all drugs at the thirtieth potency, which corresponds to a concentration of 1 part in 10^{60} parts. This works out to a content of 1 molecule of drug in a sphere with a circumference equivalent to the orbit of Neptune" (Modell 1976, 9). If the dose contained no drug, its effectiveness was explained as due to a spiritual energy diffused throughout the medicine when shaken, or due to an "imprint" left behind on the solvent or excipient by the active molecules (Laurence and Bennett 1987). The homeopathic pharmacy contained many preparations that are as strange as those prescribed by ancient practitioners. Listed in the materia medica are "luna or moonlight," pediculi (lice), "flavus irides" (yellow ray of the spectrum), "albuminurea" (renal albumen or diseased urine), "adenia" (glands from a person suffering from Hodgkin disease), and many other such preparations (Reyburn 1990). Successful homeopathic and allopathic treatment illustrates the therapeutic benefit of the placebo effect and spontaneous improvement.[6]

The practitioners of eclecticism, a third system originating in the early nineteenth century, were defined as "those who subject and adopt in practice whatever is found beneficial, and who change their prescriptions according to emergencies, circumstances, and acquired knowledge" (Kremers and Urdang 1940, 161). It used a pharmacological smorgasbord, a combination of drugs that seemingly had a beneficial effect on illness but resulted in overtreatment and toxic effects.

---

6. See the review of the status of homeopathy and critical discussion of several somewhat controlled studies in *Consumer Reports* (Anonymous 1994a).

In regard to the use of drugs, Oliver Wendell Holmes commented: "Throw out opium" for pain, "throw out wine" for anesthesia, "and use a few specifics" such as quinine, mercury for syphilis, digitalis for heart disease, colchicum for gout, iodine for goiter, and ipecac for dysentery, "which our art did not discover." "If the whole materia medica . . . could be sunk to the bottom of the sea, it would be all the better for mankind and all the worse for the fishes" (Holmes 1891, xv).

Another recommended treatment was to suspend a patient by the feet or the head. Suspension by the feet, allowing the blood to flow into the head, was reported by Dr. Fulgence Raymond at the Salpêtrière in Paris to cure 70 percent of patients suffering from various diseases, including tabes. A similar success rate in a variety of organic and nervous diseases was reported by Dr. Haushalter, a collaborator of Bernheim, who suspended patients by the head (Volgyesi 1954). An interesting aspect of these studies is that the results for the two treatments were compared. The empirical comparison of results was clearly different from physicians' previous reliance on theory and venerable authorities to determine which therapies work.

By the end of the nineteenth century, physicians had become increasingly skeptical about medical treatment and were quite nihilistic about drug treatment (Medical Research Council 1950; Modell 1976; Coleman 1987). Osler, with more sophisticated views than were common at the time, characterized medicine at the end of the nineteenth century as "the New School of Medicine":

> The battle against poly-pharmacy, or the use of a large number of drugs (of the action of which we know little, yet we put them into bodies of the action of which we know less), has not been fought to a finish. . . . The characteristic of the New School is firm faith in a few good well-tried drugs, little or none in the great mass of medicines still in general use. . . . It is more concerned that a physician shall know how to apply the few great medicines which all have to use, such as quinine, iron, mercury, iodide of potassium, opium and digitalis, than that he should employ a multiplicity of remedies the action of which is extremely doubtful. (Osler 1932, 254–55)

chapter two

The Semantics of the Placebo

When I use a word . . . it means just what I choose it to mean—
neither more nor less.
HUMPTY DUMPTY, IN LEWIS CARROLL'S
"THROUGH THE LOOKING GLASS"

Definitions of the placebo have proliferated since the term *placebo* was first defined in a medical dictionary in 1785. This chapter focuses on the history of the
word, changes in its definition over time, and unknown or misunderstood semantic factors responsible for some of the diversity of opinion about the definition. It then proposes a definition fulfilling etymological, semantic, methodological, and heuristic criteria.

Etymology and Original Definitions

The history of the placebo begins with the Hebrew Bible. Psalm 116:9 begins
with the word *ethalekh,* which means "I will walk before." When the Bible was
translated into Latin, *ethalekh* was translated as *placebo,* the first-person singular,
future indicative active of the Latin verb *placere. Placebo* took on liturgical meanings when it became associated with a popular Catholic rite. It was the initial
word of the first antiphon and the name commonly given to Vespers in the Office
for the Dead, or Vespers for the Dead, a custom that is no longer used and whose
meaning has become obscure (*Catholic Encyclopedia* 1911). The entire sentence,
"Placebo Domino in regione vivorum," is translated as "I will please the Lord in
the land of the living," or "I will walk before the Lord in the land of the living"
in the King James version. With this usage, *placebo* entered the English language
in the thirteenth century, translated as "to please, give pleasure, be approved, be
pleasing, be agreeable, acceptable, to suit, satisfy." It was also used to denote win-
ning the applause of an audience (Lewis 1953).

   Placebo took on a secular meaning in the fourteenth century, and its conno-
tation became progressively derisive over the next several centuries: "to sing (a)

play (with), make, be at the school of placebo, etc.: to play the sycophant, flat-
terer, be servile or time serving, Obs." (*New English Dictionary* 1933). This usage
derives from derogation of the professional mourners who were paid to "sing
placebos"at the bier of the deceased in lieu of the family, whose role this was originally. The professional mourners probably were derogated because of their low
social status, because they derived income from the dead, and possibly because
they were a convenient object upon which the living could project their guilt.

A third use of the word has even more contemptible connotations: "a flat-
terer, sycophant, parasite" (*New English Dictionary* 1933) and "one who servilely
echoes another, a toady" (*Webster's New International* 1934). Chaucer used *Placebo* as the name of a character of this sort. This usage appears in various phrases
between 1388 and 1572.[1] In this etymological setting, the placebo as used in
medicine was born. Introduction of the word *placebo* to describe a class of treatments not previously specified was an important development in the history of
methodology and medicine.

A New English Dictionary on Historical Principles (1933) is the principal reference in the English language for the origin and history of the word *placebo*. Its
history of the term has two errors. The first definition of *placebo* was attributed
erroneously to Hooper's *Quincy's Lexicon-Medicum* (1811): "Placebo . . . an epithet given to any medicine adopted more to please than to benefit the patient."
This definition actually appeared eight years earlier, in Fox's *New Medical Dictionary* (1803). More serious is the omission of a definition that appeared even earlier. This omission has contributed to some of the subsequent confusion about
the definition.

A New English Dictionary on Historical Principles (1933) was the only reference
source for the history of the placebo until 1945, when Pepper published his now-
classic paper on the placebo.[2] Pepper corrected an important error in the *New
English Dictionary:* he noted an earlier definition that appeared in the tenth edition of Quincy's *Lexicon Physico-Medicum* (1787). A minor error was Pepper's failure to note that this definition had actually appeared two years earlier, in the sec-

---

1. 1388 Chaucer *Merch.* "Placebo seyede o Januarie brother (etc.)." 1426 LYDG. *De Guil
Pilgr.* "Ffletergny . . . Somme callen, hir Placebo, ffer sehe kan maken an Eccho Answere
euere ageyn the same." 1572 Knox Hist. *Ref. Wks.* "The Bischop . . . having his placebos
and Jackmen in the toun buffatted the Frier, and called him Heretick." 1651 Calderwood
Hist. Kirk. "Placeboes and flatters went to court."

2. Pepper's eloquent "Note on the Placebo" (1945) was one of the earliest papers devoted exclusively to the placebo effect, and the first to include the word *placebo* in the title.
The paper marked the beginning of interest in the placebo effect. It is a gem of medical reporting and is probably the most cited paper in placebo literature.

ond edition of Motherby's *New Medical Dictionary* (1785). But more important, Pepper, and those who followed, misquoted this definition as "a commonplace method of *[sic]* medicine." The actual definition, in Motherby, Quincy, and others, was "a commonplace method or medicine."

The distinction between *of* and *or* is important. The former limits the definition to medicine, whereas the latter includes methods *or* medicines. Thus, these early definitions classify as placebos not only medicines, or active drugs, but also methods—which could be types of nondrug treatment such as magic, talking, hypnosis, and psychotherapy. It is noteworthy also that early definitions did not classify placebos as inert substances.[3]

The Medical Definition of "Placebo"

The reasons for the introduction of the word *placebo* into medicine in 1785 are largely unknown. It is known, however, that placebos in the form of intentionally administered inert substances were not used clinically before 1785. Treatment included standard combinations such as cathartics, sweating, and bleeding, which were believed to be effective. With increased skepticism about the effectiveness of treatment, the term *placebo,* defined by Quincy (1787) as a "commonplace medication or method," began to be applied to some treatments.

Contempt and derogation characterized the premedical etymology of *placebo* and are reflected in the use of *commonplace* in the original medical definition. *Commonplace* refers to that which is common, trite, and pedestrian (*Webster's American* 1838), or "a cliche, superficial, used often, without originality or freshness, ordinary, dull, trite and stale" (*Webster's Third New International* 1961). The derisive intent was reflected in the first change in the definition of *placebo,* which

3. We wrote to the editors of the first edition of *The New English Dictionary on Historical Principles* (1933) in 1968 to correct their errors and clarify the history of the word *placebo* as described previously in this chapter. The corrections were acknowledged by the editors but did not appear until 1989, when the second edition of the *Oxford English Dictionary* was published. We were gratified, after all the years of disputing our definition with colleagues, to see how similar the definition in the 1989 edition is to the definition we proposed in the 1960s and in this chapter: "a substance or procedure which a patient accepts as a medicine or therapy but which actually has no specific therapeutic activity for his condition or is prescribed in the belief that it has no such activity. Freq. attrib., esp. in placebo effect, a beneficial (or adverse) effect produced by a placebo that cannot be attributed to the nature of the placebo." Thus, the 1989 *Oxford English Dictionary*'s definition of the placebo now includes inert and active medications, surgery, electricity, machines, methods, psychotherapy—in fact, any type of therapy, whether or not its ineffectiveness is known to the healer who prescribes it or the individual who uses it.

appeared in dictionaries by Motherby (1795, 1801) and later Parr (1809, 1820): "a commonplace method or medicine calculated to amuse for a time, rather than for any other purpose."

As discussed, although the definition of *placebo* changed slightly, to "a medication given to please," references to the placebo as medication were retained in major medical dictionaries until 1951. The placebo was first defined as inactive or inert at the end of the nineteenth century in Foster's (1894) dictionary; it was defined, idiosyncratically, as "an inactive substance" in *Taber's Medical Dictionary for Nurses* (Taber 1905) and as "inert" in *A Simplified Medical Dictionary for Lawyers* (Maloy 1942) and in the 1951 edition of Dorland's *American Illustrated Medical Dictionary*. Foster (1894) defined *placebo* as "a makebelieve medication." This definition was copied in several editions of *Appleton's Medical Dictionary* between 1904 and 1915, and although Dorland's dictionaries had defined placebo as "a medication given to please" in editions published between 1900 and 1944, the "makebelieve medication" surprisingly reappeared in Dorland's 1947 edition. In the 1951 edition of the *American Illustrated Medical Dictionary* the placebo was defined as "an inactive substance." Subsequently, other dictionaries and papers on the placebo effect began to define *placebo* as inactive or inert.

The word *inactive* first appeared in the definition of *placebo* in a nonmedical dictionary, when it was added parenthetically to the traditional definition in the second edition of *Webster's New International Dictionary* (1934): "a medicine, or preparation, especially an inactive one, given merely to satisfy a patient."[4]

Thus, for most of its history, from 1785 to 1951, the placebo was defined as a medication (such as cimicifuga nigra, condurango blanko, tincture of strychnine, valerian, or placental or orchic substance) or a method (such as Perkins's tractors and Mesmer's group hypnosis). Idiosyncrasy rather than substantive semantic or methodological principles largely contributed to the placebo's frequently being viewed as inactive or inert. According to its original definition and the definition used during most of its history, the word *placebo* describes a medication, often commonly in use, knowingly prescribed by a physician "to please a patient" rather than for its specific effect on a symptom or illness. Possible major contributing reasons for the changed definition are scientific progress in medicine, the defensiveness of physicians, the increased frequency of the use of inactive placebos in single- and double-blind studies, and the

---

4. This definition comes close to defining the placebo as an inactive or inert substance. According to Kay, who was the editor of *Webster's* dictionary in 1963, this definition stems from the late Dr. Esmond Long, of the Henry Phipps Institute at the Johns Hopkins University (Kay 1963).

marked increase in the number of papers on the placebo effect in the 1950s.

Defensiveness might have contributed to the original definition of *placebo* (Shapiro 1960a, 1960b). Despite medical advances, the vast majority of treatments were ineffective or placebos (Shapiro 1959, 1960b). It was not easy to differentiate between quack and physician on almost any criterion (Walker 1959), secret remedies characterizing the treatments of both (Garrison 1921). Physicians occasionally rejected important contributions by quacks, who often received official recognition by reigning royalty (Duran-Reynals 1946; Walker 1959). There was heated disputation; physicians vehemently railed against quacks and other physicians (Garrison 1921; King 1958; Shapiro 1960b). If the term *placebo* arose, in part, as a way for physicians to deprecate the treatments of quacks, the derogation rebounds on the physicians, because their own treatments were probably not much better and at times were actually more harmful (King 1958). Physicians may have become sensitive to the inadequacy of their ministrations. The derisive character of the epithet *placebo* suggests that it was a defensive appellation applied to the treatments used by others, much as today physicians attribute the use of placebos not to themselves but to other physicians (Hofling 1955; Shapiro 1960a; Shapiro and Struening 1973a, 1973b, 1974). Implying that the patient is amused, pleased, or humored by a placebo suggests a projective mechanism in which the physician disowns feelings of impotence, hostility, or guilt by portraying patients as foolishly requesting and responding to placebos (DeMaar and Pelikan 1955; Whitehorn 1958; Frank 1958; Shapiro 1959, 1960a, 1960b, 1963, 1969, 1971; Shapiro and Morris 1978).

Although the original definition characterized the placebo as a treatment knowingly prescribed for its psychological effect, it is likely that the knowing use of placebos was infrequent. It is probable that physicians denied their use of placebos and attributed this practice to derogated colleagues.

Placebo was a pejorative and not a scientific term. This may explain why it was used so infrequently in the past. Although the term is commonly used in medicine today, it was hardly used during the first hundred years of its existence. We have not been able to find any reference to its use in medicine, other than in dictionaries, until 1887. Although as early as the nineteenth century many papers discussed what we would refer to now as the placebo effect, the word *placebo* was infrequently used, and the term *placebo effect* has been used only since the mid-1950s.[5] In clinical treatment of patients, the knowing prescription of placebos

---

5. The term *placebo effect* appeared in medical literature concurrently with the use of the term *double blind* and the widespread introduction of controlled methodology in the evaluation of treatment.

(i.e., inert substances such as lactose) has not been used in medicine for many years.

The most frequent use of the placebo (a drug that does not have a specific effect on the condition being treated) was in the prescription of a drug that, unknown to the physician, was in fact a placebo, or in the prescription of a drug at a low dosage that does not have a specific effect (Modell 1955a).

The Scope of the Original Definition

There was no implication in the original definition, or in those that followed for a hundred years, that the term *placebo* was limited to, or even should be applied to, inert or inactive substances. In fact, it is doubtful that there was any significant deliberate prescribing of inert medication such as sugar pills. Such substances do not appear in the formularies or pharmacopoeias of the period. It is probable that if placebos were knowingly used, they were chosen from a group of drugs believed to be active but not very active. The judgment that the medications used in the past were placebos is that of hindsight and not that of the physicians who used the medications (Pepper 1945; DeMaar and Pelikan 1955; Shapiro 1959, 1960a).

The inclusion of treatment other than medication in the original definition may have derived from the eighteenth-century use of methods such as Franklinism, Galvanism, Mesmerism, celestial beds, laying on of hands, Perkins's tractors, and so forth.

The Narrowing of the Definition

During the nineteenth century, definitions of the placebo were increasingly limited to medicines. Methods disappeared from the definition entirely, although vague entities such as "treatment" and "anything" did continue in some definitions. The probable reason for this change was that nondrug treatment declined in importance during the first half of the nineteenth century, and medical practice became characterized by drug treatment. This was reflected in the treatments used by quacks, who usually follow and exploit those areas legitimately developed by scientific medicine (Garrison 1921; Walker 1959). The nineteenth century has been described as the great age of the patented, secret preparation, or nostrum, and the predominant quack activity during that period was the use of these drugs (Garrison 1921; Young 1961). As a parallel development, placebo definitions gradually became limited to medicines.

The first allusion to the placebo as inert occurred during the last decade of the nineteenth century. The details of this change and the possible happenstance contributing to it were described above. Other factors were even more important: scientific medicine began in the late nineteenth century, and therapy became more rational and effective. Physicians probably became more confident, but at the same time somewhat self-conscious about their impotence and pretensions. The first Food and Drug Act was passed in 1906 (Young 1961). Polypharmacy was bitterly denounced, and the use of senseless remedies decreased (Cramp 1911, 1913, 1921, 1936; Sollmann 1912, 1916, 1917, 1930; Osler 1932). Fewer medicines were available for simple psychological treatment, and substances that were clearly inert could perhaps better perform this function. Psychological factors in illness and treatment became more evident after the remarkable success of Christian Science (Twain 1899; Janet 1925), the impact of homeopathy (Holmes 1891), the study of hypnotism and suggestion (which was termed the stage of scientific psychotherapy by Janet [1924, 1925] and Bernheim [1889]), and the introduction of moral, persuasive, suggestive, and insight psychotherapies that followed (Parker 1908–9). Perhaps a preference for uncontaminated or inert drugs developed because of a belief that they differentiated their prescriber from the homeopathist. But during this period the placebo was inert by implication only. It did not become popularly or medically characterized as inert until about the second half of the twentieth century.

Ironically, the major determinant of this limited definition (defining the placebo as inert) was the introduction of scientific methodology in which inert placebos were used in the evaluation of treatment and the conduct of clinical trials. Medical journals increasingly published more controlled than uncontrolled clinical studies. Beginning in the 1950s, controlled clinical trials, double-blind procedures, and statistical analyses, almost nonexistent before 1950, increased dramatically in number. It is too early to say whether future historians will consider this development the major medical advance during the 1950s.

Early in the development of controlled clinical trials, inert placebos were given as single-blind controls. This proved to be inadequate, and the double-blind procedure evolved as a more adequate method of controlling bias. The rationale was that the inert placebo, under double-blind conditions, would provide a control for spontaneous change and psychological and other variables and would permit clear-cut differentiation between active and inactive treatments (Gold 1946; Greiner et al. 1950; Modell and Houde 1958; Shapiro 1978). Placebos have received considerable publicity through their increased use in major studies such as the Medical Research Council study of tuberculosis in England (1948), the poliomyelitis study in America during the 1950s, and many studies of the placebo effect (Shapiro 1971; Shapiro and Morris 1978; Shapiro and Shapiro 1984b;

White et al. 1985). With these developments the placebo became increasingly identified with inert substances.

Concurrent with these advances in methodology, clinicians and behavioral clinical researchers became interested in the placebo effect. Placebo literature, almost nonexistent previously, became voluminous (Shapiro 1960a, 1960b, 1971; Shapiro and Morris 1978). More papers have probably been written about the placebo effect in the last twenty-five years than in all previous years combined. The American Psychiatric Association held its first roundtable meeting on the placebo in 1959, and many journals have reviewed the subject: *Physicians Bulletin* (Anonymous 1955a, 1955b), *Spectrum* (Anonymous 1957a, 1957b, 1960b), the *New York Herald Tribune* (Ubell 1959), the *New Yorker* (Roueché 1960), the *Psychiatric Reporter* (Smith Kline and French 1962), the *Medical Times* (Anonymous 1962), *Hospital Focus* (Anonymous 1964b), and *Medical Science* (Anonymous 1964a, 1964c). All contemporary dictionaries contain definitions of *placebo*.

But further refinement of the double-blind procedure has lagged behind other advances in the conduct of clinical trials. For example, it now has become apparent that inert placebos frequently are inadequate controls in double-blind studies (see chapter 9). Inert placebos can be differentiated from active drugs by patient and physician, and the procedure may become single blind or nonblind. The incidental physiological effects of an active agent may have profound psychological effects on patients, physicians, and evaluators. Today it is known that an adequate placebo should mimic the telltale effects of the active agent under study and be carefully formulated and matched so that patients and physicians are unable to detect physical differences (Blumenthal et al. 1974). To mimic the effects of the active agent necessitates the use of an active substance as a placebo control (Modell and Houde 1958; Nash 1959; Shapiro et al. 1960; Shapiro 1963, 1964a; Blumenthal et al. 1974). The limited definitions in dictionaries reflect this lag in knowledge.

The question of inert versus active placebo is academic, because there is no such thing as an inactive substance. Even substances such as distilled water and lactose can cause bodily changes. (Nevertheless, in this book, particularly when describing other researchers' studies, we often make the conventional distinction between "active drug" and placebo.)

Attempts to differentiate between active and inactive dosages of a drug are often difficult and arbitrary. Just as homeopathists believe their dosages to be active, many physicians unknowingly prescribe inactive dosages of tranquilizers, such as trifluoperazine, 1 mg twice a day, or meprobamate, 200 mg three times a day (Shapiro 1964a). The continuum from inert to active cannot be easily dichotomized. Many drugs are prescribed in a range of dosages in which it is difficult to specify when the drug is active or inactive, and when psychological factors and placebo effects become important variables and determinants of drug response (Shapiro 1963, 1964a, 1978).

Limiting the definition of *placebo* to inert medication is historically inaccurate, not in keeping with modern usage, and irrelevant, arbitrary, and heuristically useless.

The Broadening of the Definition to Include Psychotherapies

Definitions of the placebo were not included in psychological and psychiatric dictionaries until recently. The first definition of *placebo* in a psychological or psychiatric dictionary appeared in the *New Dictionary of Psychology* (Harriman 1947). *Placebo* was defined traditionally, as "a pill or a liquid given to humor the patient with a psychoneurotic disorder. Its therapeutic effects, if any, are psychological, not physiological." A more comprehensive review of psychiatric definitions is given in Shapiro 1968.

Considering the long history of medicine, the history of the placebo is recent. The meaning and definition of *placebo,* like those of most other words, have changed during its brief history. There have been periods during which the term was hardly used. Recently, *placebo* has become a popular word and an important methodological concept. It has replaced terms such as *suggestion* and *dummy preparation.* The meaning and definition of the term will probably continue to evolve as a function of changes in medical practice, knowledge, and theory.

This leads to the semantic question of whether new treatment methods should be included in the definition of *placebo.* Psychotherapy and psychoanalysis are the most recent treatments to be considered for inclusion, but psychotherapists frequently reject the inclusion of these treatments in the definition. Their reactions are defensive, and similar to those of physicians and healers of the past when the effectiveness of therapeutic methods was challenged (Shapiro 1960a; Shapiro and Struening 1973a, 1973b, 1974). The arguments against including psychological treatment in the definition include: psychotherapy is not a drug and therefore cannot be a placebo; psychotherapy is the application of psychological principles and does in a scientific way what the placebo attempts to do unscientifically, and therefore is not a placebo; and psychotherapy was not included in the original definition (see also the discussion in chapter 5).

It is true that psychotherapy was not included in the original definition. But the reason for this exclusion is that no such treatment formally existed at the time. Retrospectively, however, it can be included in the definition because any type of therapy can and should be included. Not to include it would render logic and scientific methodology meaningless and would emphasize the essential defensiveness of such a position.

If a specific psychological therapy, tested under controlled conditions, resulted in a nonspecific benefit no different from that resulting from nonspecific control therapies, it is incontestable that this benefit would have to be attributed to what is now referred to as the placebo effect. This operational definition has been advocated in many of the papers referred to in previous sections.

The Use of the Term "Placebo" in Research

The term *placebo* has been reserved for agents or procedures used as controls in experimental studies, whether or not the research includes evaluation of a therapy. British authors occasionally use the word *dummy* to describe an agent used as a control in research, and *placebo* to describe an agent used in therapy (Gaddum 1954; Wilson 1962). The rationale for this differentiation is unconvincing (Beecher 1956), and the word *dummy* appears infrequently in the literature.

The Inclusion of Mechanisms of Action in the Definition

Several authors have defined the placebo operationally by including in the definition explanatory mechanisms such as expectation, transference, conditioning, mobilization of hope, faith, and so forth (Whitehorn 1958; Hinsie and Campbell 1960; Frank 1961; Hahn 1985; Plotkin 1985; Wickramasekera 1985). But none of the mechanisms has been experimentally verified as the major variable. An operational definition is therefore premature. Such definitions may have heuristic value, however, and provide models for further experimentation.

The Distinction between Placebo and Placebo Effect

It has been proposed that the placebo be defined as the agent or procedure and the placebo effect as the response to the placebo (Fischer and Dlin 1956; Lesse 1962). The placebo effect may be positive (a favorable response), or negative (an unfavorable response), or absent (no response). Since placebos are medications or procedures, the implication is that placebos are only used knowingly and deliberately, and the placebo effect, if it occurs, may be known or unknown to the prescriber of the placebo. Although this distinction has merit, it leads to a logical inconsistency. If a treatment is prescribed by a physician in the belief that it is specific and not a placebo, and a placebo effect occurs unknown to the physician, the treatment cannot then be considered a placebo treatment. This awkward inconsistency can be parsimoniously resolved by defining the placebo effect in terms of the placebo. Such a definition also can fulfill other historical and heuristic criteria.

Other authors have proposed a distinction between placebo response and placebo effect. For Michael Jospe (1978), the placebo response is the behavioral change of subjects receiving placebos, while the placebo effect is only the portion of behavioral change that is attributed to any therapeutic procedure that lacks specific activity for the condition to be treated, and not that portion related to other "spontaneous" influences or the passage of time. Sherman Ross and L. W. Buckalew (1985) saw a difference between a response and an effect. An effect, they wrote, is part of the response domain and is directly attributable to the specific action of a drug or placebo.

A distinction should be made, however, between suggestion and the placebo effect. The terms *placebo* and *placebo effect* should be reserved primarily for therapies and therapeutic effects. Suggestion is associated more closely with laboratory experiments and hypnosis. There are historical, linguistic, and methodological reasons for this distinction. Some of the factors that are important in the therapeutic situation are not present or are minimized in the experimental situation, which includes an experimenter rather than a therapist, a subject rather than a patient, and a laboratory experiment rather than a clinical treatment (Shapiro 1960b, 1963, 1964c, 1971, 1978). Other factors that are absent in the experimental situation include the physician-patient relationship, the physician's interest in the patient and the patient's clinical condition, professional and therapeutic commitments, the optimistic needs of the physician, the patient's expectations, clinical anxiety (as distinct from experimental anxiety), and many other variables (Shapiro 1969). In addition, there is little correlation between tests of suggestibility in a laboratory situation and the placebo effect in a clinical setting (Shapiro 1960b, 1963, 1964b, 1964c, 1971, 1978).

Autosuggestion and posthypnotic suggestion during hypnosis are included in the same category as suggestion. However, if they are used as a therapeutic technique with expectations of therapeutic benefit, the procedure may be a placebo and result in placebo effects.

A Proposed Definition of "Placebo"

The original definition of *placebo* included medicines and methods. Therefore, all types of therapy were included in the first definition. Later, definitions of the term became limited to medicine, and recently to inert substances. These changes paralleled changes in medical theory and practice. Recent advances in medicine and experimental methodology justify another revision of the definition: it should once again include any method of therapy. The definition should also provide a unified concept that operationally can include both physiological and psychological therapy. It should include, for example, active medication such as vitamins for neurasthenia (Anonymous 1955c), surgical procedures such as mammary artery ligation for angina pectoris (Wolf 1959a, 1959b; Beecher 1961), and relatively recent treatments such as psychotherapy. Limiting the definition of *placebo* to medicines is unjustified historically, linguistically, and methodologically.

Placebo was used originally as a derisive epithet to describe the treatment provided by nonphysicians and not knowingly or deliberately prescribed by physicians. The criterion for placebo treatment should be based on principles of scientific methodology. Nevertheless, it is clear from statements published in the literature that there are many different, strongly held views that vary between and within medical specialties, and that the attitudes of psychiatrists are different from those of nonpsychiatrists. These differences were surveyed in 1960 (see discussion in chapter 8). The difficulties in determining what should be included in the definition of *placebo* were discussed in this survey.

Inadequate definitions of the placebo and the placebo effect can lead to erroneous conclusions and hamper research. For example, various investigators have attempted to relate placebo effects (positive, negative, and absent) to the personality of the patient. But these attempts have not been successful: personality traits found in one study differ from those reported in others. Contradictory findings can be the result of different clinical conditions, patient populations, research procedures, and settings. Some of the studies report, however, and it is commonly assumed, that (when compared with placebo nonreactors) placebo reactors are less intelligent; less educated; more frequently neurotic or psychotic; more frequently female; from lower social classes; more dependent, inadequate, immature, impulsive, atypical, depressed, religious, and stereotypic (Shapiro 1964b, 1964c, 1964f; Shapiro and Shapiro 1984b); and more likely to have symptoms of hypochondriasis, obsessive compulsiveness, anger–hostility, bewilderment–confusion, and performance difficulties (Shapiro and Shapiro 1984b). In our studies and others there appear to be no consistent data relating either these variables or demographic variables such as age, sex, intelligence, race, social class, ethnicity, religiosity, or religious background to placebo reaction. (See later chapters for a discussion of these findings.)

These personality variables probably describe patients for whom a placebo in the form of a drug is culturally appropriate. The traits are probably inherent not in placebo reactors but in patients who are drug oriented. Such patients may react favorably to a drug placebo stimulus and unfavorably, or not at all, to a psychotherapeutic placebo stimulus. The converse may occur with patients who believe in psychotherapy. They may not react, or may react adversely, to a drug placebo stimulus. In other words, a drug may be a good placebo stimulus for some patients, and psychotherapy may be a good placebo stimulus for others (Fenichel 1954; Schmideberg 1958; Shapiro 1964b, 1964d; Shapiro and Shapiro 1984b). All patients are likely to react occasionally to placebos if the placebo stimulus is appropriate; in other words, placebo reactivity is universal (Shapiro and Shapiro 1984b). Recognizing the importance of this stimulus variable is a precondition for study of the placebo effect (Shapiro 1964b, 1964c, 1964d). If research on the placebo effect is limited to drugs, the underlying mechanism may be obfuscated and the secret of the placebo reactor may continue to elude us. A heuristic definition can minimize that possibility.[6]

The conceptual schema can be illustrated by discussing the relative importance of placebo and nonplacebo effects when various doses of chlorpromazine are administered. The effect of 100 grams of chlorpromazine will be very predictable and essentially the same for all patients—hypnosis, coma, and death. By contrast, only placebo effects will occur with homeopathic dosages of 1 mg of chlorpromazine. The ratio of placebo effects to nonplacebo, specific and predictable effects will decrease with higher dosages. Not included in the schema are factors such as fluctuations in the natural course of illness, clinical bias, methodological variables, untoward side effects, and negative placebo effects.

The most predicable and highly specific effects will occur with a massive overdose of chlorpromazine. At such a dose the cortex cannot function. Without a functioning cortex, nonspecific, placebo, or psychological effects do not occur. For example, if therapeutic dosages of atropine are given to a decorticate subject, the effects on the gastrointestinal mucosa are specific and predictable. The same dosages given to a subject with an intact cortex will have variable effects that will be related to the subject's psychological state (Wolf 1959a, 1959b). Most

6. The first attempts to identify the personality of the placebo reactor occurred in studies by Lasagna and others (Lasagna et al. 1954; von Felsinger et al. 1955; Lasagna 1956). These have been extensively quoted and have stimulated other such studies. But they also contributed to the myth of the placebo personality and sidetracked fruitful research for many years. These studies can be criticized on many levels: atypical populations, use of limited settings, inadequate numbers, many uncontrolled variables, variables without evidence of reliability and validity, anecdotal and insufficient data, extensive generalizations unwarranted by the data, and so forth (see also Trouton 1957; and chapters 7 and 10 in this book). Since methodology was in a relatively primitive state when these studies were done, their shortcomings are understandable.

therapeutic agents and procedures are used in subjects with intact cortices and are useful only in a range in which psychological factors are important. Therefore, placebo and nonspecific effects are an almost inevitable concomitant of all therapy.

This schema can probably be applied to every therapeutic modality. It would include treatment with drugs such as barbiturates, digitalis, thyroid hormone, and vitamins, as well as surgical treatment, psychotherapy, psychoanalysis, and so forth.

Our proposed definition makes no assumption about which treatments are placebos or about the mechanism of placebo action. These issues are left open because the placebo effect is a multiply determined, not-yet-understood phenomenon (Shapiro 1964b, 1964c; Shapiro and Shapiro 1984b; White et al. 1985). A good definition is a phenomenological statement that avoids becoming tautological. It provides a good model for research, a structure into which variables can be put for testing, and it makes possible independent assessment about which everyone can agree.

We believe that the following definitions fulfill these criteria:

—A placebo is any therapy (or that component of any therapy) that is intentionally or knowingly used for its nonspecific, psychological, or psychophysiological, therapeutic effect, or that is used for a presumed specific therapeutic effect on a patient, symptom, or illness but is without specific activity for the condition being treated.
—A placebo, when used as a control in experimental studies, is a substance or procedure that is without specific activity for the condition being treated.[7]
—The placebo effect is the nonspecific psychological or psychophysiological therapeutic effect produced by a placebo.

In other words, a placebo therapy may be used with or without knowledge that it is a placebo. It may be a treatment that is given in the belief that it is not a placebo, but that actually is a placebo by objective evaluation. The placebo may be inert or active and may include, therefore, any medical treatment, no matter how potentially specific or how administered. It may take the form of oral and parenteral medication, topical preparations, inhalants, and any mechanical, surgical, psychotherapeutic, or other therapeutic techniques. It may be a treatment producing symptoms or side effects that are not specific for that treatment. A

7. We are indebted to Adolf Grünbaum for calling our attention to an error in wording in a previous version of this chapter.

placebo may or may not result in a placebo effect, and the effect may be favorable or unfavorable—that is, positive or negative.

Examples of a placebo would be the use of homeopathic dosages of digitalis for psychoneurotic anxiety, hysterectomy for irritable colon, or 5 mg of chlorpromazine for an acute psychosis. Examples of nonplacebos would be penicillin for scarlatina, digitalis for congestive heart failure, and appendectomy for appendicitis.

Although the definition proposed here may in the future prove to be too inclusive, for heuristic reasons it would be premature to make specific exclusions. It is likely that various factors contributing to the placebo effect will be reliably isolated—factors such as remission and exacerbation during the natural course of illness, regression of measures to the mean, observer bias and effects of investigators, patients' expectations, and methodological variables. When everything is known about the placebo and the placebo effect, there will probably no longer be a need for the definition, except in etymologies of obsolete terms, but this is a desideratum for the future.

chapter three

Fraud, Faith, and Fads

Unconventional Methods of Treatment

Quackery

The word *quack* is a shortened version of *quacksalver*, meaning one who boasts ("quacks") about the virtues of salves and ointments. When mercury became a fad in Europe, causing more toxic poisoning than benefit, nonphysicians began to use it. They were known as quacksalvers.

Clearly, quacks were transparent impostors and swindlers who had no hesitancy in unlawfully including narcotics or spirits in their patent medicines and in developing and touting bogus treatments. They frequently traded on their sociopathic charm, attractiveness, and magnetism to sell their fraudulent cures. Their medical quackery was extremely unethical. James H. Young (1961, 251) quoted former postmaster general Arthur Summerfield's remark that more money was being made in medical quackery than in "any other criminal activity."

Quackery has existed throughout medical history (Cramp 1911, 1936; Fishbein 1925, 1932; Young 1961, 1992). Although repeatedly condemned, disparaged, and dismissed, it never seems to go away. Young (1992, 3) quoted an observation by Francis Bacon: "The weakness and credulity of men is such that they often prefer a mountebank, or a cunning woman, to a learned physician. . . . For in all times, witches, old women, and impostors, have, in the vulgar opinion, stood competition with physicians." According to Oliver Wendell Holmes, "Quackery and idolatry are all but immortal." Despite repeated exposés of quackery's fraudulence, extensive federal regulations, law enforcement, and the belief that as people become more intelligent and medicine more scientific, quackery would disappear, quackery is more extensive than ever before. Young (1992, 26) noted that quackery "astonishingly had not proved to be a temporary irrelevancy beclouding the rational American mind but an integral and growing aspect of American behavior."

Recent exposures of many extensively used and expensive treatments of cancer include, for example, Harry Hoxsey's pink medicine (containing lactated pepsin and potassium iodide) and black medicine (containing "a botanical lax-ative in an extract of prickly ash bark, buckthorn bark, barberry root, licorice root, pokeweed, alfalfa, and red clover blossoms") (Young 1992, 235). The U.S. Food and Drug Administration (FDA) estimated that 38 to 40 million Ameri-cans spent $30 billion annually for fraudulent treatment, with 10 percent of the users suffering side effects (Henney 1993). Krebiozin, containing a white pow-der said to come from the blood of horses injected with a microorganism re-sponsible for "lumpy jaw in cattle," and Laetrile's apricot pit (costing seventy-five thousand people more than $168 million, and still being sold) have not deterred the development of more than one hundred quack cancer treatments that have taken their place. The number and cost of quack remedies purporting to cure arthritis and colds, to treat other ailments, and to promote health and nu-trition continue to soar, as does the use of vitamins (Young 1992). As pointed out by Fishbein in 1938, "public interest in vitamins has led to a more extraor-dinary exploitation than in any other field of medicine" (Young, 1992, 357).

Although quackery is a particularly malignant form of the placebo effect, its omnipresence and massive use is another manifestation of the ubiquity of that effect. Health quackery, according to Young (1992), involves exploitation of fear in the patient; the promise of painless treatment and good results; claims of miraculous scientific breakthrough; the proposal of one cause and one thera-peutic system to end confusion and doubt and to make complexity simple and comprehensible to the untutored mind; quacks' persecutory response to criti-cism (by representing themselves as pioneers and future heroes like Columbus and Galileo, who were also rejected); and quacks' conspiratorial response to crit-icism (the claim that members of the establishment dare not acknowledge their discovery because it will undermine their power and prestige and eliminate their jobs). Other characteristics of quackery are also typical of placebo therapy: con-stant changes in how the therapy works, and on what illnesses; repackaging of old treatments based on the fads of the day; and reliance on testimonials (which are always readily obtainable) about the effectiveness of treatment.[1]

---

1. Young (1992, 4), in his "Prologue: A Quota of Quotations on Quackery" cites two observations about quackery: "Strange to say, university towns are hot beds of quackery. Too often the professor thinks that because he knows a lot about mathematics or Greek, he automatically knows a lot about medicine." And "it is a most extraordinary thing, but I never read a patent medicine advertisement without being impelled to the conclusion that I am suffering from the particular disease therein dealt with in its most virulent form." See also *New York State Journal of Medicine* (1993) for a summary of health fraud and quackery.

Religious Treatment

Religiosity is one of the most universal of human attributes. The sociobiologist Wilson (1978) characterized the drive to religious belief as a complex and powerful force in the human mind and perhaps an ineradicable part of human nature. So too may be the need for the priest, magician, and medicine man, who were one and the same in all primitive societies (Garrison 1929). A corollary of religiosity is its association with treatment. In the Middle Ages, the Church emphasized the healing powers of Christ to weaken beliefs in Asclepius and in pagan rituals. Early Christians tended to scorn medical treatment of disease as interference with God's plan. Christ was referred to as the Apothecary of the Soul in the Middle Ages, treatment of the soul being thought more important than treatment of the body. The laying on of hands and exorcism were the primary treatments to rid the person of affliction.

"In every epoch, in every land, and in most religions, there have been well-known holy places where miraculous cures were promised, and usually attributed to the action of God" (Leuret and Bon 1957, 36). Of the thousands of shrines and sanctuaries, Lourdes is the quintessential example, receiving up to 5 million pilgrims annually (Marnham 1981). In a beautiful thirty-acre verdant setting surrounded by two crystal-clear languorous flowing rivers, up to twenty thousand pilgrims from all over the world participate each day in an extraordinary, well-orchestrated program of miraculous healing. During a visit to Lourdes in 1968, we saw several hundred of the most cachectic and moribund persons on stretchers, and many with what appeared to be severe neurological disorders in wheelchairs. Most of the other pilgrims appeared well outwardly, but an inward harboring of some distress was evident by their single-minded rushing from one healing ceremony to another. Each activity was followed by another: morning and afternoon baths at the grotto, drinking of waters, prayers in certain places and before certain statues, processions, singing of hymns, and listening to sonorous baritone songs and prayers by priests in many languages, made even more impressive by a booming crescendo of what sounded like "Amen" and "Ave Maria" by thousands of pilgrims. The mood was infectious, and we found ourselves caught up in the atmosphere, even to the point of acceding to our children's request to buy white candles so they could participate in the evening torchlight procession of thousands of pilgrims whose candles lit a path around the enclave. It was the most magnificent group therapy session we had ever experienced.

Lourdes impressed even Freud, who said, "I do not think our cures can compete with those of Lourdes. There are so many more people who believe in the miracles of the Blessed Virgin than in the existence of the unconscious" (Janet 1925, 196). Despite the popularity of, interest in, and curiosity and testimonials about the curative effect of faith healing at Lourdes, Louis Rose (1971), in his twenty-year study of faith healing, never observed anyone who grew up as a child in the village of Lourdes who had been cured of anything at the grotto of Lourdes as an adult.

Religious therapy has also taken the form of a major medicoreligious movement. Phineas P. Quimby, whose famous patient was Mary Baker Eddy, the founder of Christian Science, was a prominent nineteenth-century healer in New England. In 1859 he made a cogent observation: "But through a great many mistakes, and the prescription of a great many useless drugs, I was led to re-examine the question, and came in the end to the position I now hold: the cure does not depend upon any drug, but simply upon the patient's belief in the doctor or the medicine" (Janet 1925, 85). The importance of faith is reflected in the spread of Christian Science, primarily appealing to the middle classes. Although its proponents are one of the best-educated major religious groups in the United States, they are able to deny the rational efficacy of any treatment or medicine and to assign all treatment benefits to faith. An enormously wealthy sect, by 1990 they had about three thousand churches worldwide and eight hundred radio stations to carry their broadcasts. The only statistics allowed by the church were based on the 1936 census, which reported 268,915 adherents. No recent figures are available (*Dictionary of Christianity in America* 1990).

Throughout history there have been faith healers and psychic healers, some associated with established and marginal religions, others not formally associated with any religion. They number in the hundreds of thousands. Rose (1971) estimated that in 1970 there were probably more than ten thousand healers in England and more than forty thousand unorthodox healers (predominantly homeopathic) in France. It is ironic, however, that faith and psychic healing may have been more effective than traditional medical treatment in the past because they allowed nature to take its course, thus possibly doing no harm, whereas traditional medication not only was largely ineffective but also often harmed patients and even hastened their demise.

This is no longer true. Although much is still unknown, medicine is now on a scientific footing, many effective and specific treatments are available, and methodology can differentiate effective treatments from ineffective ones and safe from unsafe treatments. The effectiveness of religious healing, however, is based not on controlled studies but on faith, and if it works, it is highly likely that this is due to the placebo effect.

Quackery and religious treatments are similar because both rely on the placebo effect. In another way, however, they are different. Quackery is fraudulent treatment by untrained mendacious individuals without controlled studies of efficacy, whereas many of the practitioners of innumerable religious healing cults who rely primarily on faith do not seem to be deceitful scoundrels.

In addition to mystical religious healing, religious healing now includes extensive pastoral counseling provided by clerics who are trained in the traditional methods of psychotherapy. It is probable that a controlled study comparing pastoral counseling to traditional psychotherapy would find both equally effective, except that pastoral psychotherapy might be less effective for patients who were atheists and more effective for religious patients.[2] The ultimate question of whether both are largely placebo treatments is part of the ongoing controversy about whether all forms of psychotherapy are placebo treatments.

Unorthodox, or "Alternative," Therapies

Unorthodox therapies may also be referred to as alternative, complementary, or unconventional medicine (Eisenberg et al. 1993). These therapies are classified as cults because they follow dogma or principle based on theories or beliefs, to the exclusion of demonstrable scientific experience and evidence (Laurence and Bennett 1987). Some of these treatments clearly fit the quack category. For example, Young (1992) cited alternative medicine as including homeopathy, reflexology (correction of body problems by foot manipulation), and iridology (examination of the irises of the eyes in order to diagnose an impending heart attack; back, lung, or sinus trouble; acidic, arthritic, or anemic conditions; prolapsed colon; backed-up lymph system; underactive or overactive glands; and cancer).[3]

David M. Eisenberg and colleagues (1993, 246), in a study of the prevalence, costs, and patterns of use of unconventional therapies, described them as a broad spectrum of practices and beliefs not in conformity with the standards of the medical community and defined them "as medical interventions not taught

2. A study by Propst et al. (1992) indicated that cognitive behavioral therapy with religious content and pastoral counseling was significantly better for fifty-nine depressed religious patients than was cognitive-behavioral therapy without religious content.

3. The World Health Organization (Bannerman et al. 1983) listed other unorthodox therapies, such as anthroposophical medicine, applied kinesiology, Kirilian photography, reflexology, osteopathy, chiropractic, impact therapy, Rolfing, breathing, cymatics, psionics, radiesthesia, radionics, orgone therapy, pyramid therapy, naturopathy, Dianetics, aromatherapy, flower therapy, biochemics, orthomolecular medicine, and bioenergetics. See Laurence and Bennett (1987) for a discussion of cults.

widely at US medical schools or generally available at US hospitals." The sample comprised a random sample of 1,539 subjects. The sixteen therapies selected for the study included relaxation techniques, chiropractic, massage, imagery, spiritual healing, commercial weight-loss programs and lifestyle diets (e.g., macrobiotics), herbal medicine, megavitamin therapy, self-help groups, energy healing, biofeedback, hypnosis, homeopathy, acupuncture, folk remedies, exercise, and prayer.

The study reported that unconventional therapies, excluding exercise and prayer, had been used in the past twelve months by 34 percent of the 1,539 subjects, and that this use was unrelated to sociodemographics, sex, and health insurance status. The use of these therapies was more common among people between twenty-five and forty-nine years of age with some college education and annual incomes over $35,000; more common among people living in the West; and less common among African Americans. For the ten most common medical conditions, 25 percent used unconventional therapy, and 10 percent of the subjects studied were using such therapy for a primary medical condition. The most frequent conditions were back problems (36%), anxiety (28%), headache (27%), chronic pain (26%), and cancer (24%). The most frequent unconventional therapies were relaxation techniques, chiropractic, and massage. Extrapolation to the U.S. population in 1990 suggests that an estimated 61 million used at least one of the sixteen unconventional therapies; 22 million saw unconventional providers for a primary medical condition; fourteen of the therapies were used by more than 1 million people; 452 million visits were made, costing $11.7 million for visits (excluding the cost of herbs, etc.); $2 billion was spent for diet formulas, prepackaged foods, and diet pills; and the total cost for all expenses was $13.9 billion. Out-of-pocket expenses were $10.3 billion, which contrasts with out-of-pocket expenses of $12.8 billion for all hospitalizations in the United States and is nearly half as much as the $23.5 billion spent out of pocket for all physician services.

An Office of Alternative Medicine was established in 1993 at the National Institutes of Health to use conventional controlled-study methodology to evaluate the effectiveness of unconventional medical practices. The subjects to be considered include diet (macrobiotics, megavitamins), nutrition, and lifestyle changes; mind/body control (art therapy/relaxation, biofeedback, counseling, guided imagery, hypnotherapy, and sound/music therapy); traditional medicine and ethnomedicine (acupuncture, Ayurvedic medicine, herbal medicine, homeopathic medicine, Native American medicine, natural products, and traditional Oriental medicine); structural manipulations and energetic therapies (acupressure, chiropractic medicine, massage, reflexology, Rolfing, therapeutic touch, Qigong); pharmacological and biological treatments (antioxidants, cell treatment, chelation therapy, metabolic therapy, and oxidizing agents); and bioelectromagnetic applications (diagnostic and therapeutic applications of electromagnetic fields, e.g., transcranial electrostimulation, neuromagnetic stimulation, electroacupuncture). We list them to indicate the unbelievable number of alternative therapies being used, all so designated because there is no evidence from controlled studies that they are effective. How many therapies are likely to survive such studies? Or, even if they are not evaluated, how many are likely to simply disappear, only to be replaced by a newer, more fashionable placebo therapy, as do most treatments that rely on the placebo effect?

The most fashionable therapies today are referred to by Young (1992, 243) as New Age therapies, which stress "lifestyle changes . . . restoring life to more rational patterns where patients could play an active role in their own healing." As society becomes more intricate, technological, and difficult to understand, knowledge becomes more specialized. In reaction to this development, there has been a movement toward individual responsibility and an increasing desire to determine and control one's health. Recent therapeutic trends include psychotherapeutic treatment by clerics, nurses, laypersons, and gurus; a multitude of self-help modalities; and, most recently, interest in holistic medicine and behavioral health, exemplified by the use of jogging, megavitamins, nutrition, organic foods, vitamins, and stress reduction; the rise of speculative beliefs about how the mind affects the body; and immune therapy, such as mentally and visually imagining and encouraging the growth and strength of good white blood cells in order to immunologically destroy bad, malignant cells.

The universal quest for tranquillity, healing, immortality, and freedom from dysphoria and disease continues unabated and constantly changes, influenced by culture and the failure of older therapies. A renewed interest in these therapies and their new respectability is reflected in two featured articles that appeared one week apart in the *New York Times*.

The first article discusses ecopsychology, or ecotherapy, probably flowing from Rousseau and Thoreau, and the biophilia hypothesis of Edward O. Wilson (1984) and Stephen O. Kellert and Wilson (1993). This therapy is based on the belief that humans have a deep, genetically based emotional need to affiliate with nature. Although Kellert and Wilson acknowledged that these ideas are unproven, diverse healers have romanticized the concept and have launched a new therapy (Goleman 1993; Stevens 1993). Healing relies on extended pilgrimages to commune with nature in the wilderness, establishing an emotional bond with the natural environment, restoring harmony with the natural world, and establishing a pertinacious bond between our species and the planet. Such retreats purport to disrupt people's normal sense of themselves, opening the way to change. Pilgrims may get up in the middle of the night and climb a mountain by moonlight, and remain silent for three to four days. A psychologist reported having taken more than fourteen hundred people into the wilderness for up to four weeks, and described profound changes in personal relationships, work, and awareness, as well as power and energies that had been obtained from nature. The program for business executives emphasizes leadership and team building; programs for others (e.g., juvenile offenders, battered wives, and alcoholic persons) emphasize bolstering self-confidence or can be tailored to heal whatever ails you. Some refer to ecotherapy as the wilderness program, and its practitioners include a growing number of psychologists. It is even being taught at a dozen universities.

Would a study comparing a sample of lifelong urbanites with people who lived in the wilderness all their lives or people in ancient societies show the non-urban groups having less distress and dysphoria? We doubt it. Moreover, the principles of ecotherapy have been used repeatedly in essentially similar forms since ancient times (Ellenberger 1970).

One week after the article on ecotherapy appeared, the *New York Times* (O'Neill 1993) featured a nurse practitioner who described herself as a meta-physician: *meta* reflecting the psychic, mental, or spiritual component of disorders, and *physician* reflecting the physical component. Her treatments blend the use of astrology, Tarot, the I Ching, the cabala, reflexology (detecting energy blockage by prodding a patient's feet and treating with foot massage), herbal teas, the ability to recognize colors corresponding to the body's seven chakras or energy channels (which, when blocked, cause physical symptoms), and occasionally Western medicine. She treats thirty patients each week, only by referral, and is booked months in advance. Her clients include writers, actors, movie producers, lawyers, stockbrokers, and an investment banker. Her Greenwich Village studio contains flickering white and purple lights, a portrait of her mentor (the late Ruth Weiner, a renowned reflexologist), along with a crucifix, a star of David, and a library of esoterica and theology.

Herbal medicine, witch doctoring, treatment by barefoot healers, and other forms of unorthodox treatment are passively tolerated and encouraged in economically deprived nations of the world where scientific medicine is inaccessible and trained physicians are not available (Laurence and Bennett 1987). This is reminiscent of the early years when a scarcity of physicians led to extensive treatment by apothecaries and clerics in England. Although scientifically trained physicians in Africa, China, and the former Soviet Union acknowledge that these therapies function as placebos, they tolerate them as a temporary expedient.

The common attitude is that placebos are better than nothing. Even in the United States and other advanced countries, as medicine becomes more scientific and useful, and as expensive diagnostic instruments and treatments are developed, there is a tendency to passively support unorthodox healing to curb the excess drain on the economy and provide care for those unable to afford costly treatment. In a way, since most conditions are self-limited and spontaneously wax, wane, fluctuate, and remit, this policy causes little harm, patients are reassured and hopeful, and the costs go down. However, as has been documented repeatedly, if the medical condition is serious, these therapies can result in calamities. A further caution is that by creating an Office on Alternative Medicine to evaluate these unconventional treatments, the federal government has given its imprimatur to such techniques, thereby encouraging deception.

Humans are remarkably creative in repeatedly generating new but essentially repackaged treatments to mobilize hope. The principles underlying these therapies are essentially similar, as are the formal aspects of their introduction, development, and demise; controlled studies to prove their effectiveness are never provided. The media provide the public with sensational accounts of the benefits of such therapies without any scientific evidence. This poses a danger to desperate patients, who spend billions of dollars on alternative therapies. When illnesses are not serious and spontaneously disappear—and most illnesses or symptoms for which help is sought are of this type—no harm will be done. But if a serious illness can be treated or prevented by early detection and crucial medical treatment, there is the danger that, as Benjamin Franklin said, "he that lives upon hope will die fasting."

Quackery, religious healing, alternative healing, and the placebo effect of conventional medical therapy are universal throughout medical history and continue to prosper in the current period of scientific medicine. Their long life and omnipresence indicate the extensiveness of the placebo effect and attest to its therapeutic potency.

Whenever physicians have no specific treatment for an illness, the door is opened to nonspecific treatment and placebo effects. If treatment is nonspecific or placebo based, many nontraditional, unorthodox, nonphysician practitioners and quacks can capitalize on the placebo effect, enter the therapeutic arena, and dispense whatever placebos are fashionable. When the etiology and especially the treatment for an illness are known, however, only physicians—and frequently, specialized physicians—dispense treatment, and quacks withdraw from the therapeutic marketplace. For example, appendicitis is no longer treated by massage or high colonic irrigation but is treated only by surgery. There are many such examples in history.

A close examination of quackery, religious healing, alternative medicine, New Age therapies, the placebo component of medicine and psychiatry, religion, and other such institutions and beliefs would reveal a common underlying theme. Fielding Garrison (1929, 44) recognized this when he compared mankind's desire to seek medical assistance for sickness or injury "to the emotional element in religion, both being based upon 'a deep-lying' interest in human nature that relief from suffering is an obtainable good." Thus, he noted, "The history of medicine is also the history of human fallibility and error . . . the folk-ways of medicine are inevitably the same and independent of time and place and circumstance" (45). The same theme, a basic instinctlike drive, is mentioned by Holmes (1891, 378–79): "There is nothing men will not do, there is nothing they have not done to recover their health and save their lives. They have submitted to be half-drowned in water, and half-choked with gases, to be buried up to their chins in earth, to be seared with hot irons like galley-slaves, to be crimped with knives like codfish, to have needles thrust into their flesh, and bonfires kindled on their skin, to swallow all sorts of abominations, and to pay for all this as if to be singed and scalded were a costly privilege, as if blisters were a blessing and leeches a luxury."

Catharsis: A Common Element in All Therapies

An important curative factor underlying all treatment is the concept of catharsis (Scheff 1979). *Catharsis* (derived from the Greek *katharsis*) is defined as a cleaning, purification, or purging of the body, the mind, or the soul. Catharsis of the body refers to "purgation of the excrement of the body, the bowels, evacuation, vomiting, relief of dropsy, a medicine producing purgation or evacuation, a laxative." Catharsis of the soul is reflected in "the spirituous body cleansed by cathartic vapors" (*Compact Edition of Oxford English Dictionary* 1971, 356). Catharsis of the mind has three definitions: 1. "any purification or purgation of the emotions (as pity or fear) . . . 2. that brings about a spiritual renewal or a satisfying release from tension . . . release of the body from terrible memories and emotions . . . 3. bringing repressed ideas and feelings into consciousness by the technique of free association, drugs, or hypnosis" (*Webster's Third New International* 1961, 353). "Bringing traumatic experiences and their affective associations into consciousness . . . psychiatric symptoms or symbols are looked upon as disguised representations of forgotten and repressed ideas or experiences [and are] brought back into the sphere of consciousness and lived out fully (in a therapeutic sense)" (Hinsie and Campbell 1970, 113).

The term *catharsis* is used broadly to indicate the expunging, externalization, or removal of unacceptable aggressive, sexual, or evil impulses and conflicts, or unacceptable thoughts about the body, mind, or soul of a patient by a therapeutic procedure, because the therapy provides reassurance, forgiveness, atonement, expiation, or some other reduction of guilt. The response may be physical or emotional, or may be experienced as something frightening, evil, bad, emotionally dysphoric, or threatening to well-being, life, or afterlife. Using this broad definition (although the psychodynamic formulation does not have acceptable experimental support, and the symptoms and therapy appear to change over time), we can heuristically interpret the history of medical treatment as largely comprising cathartic methods of treatment.

Treatment in primitive cultures did not differentiate among physical, emotional, and spiritual illnesses. Treatment was spiritualistic and relied on magical incantation by primitive healers and propitiation of the gods by priestly healers. From our current perspective, none of the treatments was specific: all fell into the domain of the placebo effect. The treatments were activities or procedures that reduced guilt and/or provided an explanation for the problem, offered propitious priestly intervention with the gods, or involved an expression of atonement by the patient or some other form of catharsis. This primitive approach was superseded by the more rational humanist Greek-Hippocratic-Galenical approach to treatment, with its focus on rebalancing aberrant humors, and Galen's elaborate pharmacopoeia, primarily designed to remove bad things from inside the body and mind. Following this was a return to religious treatment, with Christ becoming Apothecary of the Soul, removing guilt and exorcising incubi. More direct methods of removing evil from the body grew in importance during the Middle Ages and after the Renaissance. These included dehydration methods such as phlebotomy, clysterization, stomachics, vomachics, purgation, sweating, leeching, scarification, and removing stones from the head and every orifice; these methods were followed by the continuation of all types of empirical, eclectic, allopathic, homeopathic, and placebo remedies reaching into the second half of the twentieth century and likely to continue into the twenty-first.

Cathartic treatment, in many forms (dehydration being only one), was probably the major treatment modality used throughout medical history for both somatic (physical) and psychological illnesses. Somatic and psychological illnesses were inexplicably intertwined and were difficult to differentiate. The underlying theme for all cathartic treatment was the removal of the bad, evil, or diseased, which reassured the patient, increased hope, and made the patient feel better. In addition, since the language for expressing emotional problems was limited and was displaced onto physical complaints, it is likely that psychological problems were expressed symbolically by somatic complaints. For example, depressive symptoms could be experienced somatically as exhaustion, abdominal distress, insomnia, or decreased libido, and were treated with purging, bleeding, enemas, or religious expiation. The treatment would serve the psychological function of catharsis by symbolically expressing, expelling, or reducing guilt, conflict, evil thoughts, and impulses, and would result in clinical improvement, which could seen as exemplifying the placebo effect.

With scientific and medical progress in the twentieth century, a better-educated laity, and the failure of traditional religious and medical explanations for emotional problems, there arose a more direct approach to psychological conflicts, ego-alien impulses, guilt, interpersonal relationships, and self-understanding. However, understanding the cause and treatment of psychological problems is complicated, and attempts to do so are invariably inadequate. This often results in guessing, and the use of imagination, speculation, and fantasy. Although the syntax, parlance, concepts, and explanations of the cause and treatment of psychological illness may change over time and usually are expressed in conformity with the most recent paradigm, symptoms essentially do not change, and responses to treatment are governed by the same basic principles of the placebo effect.

This is illustrated in a plaque from an Asclepian temple depicting the interpretation of a dream. A patient asleep on a cot, with a benign and compassionate orderly in attendance at the head of the bed, dreams that a serpent (an ancient magical symbol of renewal, since it is capable of shedding its skin and growing a new one) is licking his shoulder. In the corner, Asclepius, majestic and larger than life, is seen treating the patient. The methods of dream interpretation used at the time would foresee a propitious outcome, since the dream included both the ministrations of the god-physician Asclepius and the presence of the magical symbolic serpent. A Freudian interpretation might be that the dream expressed a denial or repression of a latent or unconscious fear of or wish for a sadomasochistic homosexual assault.

When psychoanalysis and psychotherapy became an institutionalized outlet for the expression and resolution of conflict in the twentieth century, placebo effects, formerly associated with physical illness and medical treatment, could be expressed and experienced through psychological treatment. Instead of being expelled by symbolic physical methods, the evil could be treated by symbolic verbal cathartic methods. Today, in the era of biological psychiatry, the dream might not be interpreted at all: it might be attributed to excessive dopamine and treated with a dopamine blocker.

Despite obvious differences between treatments given in Asclepian temples, the depletion therapies used for several thousand years, psychoanalysts' attempt to cure by making ego where id once was, and the recent focus on correcting chemical imbalances, the placebo effect is a more important curative factor than any of these treatments, or at least a significant factor contributing to a cure, accounting for significant improvement in many psychological and biological therapies.

Healers and the Placebo Effect

Physicians' Rejection of Useful Treatment

The tendency for healers to overvalue the verity of their clinical diagnosis and treatment is a major factor contributing to the placebo effect and is so powerful that it can cause physicians to reject effective treatment, especially if a new remedy does not fit the dominant medical theory or was created by nonphysicians or by other physicians. Examples are the introduction of cinchona bark for malaria by the Jesuits, the use of lemons for scurvy, and the use of tar-water.

In eighteenth-century England, the demand for medical treatment could not be met by the fewer than one hundred physicians accredited by the College of Physicians and was largely filled by clerics and apothecaries. One such cleric was the philosopher Bishop George Berkeley, whose most famous remedy was tar-water. This concoction was made by shaking a gallon of water with a quart of tar, allowing it to stand for three days, then pouring off the supernatant. Berkeley (1744) wrote metaphysical tomes about the virtues of tar-water. It was widely used by empirics but was referred to by others as quackery; Oliver Wendell Holmes (1891, 2) wrote of "the Tar-water mania of Bishop Berkeley." Berkeley claimed superior effects: "From my representations for tar water as good for many things, some perhaps may conclude it is good for nothing. . . . Men may censure and object as they please, but I appeal to time and experiment" (Holmes 1891, 13). Berkeley proposed an experiment in which patients would be "put into two hospitals at the same time of year, and provided with the same necessities of diet and lodging; for further care, one patient would have a tub of tar-water and an old woman, and the other hospital what attendance and drugs you please" (King 1958, 43).

If the experiment had been done, a proposal that was far ahead of its time and showed an understanding of experimental method, the controlled clinical trial, tar-water would have proven superior to all the treatments of the best physicians of the time. The reason is obvious today: medical practice was under the influence of humoral theories, and treatment was largely based on depletion, evacuation, and dehydration—such harmful measures that if the patients were not killed by the original illness, they would be by the treatment.

The history of tar-water illustrates three important behavioral traits of physicians. Two were mentioned previously—namely, the tendency to reject new treatments created by nonphysicians, and the tendency to reject new therapies that conflict with previously established theory or clinical custom. The third involves the use of treatment that is believed to be beneficial but that is in fact harmful.

Healers' Awareness of the Placebo Effect

Another lesson from medical history is that although all healers, therapists, physicians, and even quacks are aware of and sensitive to the placebo effect of treatment, this knowledge is no guarantee against each becoming subject to a belief in his or her own placebo. Healers' awareness of the placebo effect can be illustrated by Galen, who observed that "he cures most in whom the people have the most confidence" (Osler 1892, 117), that "the temples of Asculapius furnish us with proof that many serious diseases can be cured by nothing more than a shock to the mind" (Janet 1925, 49), and that 60 percent of patients consult physicians for symptoms with underlying emotional rather than physical origin—a figure close to contemporary estimates.

Maimonides, a famous twelfth-century philosopher, physician, and rabbi known as the "second Moses," referred to senseless beliefs and degenerate customs as diseases of humanity, but despite his astuteness he recommended urination into a hollow carrot as a treatment for impotence in *Treatment of Sexual Disorders* and was the keeper of theriac in Cairo (Baruk 1957). The Italian philosopher Pietro Pomponazzi observed in the sixteenth century: "We can easily conceive the marvelous effects which confidence and imagination can produce. . . . The cures attributed to the influence of certain relics, are the effect of this imagination and confidence. Quacks and philosophers know that if the bones of any skeleton were put in place of the saint's bones, the sick would none the less experience beneficial effects if they believed that they were near veritable relics" (Tuke 1886, 193).

Paracelsus, in the fifteenth century, vigorously opposed the senseless polypharmacy of his day, observing that medicine killed and nature healed. He noted, "Whether the object of your faith be real or false, you will nevertheless obtain the same effects. Thus, if I believe in St. Peter's statue as I would have believed in St. Peter himself, I will obtain the same effects that I would have obtained from St. Peter; but that is superstition. Faith, however, produces miracles and whether the object of your faith be real or false, you will nevertheless obtain the same effects" (Charpignon 1864, 192). Despite these and other insights, Paracelsus clung to his own incredible placebos, such as "sympathetic powder," purported to cure the injuries of a wounded person when applied to the blood-stained garments and weapon, and "sympathetic ointment," which was applied to the inflicting instrument (Garrison 1929). Despite the irrationality of this treatment, Henry M. Pachter (1951) suggested that leaving the wound to heal naturally rather than subjecting it to dressings with noxious ointments or to treatment with scalding oil or the branding iron probably saved the lives of some wounded soldiers. Ambroise Paré contributed to the abandonment of Egyptian mummy, unicorn horn, and bezoar stones, and of boiling oil for the cauterization of wounds. However, for the last he substituted his own placebo: "fat of puppy dogs," which he applied to wounds (Garrison 1929). In keeping with medical lore at the time, he believed in venesection, cupping, leeches, cures by saints, and the effectiveness of the royal touch for the King's Evil or scrofula, and he believed that stars influence the course of disease, witches cause misfortunes, and divine will causes plague (Major 1954).

Similar insights, marred by credulity, were expressed by Armand Trousseau (1833, 196), who urged physicians to hurry and use the new drugs while they worked, but at the same time was able to say, "As for us, who have sometimes made use of the magnet, we can state that this therapeutic agent exercises an influence which it is impossible to refer to the patients' imagination," and claimed that diseases such as neuralgia, nervous dyspnea, angina pectoris, and rheumatism could be modified, rapidly checked, and cured by magnetic armatures.

Oliver Wendell Holmes first presented in 1842 his lecture "Homeopathy and Its Kindred Delusions," in which he discussed the royal cure of the King's Evil, the weapon ointment, sympathetic powder, the tar-water panacea of Bishop Berkeley, and Elisha Perkins's metallic tractors (Holmes 1891). He declared that patients can benefit "through the influence exerted upon their imaginations," and that they "all display in superfluous abundance the boundless credulity and excitability of mankind upon subjects connected with medicine" (Holmes 1891, 3). He examined these phenomena to illustrate the ease with which numerous facts are accumulated to prove the most fanciful and senseless extravagances, and the inefficiency and incompetence of persons who lack medical knowledge despite having wisdom, honesty, and accomplishment. He was aware of the role of spontaneous remission in the natural course of disease, citing a 90 percent recovery rate in patients seen in general practice "provided nothing were done to interfere with the efforts of nature." He was familiar with probability theory and mentioned several primitive attempts at controlled studies. Although Holmes relegated the majority of drugs then in use to the bottom of sea, he addressed the abuses of the past and those at the periphery of medicine, and not the overwhelming use of placebos by the mainstream medicine of his day.

Sir William Osler, a therapeutic nihilist critical of irrational polypharmacy, observed, "Faith in the gods or in the saints cures one, faith in little pills another, hypnotic suggestion a third, faith in a plain common doctor a fourth. . . . Faith in our drugs and methods, is the great stock in trade of the profession. . . . the touchstone of success in medicine. . . . and must be considered in discussing the foundation of therapeutics. . . . [It is] a most precious commodity, without which we should be very badly off " (Osler 1932, 258–60). He also observed that physicians do not enjoy a "monopoly in the faith business. . . . While we doctors often overlook or are ignorant of our own faith-cures, we are just a wee bit sensitive about those performed outside our ranks" (259). At the same time, Osler used cupping, leeching, venesection, and questionable drugs, and recommended that in the treatment of pneumonia "a timely venesection may save life . . . relieving the pain and dyspnoea, reducing temperature, and allaying cerebral symptoms" (260).

Pierre Janet (1925, 43) observed that, as discerned by all sensitive clinicians, "it is only too easy to make fun of stories of miraculous cure. Not merely are skeptics prone to use this weapon of ridicule, but the faithful do the same thing. The devotees of a religion are strongly inclined to attack kindred superstitions. Nothing will persuade the adepts of Lourdes that the miracles worked at the shrine of Aesculapius were genuine. Who could induce the admirers of animal magnetism to take a serious view of such miracles as those of Lourdes: Each one attacks his neighbor, and is quite aware that his criticism rebounds upon himself." All this despite Janet's own bevy of placebo psychological treatments. Psychoanalysts attribute all cures short of those due to a full psychoanalysis to *transference,* their word for the placebo effect.

Clinicians and the Effectiveness of Treatment

An important conclusion to be drawn from review of the placebo's role in medical history is that the overwhelming majority of clinicians, including the gifted ones, were astonishingly and abysmally wrong. Intelligence, learnedness, professional status, and elaborate theorizing are no guarantee against the placebo effect and have invariably produced the most elaborately ineffective remedies—often those with monstrous potential for harming or killing patients.

This tendency is true even of nonphysician scientists, as noted by Walter Modell about Robert Boyle, the founder of modern chemistry:

Mankind applies its powers of reason in a curiously erratic manner. In some subjects, such as pure chemistry and physics, the implications of the exist-

ing knowledge are explored promptly and confidently, but on other subjects, of which therapeutics is an outstanding example, there has been extreme hesitation to apply scientific methods. This difference often results in
contrasts that are glaring and absurd. For example, Robert Boyle's work *The
Sceptical Chemist* (1661) provided the foundation for modern chemistry and
was particularly characterized by the bold and critical reasoning it contained. The same author, however, when dealing with therapeutics (*A Collection of Choice Remedies,* 1692) was content to describe and recommend a
hodgepodge of messes with ingredients such as worms, horse dung, human
urine and moss from a dead man's skull. The great scientist, when he ap-
proached therapeutics ceased to think, and was content to be a collector of
semimagical folklore. (Modell 1976, 7–8)

The history of medical treatment is characterized by the introduction of new
placebos by successive generations of physicians, often accompanied by vehement and vituperative denunciation of opposing physicians who preferred other placebos. The strong beliefs of physicians, objectively unjustified, suggest that
they have been as defensive about their treatments throughout medical history
as they are today. This conclusion is supported by studies that demonstrate that
physicians attribute the use of placebos to other physicians three times as often
as they attribute it to themselves (Hofling 1955; Shapiro 1960a; Shapiro and Struening 1973a, 1973b, 1974). In addition, in a series of questions on what should
be included in a definition of placebo, physicians tend to exclude their own therapies from the definition: surgeons exclude surgery, internists exclude active
medication, and psychotherapists and psychoanalysts exclude psychotherapy and
psychoanalysis.

No Treatment Is Often the Best Treatment

Many treatments have helped simply because they did no harm to patients and
let nature heal. The sympathetic powder and ointment used by Paracelsus was a
far better treatment than smearing the wound with highly infectious concoctions of feces, spiderwebs, and vipers. Tar-water avoided dehydration. Homeopathy was a better treatment than allopathic treatments and other harmful treatments of the time because it did little to disturb the natural course of illness.
Even Christian Science in the past was a better treatment, because it involved no
harmful treatment.

Astute observers of their time, such as Maimonides, characterized the perfect
physician as one who judges it better to abstain from treatment rather than pre-

scribe a treatment that might perturb the course of the malady (Baruk 1957). Montaigne, in the sixteenth century, observed that physicians, in general, were a danger to their patients (1946). Shakespeare's sensitivity is revealed by the comments of his characters: Helena, in *All's Well That Ends Well* ("Our remedies oft in ourselves do lie" [1.1.202]); a physician in *Measure for Measure* ("The miserable have no other medicine but only hope" [1.2.111]); and Warwick, in *Henry IV* ("a body . . . distempered . . . to his former strength may be restored with good advice and little medicine" [4.3.39]).

The Effectiveness of Primitive Medicine Is Exaggerated

The treatments discussed above were not extreme exceptions to rational treatment; they were characteristic of most medical treatment until recently. Therapy rested on placebo foundations, despite the tendency of most historians to glamorize, sentimentalize, and exaggerate the significance of primitive and prescientific medicine. Although it is likely that ancient healers occasionally stumbled upon useful drugs, the inability to scientifically evaluate the specific usefulness of these drugs contributed to their inconsistent use or their loss to future generations.

Medical historians seem to be entranced by the presumed perspicacity of ancient healers and predisposed to cite any substance that remotely could have had an effect, whether significant or not, as well as drugs that may be used today for nonmedical purposes. Major (1954) cited a number of drugs used in Babylonian-Assyrian medicine as having "had a definite therapeutic value." Many were carminatives for expelling gas (anise, also used for flavoring; cardamom, also used as spice and condiment; coriander, also used for flavoring and seasoning; asafetida, an ill-smelling substance, also called "devil's dung," also a potent laxative and an ingredient in Worcestershire sauce). The laxatives and cathartics included drastic ones (colocynth, castor oil) and milder ones (elaterium; pomegranate, also a vermifuge; and aloe, also an astringent). The Babylonian-Assyrian drugs that are used today as flavorings, seasonings, and condiments include cassia or its substitute, cinnamon; licorice; mint; mustard (also a counterirritant); garlic; myrrh (also used as an astringent and used in perfume and incense); and juniper (a flavoring for gin). Mandragora (the European mandrake, containing hyoscyamine, scopolamine, and mandragorine) and henbane (hogbean, the killer of hogs, a poison containing hyoscyamus) have not been used for a long time. The use of cannabis for depression and neuralgia could cause more harm than benefit. Poppy might have been effective for pain, but not if the seeds were used. Belladonna is cited as an effective anodyne, used for soothing or alleviating pain and for checking the flow of saliva, bladder spasms, dysmenorrhea, bronchitis, and asthma. But it is hard to know what drug is referred to when prescribed in the past. The name *belladonna* means "pretty woman" in Italian, a language not in existence at the time. It was given that name because Italian, Spanish, and other women used it to constrict their pupils, enlarging the iris, which resulted in startlingly large black eyes but rendered the women half-blind. This effect can be observed in Goya's paintings of women. Belladonna consists of a mixture of more than five cholinergic agents that may be present in different concentrations with unpredictable action, especially depending on the time of year and which parts of the plant were harvested, how the drug was extracted, stored, and prescribed, and whether the compound was counterfeited. It is a tricky drug that requires careful titration to be effective without serious side effects.

Another example is Major's citation of Egyptian drugs: "The prescriptions in the Papyrus Ebers resemble those of the modern era. . . . The medicines . . . constitute an imposing list of substances. . . . While many of the substances are of no known therapeutic value and some cannot be identified, others are of unquestioned value and hold their place after millenniums of experience" (Major 1954, 50). Three—colocynth (a drastic cathartic), castor oil, and senna—are purgative or cathartic. Three—turpentine, hyoscyamus, and pomegranate (not when eaten fresh but only if enough of the active substance, pelletierine tannate, could be successfully extracted and administered)—were taeniafuges (for expelling tapeworms) or vermifuges (for intestinal worms). Ox liver is cited for night blindness; tannin-containing plants, as astringents; and acacia tips (unclear whether they are stems, twigs, or the gum, called gum Arabic), for contraception. (According to Major, in the vagina acacia forms lactic acid, which is present in many contraceptive jellies.) Acacia is used today as a solvent and flavoring agent and for its emulsifying and suspending properties.

Haggard (1933) credited the ancient Chinese with giving ground dragon (dinosaur?) bones for convulsions, unaware that the calcium might have been helpful only for children with infantile tetany; and with giving burnt sponge, which contains iron, for lumps that might have been goiters. Major (1954, 95) added ground sheep thyroid in goiter and cretinism, and adds that Li Shi-chen comments, "The liver stores blood, and is therefore beneficial for all diseases of the blood." Neither author cited original sources for these treatments or identified how they were used and for how many (probably numerous) conditions they were prescribed. If we add poppy and mahuang to the list of possibly effective drugs, we end up with six drugs, or only 0.03–0.04 percent possibly effective drugs from a total of two thousand times drugs were mentioned and sixteen thousand prescriptions used in Chinese medicine, a percentage far below the number of effective drugs expected by chance alone.

Ilza Veith (1972), in her *Yellow Emperor's Classic of Internal Medicine,* concluded, as do many historians seduced by the drama of antiquity, that the maintenance of these cumbersome and probably painful methods of treatment must indicate that they possessed healing power, in spite of the condescension with which Westerners are apt to speak of pulse diagnosis, acupuncture, and moxa treatments. Did the Yellow Emperor inadvertently propose a better explanation? "The ancient sages did not treat those who were already ill; they instructed those who were not ill. . . . When the body is worn out and the blood is exhausted" it is not possible "to assure good results . . . because there is no more energy left. . . . If man's vitality and energy do not propel his own will his disease cannot be cured" (152). His advice provides a primer for placebo effects: treat only those patients who are not seriously ill, those likely to improve spontaneously and to benefit from nonspecific or placebo treatments.

Guido Majno (1975) cited several other examples of historians exaggerating the usefulness of drugs described in Egyptian papyri. He cited James H. Breasted, a prominent Egyptologist, commending willow leaves, which contain salicin, for antisepsis. However, willow leaves contain very little salicin, and if used for treatment would be as ineffective as putting traces of aspirin on wounds. As previously noted, the ancient Egyptian healers were fond of dung, recommending excrement from humans and eighteen other animals. Other historians cited the use of flyspecks scraped from walls, mentioned in the Ebers Papyrus, as an insightful use of penicillin, and placebos made of stale bread as containing antifungals.

Corroboration of the effectiveness of these remedies would require controlled studies describing how, when, and from where they were collected; the method of extracting the essential ingredient; how the active moiety was stored, evaluated, and prescribed (orally, topically, or parenterally, once a day or periodically); and how long the effect or the half-life lasted. Considering how complicated drug manufacturing is today, it is unlikely that any of these concoctions would be judged a useful remedy after sophisticated methodological evaluation. Many older drugs cited as effective have never been evaluated. Although pennyroyal, recommended by Galen, sometimes induced successful abortions and became a fad in the midwestern United States during the 1970s, its popularity was brief because it often caused the death of the mother. Many other therapeutic claims would not be substantiated.[4]

---

4. Other exaggerated claims about the effectiveness of ancient remedies include those of Jayne (1962) for Egyptian remedies ("time having proved the value of a goodly number . . . such as castor oil, aloes, mint, myrrh, copper, lead, slat, goose oil and fats, opium, co-

Treatment recommendations were too general, and the medications were applied in an undisciplined way to illnesses—for example, one hundred different prescriptions for epilepsy and another hundred for phthisis in ancient Indian medicine, usually in mixture with many other substances (Major 1954). In addition, medications were not limited to the specifically useful indication (e.g., quinine for malaria but not for other fevers of unknown origin). Another problem is the difficulty of translating the names of drugs mentioned in ancient languages into the names of drugs known to us. Moreover, no information or insufficient information is available about how ancient drugs were prepared and administered. Poppy is frequently mentioned, but if the seeds were used the preparation would be useless. In addition, since every known organic and inorganic substance was used as medicine at one time or another and the same substance was prescribed for scores of different symptoms, selecting only those for which a possible indication can be found today would not be difficult and would be entirely a chance event. In fact, by chance alone one would expect that many more useful remedies would have been found. Considering the thousands of treatments used throughout history and how infrequently useful remedies were discovered, it is likely that there were many factors operating against chance discoveries. It is striking that with 370 drugs from Mesopotamia, 1,871 different therapeutic agents (e.g., metals, minerals, and trees) and 16,000 prescriptions from China, 600 drugs from India, 195 to 400 in Hippocratic medicine, 1,000 listed by Pliny, and 820 for Galen—a total in excess of 5,000 drugs and 20,000 prescriptions—so few effective drugs were found. It is obvious that the number of effective drugs—even if we are imaginative, indulgent, charitable, and credulous about labeling drugs effective—is surprisingly, pathetically, and significantly low. Why?

There are many interacting factors, among which are the limits that overriding theories imposed on clinical observation; reliance on authority; the absence

---

riander, turpentine, cedar, hyoscamus, and others") (44); and for Greek remedies ("All healing sanctuaries were abundantly supplied with water . . . and some of these waters appear to have had definite medicinal properties") (232).

The drugs with real pharmacological activity used in ancient Egyptian treatment include antiseptics (copper salts); astringents (alum and lead salts); sedatives and antispasmodics (Indian hemp, hyoscyamus, mandrake, opium); laxatives (colocynth, ricinus, aloes, senna, tamaris, figs, colchicum); digestives and carminatives (camomile, coriander, aniseed, cumin, mint, fenugreek, thyme, saffron); eupeptic appetizers (gentian, coriander); stimulant carminatives (absinths, nutmeg); demulcents (almond); eye koh-cassia-abus; scalp stimulant (castor oil); and molds that cover bread or wood long soaked in water, which provided antibiotics extracted from the fungi.

of methodology to evaluate treatment adequately; the spontaneous waxing, waning, fluctuation, and remission of symptoms and disease; and the power of the placebo effect. For brief periods, useful remedies were employed, but they did not last, because the methodology to establish their specificity did not exist, nor did methods exist to communicate their value to future generations. The remedies, used for too many illnesses, lost their usefulness, and the powerful placebo effect obfuscated their specific effect.

Poppy

Of the many ancient hallucinogens and narcotics—mandrake, henbane, hellebore, cannabis, nepenthe, bufotenine, and other unknown hallucinogenic substances (Caldwell 1970, 1978)—the poppy, or opium, is the earliest effective and most consistently used ancient drug. It is frequently cited as an exception to the concept that the history of medicine is largely the history of the placebo effect. Although this is true to some extent, opium's usefulness tends to be exaggerated.

The medicinal use of the poppy is said to extend back into remote antiquity. However, the evidence is indirect and tangential, based on archaeological artifacts—such as containers, pendants, pottery, jewels, and clay offerings to the gods—resembling the poppy capsule (Terry and Pellens 1928; Jaffe 1970; Majno 1975). The poppy was possibly first referred to as *hul gil,* translated as "joy plants," in Sumerian ideographs dating back to about 4000 B.C. It is mentioned as *arat pa* in the Assyrian medical tablet in the seventh century B.C., as red shepenn in the Smith Papyrus in about 1700 B.C., and as red shepenn, to which flyspecks scraped from a wall were added to placate a crying baby, in the Ebers Papyrus in 1550 B.C. The Greek goddess of the poppy dates from about 1300–1325 B.C., at the time of the Trojan War, and Helen's Egyptian potion, *nepenthes,* a drug possibly containing opium, is mentioned as a remedy for grief and pain in the *Odyssey.* Hippocrates recommended drinking white poppy juice for leucorrhea or uterine suffocation and described it as hypnotic meconion, or poppy. It is mentioned as the sleep-bringing poppy by Virgil in the first century B.C. David I. Macht (1915), however, ascribed the earliest authentic reference to the poppy to Greek and Latin literature. Theophrastus referred to the milky juice of poppy as *poppy juice* and *meconion* in the third century B.C. (The word *opium* is derived from the Greek word for "juice.") The method of procuring opium from poppy capsules is described by Scribonius Largus in A.D. 40; other attributes are described by Dioscorides, Pliny, and Celsus in the first century A.D.; and poppy was enthusiastically praised by Galen in the second century and by Avicenna in the tenth century.

Poppy may have been referred to as *ma-fei* by Huang Ti in China in about A.D. 200 (Veith 1972). It was known to Arabian physicians, who introduced it to Persia and India (where it was used for dysentery); it was first mentioned as a product from India in the sixteenth century, was possibly but not definitely compounded as laudanum in the fifteenth century by Paracelsus, was compounded in the seventeenth century by Van Heimont and Sydenham, was generally understood by the sixteenth century in Europe, and was isolated as morphine in 1903. Much of the success of many of these physicians, especially Paracelsus, is ascribed to the use of opium, usually in disguised form in a remedy that contained many useless ingredients. It has been used for more symptoms and diseases and has stimulated more discussion and provoked more enthusiasm than any other drug in the history of medicine.

One would expect that, once discovered, opioid narcotics, which have powerful analgesic properties, would have been used consistently over the centuries. This was not the case, however; only sporadic references to the use of poppy are found throughout medical history. Typically it is listed as an unimportant ingredient in elaborate concoctions, usually at unknown or very small dosages—in panaceas such as mithridatum, theriac,[5] matioli, philonium,[6] diascordium,[7] which was later referred to as pulvis catechu compositus and pulvis kino compositus and was subsequently given many other appellations (Macht 1915; Majno 1975).[8] It was used inappropriately for numerous conditions other than pain. Dysentery would have been an exception because of the constipating side

5. Galen described the panacea theriac: "It resists poisons and venomous bites, cures inveterate headache, vertigo, deafness, epilepsy, apoplexy, dimness of sight, loss of voice, asthma, coughs of all kinds, spitting of blood, tightness of breath, colic, the iliac poison, jaundice, hardness of the spleen, stone, urinary complaints, fevers, dropsies, leprosies, the troubles to which women are subject, melancholy and all pestilences" (Macht 1915, 479). The ingredients in Galen's theriac are described in chapter 1, note 1.

6. The ingredients of philonium, which was devised by Philon of Tarsus in the first century A.D., was listed in the *London Pharmacopoeia* of 1746, and remained in the English pharmacopoeias until 1867, included white pepper, ginger, caraway seeds, strained opium, and syrup of poppies (Macht 1915).

7. The principal ingredients for diascordium, concocted by Frascatorius in sixteenth-century Verona and adopted by the first *London Pharmacopoeia,* included cinnamon, cassia wood, scordium, dittany, galbanum, storax, gum arabic, opium, sorrel, gentian, Armenian bole, Leminian earth, pepper, ginger, and honey (Macht 1915).

8. Other concoctions, containing varying amounts of opium, prepared with varying extraction methods, and always containing multiple ingredients, were magisteria opii, Lancaster or Quackers's black-drop (which was three times as strong as laudanum), Elixir Asthmaticum, Elixir Paregoricum, Tinctura Opii Camphorata, Tinctura Opii Benzoica, Pilulae Opii, Pilulae Sopanaceae, Matthew's Pills, Sharkey's Pills, and Dover's Powder.

effects of opioids, although this beneficial effect would have been contravened because of the dehydration caused by the usual purgation.

Moreover, if opium was used consistently, it would be reasonable to expect that the severe and unmistaken consequences of addiction would have been cited. It was discovered at the beginning of the nineteenth century that the chief active principle of opium was morphine. But morphine's severe addiction potential was recognized only after its wholesale hypodermic use during the U.S. Civil War. Despite this knowledge, a prominent physician (Kane) listed fifty-four indications for its use in 1880 (Terry and Pellens 1928); they included fever, cholera, diabetes, polyuria, urinary incontinence, lead colic, malaria, uremia, shock, cerebral edema, meningitis, vaginismus, nymphomania, mania, and insanity. Opium was used topically as an ointment on open wounds, mixed with all manner of substances, including sizable quantities of alcohol, or used as a salve. Although opium was used topically more frequently than it was ingested orally, it is unlikely that it could be absorbed through the skin in adequate dosages.

In addition, opium could have been derived from ineffective parts of the poppy, such as the root, stem, capsule, or flowers, rather than from the effective moiety of dried sap that oozes from slits in the capsule. The complicated process of extracting the essential pharmacological moiety, the storage of the preparation, and the method of domesticating are not consistently described. Additional factors obscuring the effectiveness of opium as well as many other old drugs include fraudulent substitutes, the absence of methodology to establish a drug's specificity and utility, and the obfuscating aspect of the placebo effect. Clinical observation, even after centuries of use, does not always establish the proper therapeutic dosage of morphine: researchers in the 1950s concluded that the dosage of morphine that had previously been used was 50 to 100 percent greater than the dosage that gives maximal pain relief as well as reduced toxicity (Lee 1942; Denton and Beecher 1949; Keats et al. 1950; Beecher 1952; Lasagna and Beecher 1954).

Drugs to Promote Wound Healing

Wound healing was more advanced than the treatment of internal diseases because the effect of treatment could be more readily observed. Majno, a pathologist, evaluated the effectiveness of ancient drugs for wound healing that were described in ancient scrolls, tablets, books, and papyri (Majno 1975). He tested whether remedies used to treat wounds had bactericidal or bacteriostatic effects by plating the substance on petri dishes containing bacteria. Estes, a pharmacol-

ogist, evaluated both internal and external remedies mentioned in Egyptian papyri and added dose-response studies, with the expectation that the dosage of
the plated substance would correlate with bacterial inhibition on the petri dish
(Estes 1989).

The use of malachite and honey for wound healing are possible exceptions to the bleak landscape of effective remedies described in Egyptian papyri
(Majno 1975; Estes 1989). Malachite, which contains copper, is a bright green
mineral that was used for decorative cosmetics by the third millennium B.C. and
is the active ingredient in thirty-nine drug mixtures described in the Ebers Papyrus for the treatment of wounds and eye disorders. Copper sulfate was used as
a home remedy for infection as recently as the twentieth century, and cupric sulfate is still used as a fungicide in fish tanks and swimming pools. Honey is the
most extensively mentioned drug in Egyptian papyri. Both copper salts and honey weakly inhibit certain bacteria commonly found in wounds, which suggests
that they would inhibit bacterial growth in open wounds or allow tissue repair
to proceed normally. However, questions remain about the effectiveness of malachite and honey. If their effect had been meaningful clinically, it is unlikely that
they would have been combined with numerous other substances, many of
which were bacteriogenic and noxious. In addition, many other ineffective and
harmful drugs continued to be used for wound healing much more frequently
than malachite and honey. Wounds, and almost all else, continued to be extensively treated with diverse kinds of dung: sores were treated with dung in
Mesopotamia; wounds were treated with dung in Egypt and India, and such
treatment was also recommended in the Talmud; either fresh or dried and powdered dung was recommended by Pliny for wounds made by iron; dung was recommended for wound dressing by Celsus; and the specific use of dove dung for
wounds was recommended by Galen. Honey was not used in Greek medicine;
copper salts continued to be used (again mixed with other substances) but were
only one of many substances used for wound healing.

It is questionable whether a laboratory study in a petri dish rather than on
human wounds, without the use of randomization, controls, the double-blind
procedure, and adequate sample size, is an adequate test of the effectiveness of
these remedies. It is possible that copper and honey would be no better than a
saline control, no treatment, or merely keeping the area clean. A significant effect
of treatment with copper or honey might be the avoidance of other noxious
treatment.

Majno's conclusion that some patients may have been helped may be correct,
especially if the least amount of treatment was used rather than the most extensive and elaborate treatment. In fact, if physicians adhered to the Hippocratic tri-

ad of bleeding, purging, and starvation, rather than the simple application of one of these substances to a wound, it is likely that more patients would have died than would have been cured.

Despite the possible but weak effects of these drugs on wounds, Majno cautioned about the dangers of exaggerating the effectiveness of ancient remedies: "Regardless of which plant [one needs to ask] what part was used, how it was prepared, how much was given, with what, and for what reason? Multiply these questions by some seven hundred 'drugs,' and the problem grows to such a size that one tends to brush it off by concluding that ancient Egyptian pharmacy was tremendously advanced—whereby what stands proven, rather than ancient wisdom, is modern confusion. Once and for all, beware: *next to nothing is known about the effectiveness of ancient drugs;* and even when the drug itself is known, experimental studies are almost nil" (Majno 1975, 108). Estes too admonished against exaggerated claims for ancient Egyptian medicine: "We still do not know the exact reasoning that led him (the *swnw* or Egyptian physician) to prescribe most of his drugs . . . nor do we have any clues about the frequency with which he prescribed them, much less about their true therapeutic efficacy. Indeed, we have no good reason to believe that most of the drugs routinely prescribed by the *swnw* could have produced any substantial clinical improvement by themselves; even if some did have selective effects, such as moving the bowels, that are not beneficial effects per se (save in people who are constipated) . . . the major exceptions . . . are the wound ointments made with honey and malachite" (Estes 1989, 113). Despite this, many drugs first used in ancient Egypt continued to be used in the Hippocratic period and up to modern times, and stand as testimony to several thousand years of belief in their efficacy.[9]

9. Walter Modell, who has creditable pharmacological credentials and is knowledgeable about the placebo effect, commented (without citing references) in *Life Science Library*, a popular lay publication, that a very small minority of ancient Egyptian drugs may have been effective (Modell and Lansing 1967). He cited the Egyptian use of pomegranate extract, containing a vermifuge, for gout; ox liver, containing vitamin A, for night blindness; and juice from poppy seeds (used on bread, in food, and in the dressing of wounds, without analgesic effects) to soothe crying babies. The Greeks added mandrake, containing scopolamine, to ease an infant's discomfort (the benefit-to-toxicity ratio for both poppy and mandrake makes their use for the treatment of infants questionable); autumn crocus infusions for gout; and willow bark extracts for fever, of which aspirin is a remote descendent. The Arabs contributed mercury, a highly toxic drug, for a multiplicity of symptoms and for scabies. Establishing whether even these few drugs were effective would require the rigorous evaluation detailed previously.

Mahuang

Mahuang, also known as ephedra, ephedron, ephedrin, and ephedrine, is frequently referred to as the oldest effective drug in recorded medical history. According to legend, it was mentioned in about 2600 B.C. by Huang Ti, often described as the founder of Chinese civilization and the author of the *Huang Ti Nei Ching Su Wen (The Yellow Emperor's Classic of Internal Medicine),* the classic treatise and oldest medical book (Veith 1972). The existence of the emperor, his authorship, and the date of the treatise, however, are controversial. A more accepted date may be circa 1000 B.C., but even this date has been amended many times, and a more likely date is about 300 B.C. (Major 1954).

In our opinion, the usefulness and significance of mahuang in medical history are exaggerated and romanticized. According to K. K. Chen and C. F. Schmidt (1930), mahuang is described in the Chinese dispensary in 1596 as having value as a circulatory stimulant, diaphoretic, and antipyretic, as an ingredient in many famous prescriptions—all unsubstantiated, except a "sedative for cough" whose application is limited to cough from asthmatic bronchospasm. The drug was not mentioned in Egyptian papyri, in the Sushruta and Charaka in India, or by Hippocratic physicians, or elsewhere, until, in the first century A.D., it was described as ephedron by Pliny, who accumulated facts about it from everything he read and heard. It was also mentioned by Dioscorides as an astringent and diuretic, and as a cure for colic, dysentery, and internal rupture—again all unsubstantiated, and according to Majno (1975) it was used to staunch bleeding with a mere touch, and as a juice in the nostrils to stop hemorrhage. Mixed with fermented milk and honey (alcohol), it was used in India chiefly in religious ceremonies to induce exhilarating intoxication, probably due to the alcohol. In nineteenth-century Russia it was recommended for rheumatism, syphilis, and gout—once again being without value for these and other conditions, except possibly for some respiratory disorders. Indians and often Spaniards used it topically and internally for syphilis, gonorrhea, nephritis, pleurisy, and pneumonia, and as a tonic and blood purifier. Again, all of these uses—except for the use of mahuang in cooling beverages and in the making of bread—were inappropriate. Ephedron continued to be mentioned in a scattered and unsystematic way as a folk medicine with dubious indications (Chen and Schmidt 1930).

Other difficulties encountered in understanding the worth of ephedras in the history of medicine are that many of the ephedras used and grown throughout the world did not contain ephedrine, and yields of ephedrine diverged markedly among investigators because different parts and sexes of the plants were used, the plants were grown in different seasons and years, and extraction was difficult and complicated (Chen and Schmidt 1930). The ephedras disappeared from use until extracted from mahuang in 1885, synthesized, and in 1887 named ephedrine. However, injected animals promptly died and ephedrine was labeled too toxic and was not used again until the early 1920s (Chen and Schmidt 1930).

Schmidt, an American physician working in Peking from 1922 to 1924, systematically studied about two thousand traditional Chinese drugs for possible effectiveness. He noted repeated reference to mahuang as a treatment for asthma (Majno 1975). In collaboration with Chen and Leake, the substance was identified as the plant *Ephedra vulgaris,* from which was obtained ephedrine, related chemically to epinephrine; this eventually led to the synthesis of amphetamine, dextroamphetamine, and many other stimulants (Chen and Schmidt 1930; Leake 1958, 1970).[10] Ephedrine, now known to be a bronchodilator, mydriatic, nasal decongestant, and vasoconstrictor, provides relief from coughs arising from some allergies and asthma, relief from asthmatic symptoms, and topical vasoconstriction for superficial hemorrhage.

Mahuang is one of the drugs in ancient Chinese medicine that can be cited as effective. However, there are only vague references to its limited effects, and no information is available about how many other conditions it was recommended for, or its use elsewhere. The repetitive citation of the efficacy of mahuang, rather than providing evidence of ancient medical wisdom, appears once again to be exaggerated romanticism.

Other Treatments

Other effective treatments appeared subsequently, but erratically and at infrequent intervals. The use of cinchona (quinine) for fevers began in 1640; cinchona's specificity for malaria rather than all fevers was clarified by Thomas Sydenham and Thomas G. Morton, but its use was compromised by continued problems in growing plants with active substances, and by fraudulent counterfeits. Foxglove (digitalis), introduced by William Withering in 1776 for the treatment of renal and cardiac dropsy but subsequently established as effective only for cardiac problems, was inappropriately used for scores of conditions such as hysteria and pneumonia and was plagued by unstandardized dosages until 1937 (Gold et al. 1937). With accelerated advances with the onset of scientific medicine in the mid-1950s (vitamins, hormones, anesthesia, aseptic surgical procedures, immunization), there began a veritable inundation of highly specific and

10. Unknown in the United States, the sympathomimetic properties of ephedrine and its usefulness for asthma were described in 1917 by Japanese investigators.

dramatic treatments that continued through the second half of the twentieth century, when medicine's scientific basis markedly increased.

The Complexity of Deriving and Prescribing Drugs

An important factor weakening the hypothesis that ancient drugs were effective is the enormous complexity of collecting, preparing, preserving, packaging, and administering drugs (Tyler et al. 1976). Collecting drugs from animals, which is not discussed here, is roughly as complex as collecting drugs from plants. Almost all excretions, organs, and tissues have been used at one time or another.

The variability in the preparation of drugs from plants begins with the time of collecting. A tree or plant can yield large amounts of a drug during one season of the year, small amounts during another, and none in a third. A plant also can produce one drug, such as hyoscyamine, in the fall, and another, such as hyoscine, in the spring. Roots and rhizomes should be collected in the fall, barks in the spring, leaves and flowering tops usually at the time of flowering, flowers at about the time of pollination, fruits before or after ripening, and seeds when fully matured. Appropriate methods of collection can yield substantial amounts of active drug, whereas inappropriate methods can result in its total absence.

Appropriate harvesting includes skillful selection of plant parts, which includes skillful hand selection for digitalis and some flowers, and mowing for peppermint and spearmint, which should be left to partially dry before distilling. Leaves, herbs, and cut plants should be dried immediately and the leaf separated from stems; and fruits and seeds should be left to cure, ripen, and dry. *Garbling* is the term for the removal of unused parts of plants, dirt, adulterants, and other extraneous matter.

Appropriate drying, involving temperature control and the regulation of air flow, removes moisture, to prevent the action of molds, enzymes, and bacteria, as well as chemical and other changes. Some plants require air drying in the sun; others, air drying in the shade; some need complicated artificial procedures and equipment, which vary with the type of plant part. Absorption of moisture decreases the activity of a drug and increases enzymatic and fungal activity. Moisture concentrations as low as 8 percent can inactivate digitalis. Drugs should be stored in cool, dark places, well ventilated with dry air, shielded from ordinary and polarized light, and protected from insects, mice, and rats.

Appropriate packaging provides protection. Leaf and herbal material is baled into solid compact masses wrapped in burlap. Drugs that can absorb moisture and deteriorate, such as digitalis and ergot, are stored in moisture-proof cans. Gums, resins, and extracts are shipped in barrels or casks, tonka beans in casks, vanilla beans in tin-lined boxes, oil of rose in lead flasks, and sarsaparilla in bales covered with cowhide. Older methods included packaging of aloes in monkey skins, and curaçao in gourds, and hundreds of other, even more primitive methods.

Current pharmacological principles, which determine how drugs are used, were determined only recently. They include knowledge of the dose-response curve (the threshold dose at which the therapeutic effect appears, and the increase in therapeutic effect with increased dosage, eventually reaching a steady level, or ceiling effect, beyond which additional therapeutic effects do not occur and adverse or toxic effects may appear). The therapeutic window is the dosage range in which most therapeutic effects occur. The half-life is the time it takes for the concentration of the drug in the patient's blood to decrease 50 percent. The time-action curve is the length of time necessary to achieve an effective concentration. The duration of activity may vary from a few hours to weeks. The time needed to reach a steady state is important for long-lasting drugs; the same daily dosage increases the blood concentration over time until the concentration no longer increases. Other factors are absorption, distribution, length of time for excretion, and knowledge of the dosages that induce side effects, toxicity, and even death. Thus, the effective dosage of aspirin is half a tablet every other day to reduce strokes and heart attacks, one or two tablets every four hours for headaches, and much higher dosages for rheumatoid arthritis. Two doses of an antibiotic may be effective to prevent carditis after dental cleaning, four tablets may be taken daily for five days for a bacterial infection, and massive doses may be prescribed for syphilis or Lyme disease. The effects of a dose of certain drugs, such as methylphenidate (Ritalin) and aspirin, last only four hours, but the effects of stimulants such as dextroamphetamine (Dexedrine) last five to six hours; those of magnesium pemoline (Cylert), seven days; those of tricyclic antidepressants, twenty-four hours; those of neuroleptics, four to fourteen days; and those of MAO antidepressants and serotonin amplifiers such as fluoxetine (Prozac), two weeks. The duration of activity for benzodiazepines varies: four hours for triazolam (Halcion), six hours for diazepam (Valium), and twelve hours for clonazepam (Klonopin). Some drugs, such as Valium, work in an hour; others, such as phenelzine (Nardil) and Prozac, may take two weeks, six weeks, or even three months. Moreover, the optimal dosages for many drugs vary markedly, based on genetic factors, absorption, enzymatic activity, distribution, age, sex, weight, and interaction with food and other drugs.

These basic factors about the development and prescription of drugs, obviously so important in current medical treatment, could not have been known in the past. These factors, coupled with incorrect theory and thousands upon thousands of ineffective remedies, many with serious toxic effects, would leave an incredibly low percentage of ancient drugs that could have had any substantial beneficial effect.

Conclusion

Drawing conclusions about the effectiveness of prescientific medicine is an awesome undertaking. It must rely on those written documents that have survived, must surmount the difficulties of translation and interpretation, and must encompass many periods and cultures over thousands of years. No one person can adequately master the complexity; each is forced to focus on minutiae of medical history, which are strongly prone to errors of omission and commission. The historian's picture of the medical landscape, albeit incomplete, is scattered with thousands of treatments used over many millennia. Since many things were used for treatment, it is easy to support very different conclusions about the effectiveness of prescientific medical treatment. It is not difficult to find some treatments now known to have active chemical moieties that could have been effective if used appropriately. Equally obvious is the ease of finding many obvious placebo treatments. Thus, a preexisting bias or hypothesis may determine conclusions.

The only possible resolution is to carefully inventory the names, purposes, and methods of administration of ancient drugs, describe the ailments for which the drugs were recommended or used, translate this information into current pharmacological knowledge, and conduct in vitro and in vivo clinically controlled studies—a task not likely to be done. Despite the problem of bias and the hazards of interpretation, we propose that the available data support the overall hypothesis that the history of medical treatment up to the era of scientific medicine is largely the history of the placebo effect.

chapter four

The Placebo Effect
in the Twentieth Century

The placebo effect is a compelling explanation for many zealous conclusions about the purported effectiveness of therapies which are unsupported by experimental evidence. The placebo effect helps to explain many arcane clinical phenomena that otherwise cannot be easily understood. That it escaped scientific notice for so long is surprising. Its potency, widespread use, and therapeutic potential have not been acknowledged until recently. Study of the underlying mechanism and dynamics of the placebo effect is a relatively recent area of research.

Many authors have commented on the surprisingly belated interest in the placebo effect (Houston 1938; Pepper 1945; Dubois 1946; Findley 1953; Leslie 1954; Lasagna 1956; Wayne 1956). They have noted that placebos are administered more than any other type of treatment, that the placebo was an important therapeutic weapon, and particularly that there was a lack of study of the characteristics of placebo reactors.

Internists and physicians in other specialties first became interested in the placebo effect between 1935 and 1952. Psychiatrists soon followed, after encountering complexities in the evaluation of neuroleptics introduced in the mid-1950s.

The influence of psychiatric concepts on medicine and laypersons increased greatly after World War II. Psychiatrists affiliated themselves with medical schools and hospitals in increasing numbers. There was greater interdisciplinary contact and research. One result was the greater recognition by physicians of psychological factors, symbolism, the doctor-patient relationship, transference, and countertransference. With this came greater understanding of and interest in the extensiveness of psychological phenomena—and of the placebo effect, in particular. Another factor contributing to the increasing interest in the placebo effect was the development of controlled methodology in therapeutics.

Interest in the placebo effect could be seen in the increased number of publications about it. Between 1953 and 1957, forty-three such papers were published—more than had appeared in the entire time preceding this period; most of these papers were retrospective analyses of the data of controlled studies. After 1957 the number of published papers on the placebo effect rose steadily (Shapiro 1960b). Turner et al. (1980) abstracted nearly one thousand articles and books on the placebo and related phenomena. Another reflection of this development is the increase in the numbers of carefully controlled and clinical trial studies using statistics, placebos, double-blind procedures, and other controls.

Medicine

Nonplacebo Achievements

Modern medicine no longer relies chiefly on the placebo effect or the doctor-patient relationship. The enormous increase in medical knowledge and treatment is self-evident. Although knowledge about anatomy, physiology, biochemistry, pharmacology, histology, public health, technology, therapeutics, and all other sciences advanced slowly over time, there have been major leaps and periods of acceleration and retrogression, making it difficult to identify the major period of change in treatment. It is possible to cite a leap in medical and scientific knowledge which began in the last half of the nineteenth century and continued to World War II, and slowly led more to the rejection of ineffective remedies than to the introduction of specific remedies. The pace quickened in the 1950s as sensitivity about the placebo effect and about the need for more effective controlled clinical trials increased; this awareness became firmly established by about 1975. Technology, instrumentation, and computers strongly contributed to basic research, which was then modified by medicine and resulted in a veritable explosion in medical knowledge and treatment. For example, juvenile diabetes was a grave, uninsurable disease, with few patients surviving longer than three years, until insulin replacement therapy was introduced in 1921. Also, vitamin deficiencies such as scurvy, rickets, and beriberi are now effectively treated. Sulfonamides were introduced in the 1930s, and penicillin and streptomycin in the 1950s. Treatment of congestive heart failure improved after reliable dosages of digitalis were developed in the 1970s.

Killer diseases that decimated populations in the past can now be eradicated, controlled, and treated—with, for example, antibiotics for most bacterial infections; and vaccination for diseases such as poliomyelitis, diphtheria, pertussis, and tetanus. Smallpox, a disease that disfigured, blinded, and killed millions of people, has been eradicated, and the remaining laboratory samples of the virus are destined for destruction (Altman 1993). It is also predicted that poliomyelitis is on the threshold of being eradicated in the Americas and eventually will be known only by history (Foege 1993; Robbins 1993). Improved public health policies and an increasing number of drugs and medical procedures have been developed which have a high degree of specificity, sensitivity, and predictability.

Basic chemical parts can be precisely determined by x-ray crystallography, mass spectrometry, infrared absorption spectrometry, electron and x-ray diffraction studies, electron microscopes, the laser feedback microscope (Fox 1993), and DNA molecular procedures. Useful drugs previously derived from nature can now be synthesized in the laboratory. It is possible to map the molecular structure of bacteria, viruses, neurotransmitters, and cell receptors in the brain and elsewhere. "Designer drugs" can be designed specifically to modulate designated neurotransmitters, occupy specific receptors, or affect precise enzymatic reactions and other metabolic processes; this leads to more precise and effective drugs, with fewer side effects—for example, fluoxetine (Prozac) for depression. Opioid receptors were identified and naturally occurring opioids were then discovered in the brain, and these accomplishments contributed further understanding about how narcotic analgesics work. Of three opioid receptors, the one responsible for morphine's analgesia, tolerance, and addiction has been identified, and the genetic sequence for this molecular receptor has been unveiled (Randell 1993). Such studies and techniques may lead to solving the problem of addiction and to the development of more effective analgesics. For example, the molecular structure has been identified for epibatidine, a complicated, nonopioid, nonsedating compound from an Ecuadorian frog, which is thought to be two hundred times as effective as morphine in blocking pain. Attempts to synthesize the chemical are currently in progress (Bradley 1993). Because modern techniques can determine the molecular configuration of complicated compounds found in nature, it is no longer necessary to collect huge amounts of material from plants, animals, and humans, which increased the cost of drugs and restricted their use to very few people.

Sensitive imaging techniques, the fastest-developing techniques in biomedicine, abetted by fiber optic technology and enhanced by computers, can determine the molecular configuration of drugs and allow safe observation of internal organs and of the anatomy, neurochemistry, and cognitive changes in the brain, leading to more specific diagnosis and treatment.

Human DNA fragments have been installed in sheep, yielding valuable new treatments such as factor 9 for blood clotting in hemophilia; in pigs, offering the promise of producing AIDS- and hepatitis-free hemoglobin substitutes for blood transfusions; and in cows, producing lactoferrin to be used in formulas to help babies fight infection and making cows' milk more like human milk. Genes have even been installed in tomatoes to prevent rotting on the vine, rendering the fruits more edible and making it possible to bring them more easily to market. It is highly likely that in the near future cancer will be treated successfully, infections controlled or eradicated, and genetic defects rectified. Genetic research heralds extraordinary prospects for treatment in the future.

An increasing number of analgesic, anesthetic, antibiotic, cardiac, hypertensive, hormone, immunological, and other drugs and medical procedures have been developed that have a high degree of specificity, sensitivity, and predictability. In addition, controlled clinical trials are accepted by physicians as the *ne plus ultra* for drug evaluation, and they are required for publication in all major medical journals, for approval of grants by the National Institutes of Health (NIH), and for FDA approval of drugs for use in the United States. Medicine has become so complex that only specialists are competent to treat many illnesses adequately. It is perhaps paradoxical that as medicine becomes significantly less dependent on placebos than at any other time in medical history, its full therapeutic power will be less available because of the increasing need to curb the runaway expense of the new methodology and the cost of medicine (DeBakey 1983; Chelimsky 1993).

The Continuing Importance of the Placebo Effect

Despite the proliferation of nonplacebo drugs and procedures, placebo remedies are destined to fill the gap in knowledge as long as there are illnesses that cannot be treated adequately and the causes of illnesses are unknown. Moreover, although psychological and emotional factors may be minimized, they cannot ever be excluded. Of course, if the dosage of an active drug is high enough, all patients will react predictably with toxicity or even death, regardless of psychological factors, but this predictability is of little medical use because the majority of clinically useful drugs are prescribed in dosages far below the toxic level. Most drugs are useful only in a range in which psychological factors can occur.

Positive Placebo Effects

Psychological factors often change, modify, or suppress the usual pharmacological effects of drugs. For example, changes in mood, mentation, and sedation of medical students who were given dextroamphetamine, morphine, scopolamine, amobarbital, and sodium chloride depended more on the milieu in which the drugs were given and the expectations of the individuals taking the drugs than on the pharmacological properties of the drugs themselves (Sandifer and Hawkings 1958). In a similar study, normal volunteers and chronically ill hospitalized patients reacted to amphetamine with euphoria, and to morphine with dysphoria, while the converse was found with former addicts, who achieved a pleasurable state with morphine and a dysphoric state with amphetamine. Thus, patients may react to drugs in a manner opposite to the classic effects described in textbooks of pharmacology.

The first experimental study of the placebo effect was conducted by Stewart Wolf (1950), who demonstrated the importance of non-drug factors in a subject called Tom, who had an exposed gastric fistula, which made it possible to directly observe his gastric mucosa. Enterogastrone (Urogastrone), diphenhydramine, tripelennamine citrate (Pyribenzamine), and posterior pituitary extract inhibited gastric function when Tom's stomach was inactive at the time of administration but elicited no measurable effect when Tom's stomach was hyperactive. The variable results depended on the state of the end-organs, which, in turn, was modified by emotional factors.

Evidence that drugs' effects can be conditioned was presented in another experiment on Tom. Neostigmine (Prostigmin), given repeatedly, induced (as expected) hyperactive gastric motility, abdominal cramps, and diarrhea. On subsequent days, Tom had similar gastric effects regardless of the substances administered, which included distilled water, lactose tablets, and even atropine sulfate (a potent anticholinergic agent used to decrease gastric hyperactivity) (Wolf 1950).

In another experiment, a patient with hyperemesis gravidarum (excessive nausea and vomiting of pregnancy) was given ipecac on several occasions. Nausea and vomiting were induced repeatedly. On another occasion the patient was given ipecac again but was told that the medication would stop the nausea. Not only was the subjective complaint of nausea abolished but objective evidence of the return of normal gastric contractions was obtained. These effects, attributed by Wolf (1955) to suggestion, have been confirmed in more recent experiments involving many individuals.

The powerful and far-reaching effect of placebos was demonstrated by Henry K. Beecher (1955, 1959a), who summarized fifteen studies of more than 1,082 patients who were treated with placebos for postoperative wound and anginal pain, the common cold, clinical and experimentally induced cough, headache, seasickness, anxiety, tension, and mood disturbance. The average relief of symptoms was 35.2 percent, varying from 21 to 58 percent. Beecher, an anesthesiologist, was impressed with the results of one of his studies, in which a large dose of morphine (15 mg/70 kg) relieved severe pain in 75 percent of patients, nearly half of the effect being attributed to placebo. In another study of 162 post-operative patients, positive responders to placebo also reported more relief from morphine than those who did not respond positively to placebo.

Pierre Kissel and Daniel Barrucand (1964) summarized the placebo effects seen in studies of various medical illnesses before 1960: 28.5 percent placebo effects in twenty-five studies of analgesics, 32.3 percent in five studies of migraine, 58 percent in a study of seasickness, 41 percent in two studies of cough relief, 49 percent in eighteen studies of rheumatism, and 24 percent in four studies of dysmenorrhea and menopausal complaints.

The placebo effects associated with the placebos used as controls in studies of the effect of analgesic drugs on pain have been studied extensively. Frederick J. Evans (1985) reported that anecdotal and experimental evidence indicates that placebo treatments can be as effective as most over-the-counter analgesics for the control of pain. He estimated that placebos are about 55–60 percent as effective as active medications, irrespective of the potency of the active medications, such as aspirin, propoxyphene hydrochloride (Darvon), and codeine, and is also found in double-blind studies of nonpharmacological insomnia treatment, psychotropic drugs for the treatment of depression, and lithium.

In a retrospective review of data reported for 6,931 patients who were treated with promising new treatments for asthma, duodenal ulcer, and herpes (Roberts et al. 1993), the placebo effect or nonspecific effects exceed that reported in published reports of treatment. The clinical studies were uncontrolled, placebos were not used, and the physicians administering treatments evaluated the response. The results were reported as excellent for 40 percent of patients, good for 30 percent, and poor for 30 percent. These percentages reflect a nonspecific response by physicians and patients to presumably active and promising drugs that later proved to be ineffective. The conditions of this study would maximize the placebo effect and no doubt reflect the conditions in which most drugs and treatments are prescribed: absence of controls, enthusiastic patients and healers (both with vested interests), and healers who both treat and evaluate the treatment. Although the high percentages reported in this study require replication for other illnesses and types of drugs, they may more accurately reflect the magnitude of the placebo effect.

Placebo-Induced Side Effects

Placebo-induced side effects are invariably reported in studies using placebos. Walter A. Brown (1988) found that side effects of nervousness, xerostomia, and headache were more frequent in a placebo control group than in a group receiving small dosages of an active medication. Wolf and Pinsky (1954) reported improvement in 30 percent of thirty-two patients treated with a placebo for anxiety and tension, and described major toxic reactions in three patients: one had overwhelming weakness, palpitations, and nausea; another had a diffuse, itchy, erythematous, maculopapular rash diagnosed as dermatitis medicamentosa; and a third, ten minutes after ingesting the placebo, had epigastric pain followed by watery diarrhea, urticaria, and angioneurotic edema of the lips. Beecher (1959b) also described toxic effects attributed to placebo in his studies: warm glow, 8 percent; relaxation, 9 percent; heaviness, 18 percent; fatigue, 18 percent; drowsiness, 50 percent; sleep, 33 percent; difficulty in concentrating, 15 percent; xerostomia, 9 percent; nausea, 10 percent; and headache, 25 percent. In a review of sixty-seven publications, 23 percent (817) of 3,549 patients given placebos reported at least one side effect (Pogge 1963). Significant side effects have also been reported in studies of adrenal gland secretion, angina, blood cell counts, blood pressure, the common cold, the cough reflex, fever, gastric secretion and motility, headache, insomnia, oral contraceptives, pupil dilation and constriction, respiration, rheumatoid arthritis, vaccines, vasomotor function, and warts (Haas et al. 1959).

In our study of 1,006 patients who were given a one-hour drug placebo test, 57 percent of the subjects had one or more side effects. Interestingly, more of the patients given a placebo capsule responded with somatic complaints, whereas more of those in the control group (who were not given a placebo) had cognitive-affective complaints after just sitting in a room for an hour (Shapiro et al. 1974).

Present-Day Placebo Effects

There have been many attempts to derive overall percentages for patients having a positive placebo reaction (often including placebo-induced side effects), those having a nonplacebo reaction (usually a combined group of nonplacebo reactors and negative placebo reactors), and those having placebo-induced side effects. In addition, the percentages of placebo reaction have been reported for patients in various demographic, diagnostic, clinical, symptomatic, and psychological groups. However, the overall and subgroup percentages vary markedly, so much so that no reliable and valid estimate of placebo reactivity is currently available. Considering the different methods of administering placebos, differing time-frames (i.e., were effects measured after minutes or hours?), the different methods of measuring placebo response, and differing positive or negative attitudes toward placebos or active drug, it is understandable why there is so much dispersion in the percentages reported in the literature. Another determinant of placebo percentages is whether placebos are given in an open study, a single-blind study, or a double-blind study. A further influence is whether the placebo control in a study is an inert placebo, which reduces placebo response, or an active placebo (one with physiological effects that mimic the side effects of an active drug), which tends to increase placebo response (these factors are discussed in chapter 9). The application of meta-analysis, not yet done, would be a worthwhile technique for analysis of published literature.

Randomized double-blind controlled studies are now required by the NIH for approval of a grant, by the FDA for approval of a new drug, by scientific journals for publication of papers, by hospitals for inclusion of drugs in the formulary, and by physicians for acceptance of a drug's worth. To be considered adequate, studies now must include specifically stated hypotheses that relate specific reliable and valid independent variables to dependent variables and are clearly differentiated from subgroup or *post hoc* analyses; appropriate significance levels corrected for the number of significant tests, statistical power, statistical analyses, and adequate sample size; randomization; and the double-blind procedure. Often, thousands of patients are studied in collaborative multiple-center clinical trials, as in studies of the treatment of the common cold and of cardiac disorders, and in a recent study of more than fifty thousand patients to determine the usefulness of annual tests for occult blood in the stool.

Surgery

Nonplacebo Achievements

More nonplacebo and specific surgical treatments have been developed since 1950 than during all previous years. Some examples are the excision of epileptic brain foci and other types of brain surgery; surgery for disorders of the kidney, the bladder, and the ovary, and many other types of pathology, including malignancies; successful replacement of heart, lung, liver, gastrointestinal tract, and kidney (one organ at a time or several simultaneously); orthopedic replacement of hip joints; microscopic repair of severed fingers and hands; removal of gallbladders through small tubes inserted into the umbilicus, requiring only one day of hospitalization rather than weeks, as previously required; and hundreds of additional procedures in every surgical specialty.

The Continuing Importance of the Placebo Effect

Many medical historians suggest that surgery is less prone to placebo effects than other medical specialties. There is some support for this assertion, since the effects of some surgical procedures—such as the correction of dislocations and the setting of fractures, procedures used effectively by Hippocratic physicians—can be observed more easily and quickly than can the effects of medical treatment. However, the evidence indicates that surgery too is subject to placebo effects. Treatment of wounds by Hippocrates included some rational procedures such as rest, immobilizing the afflicted part, cleansing the wound with seawater, drying it with a sponge, and covering it with a dry linen cloth. Less rational were the medicines applied to the wound: wine, vinegar, verdigris, turpentine, myrrh, and boiled leaves of plants, often mixed with linseed. Treatment also included moderate bleeding, purgation, and the application of nonirritating substances to hasten the process of suppuration, later referred to as the formation of "laudable pus." These recommendations persisted for more than two thousand years, with reasonable modifications by Celsus in the first century A.D. and minor modifications by others. However, departure from rational treatment is apparent in the fourth century, with local application of earthworms and crushed snails mixed with flour dust gathered from a wall near a flour mill. In the eleventh century in Arabia, wounds were treated with incense, a red resin (known as dragon's blood), and quick or slaked lime, and were dressed with lime washed in sweet water and oil of roses. In the thirteenth century, Western medicine recommended the use of egg white mixed with oil of roses and an alcohol preparation.

In the fourteenth century it was believed that there was a special poison in gunpowder, and it became customary to cauterize gunshot wounds with scalding oil. In the sixteenth century it took a rustic barber's apprentice, Ambroise Paré, who later became an army surgeon, to radically change surgical practice. Some of the surgical procedures then in use had been used by physicians since the time of Hippocrates, the most famous based on the Hippocratic dictum that "diseases not curable by iron are curable by fire." Paré, after running out of the boiling oil traditionally applied to the stump of an amputated limb, observed that providing no treatment was better than singeing the stump. Paré's observation implies that previous treatment had been more harmful than it should have been. The strength of placebo effects, however, is indicated by Paré's continued use of earthworms and the boiled fat of puppydogs on amputated stumps (Garrison 1929).

With minor modifications, little change occurred in the treatment of wounds and the belief in suppuration until the rapid development of bacteriology in the nineteenth century. The concept of suppuration as essential to the healing of wounds was rapidly discounted and then disappeared after Louis Pasteur demonstrated in 1864 that there was no such thing as spontaneous generation and that fermentation and putrefaction were due to microorganisms. The contributions of Joseph Lister, Robert Koch, and Pasteur to surgery and bacteriology are referred to in chapter 1 (note 5). Other important nonplacebo developments in surgery are well known; they include the introduction of anesthetics—ether, and within five years, nitrous oxide and chloroform (1842–46)—and (as an aid against infection in surgery as well as in disease) sulfonamides in 1935 and penicillin in 1943.

Sir Zachery Cope (1958, 173), like Guido Majno, noted that "modern treatment of wounds is the exact opposite to that advised for several thousand years previously—bleeding is never produced. On the contrary in . . . severe wounds the modern surgeon makes good the depleted volume of the patient's blood by a timely and often life-saving blood transfusion."[1]

A more recent example is the history of internal mammary artery ligation therapy for the treatment of angina pectoris. It was based on the reasonable theory that occlusion of the less essential mammary artery would stimulate collateral circulation and produce increased blood flow to the heart, resulting in improvement of anginal symptoms. The surgery, reported as effective in several uncontrolled studies, was accepted enthusiastically by surgeons as highly effective (Kitchell et al. 1958). Soon thereafter, two controlled studies were done in which some patients with angina pectoris underwent a "real" operation (ligation of the mammary artery) whereas another group underwent a "sham" operation (only the skin was incised). In the first study (Cobb et al. 1959), improvement was about the same in the sham group as in the group that underwent full surgery, whereas there was no improvement with either procedure in the second study (Dimond et al. 1960).

Unlike drugs, for which evidence of efficacy and safety is required before marketing is allowed, surgery, mechanical procedures, and tests to aid diagnosis, monitor therapeutic progress, and improve treatment can be marketed without supporting evidence of efficacy and safety. This policy is responsible for the excessive use of many often unsafe and frequently expensive procedures, tests, and surgery, such as lobotomies (in the recent past), tonsillectomies, colectomies, jejunostomies, sympathectomies, hysterectomies, cesarean sections, appendectomies, and cardiac bypass surgery. A paper from an obstetrical and gynecological center published in *JAMA* cited many other examples (Grimes 1993). The author concluded that the only correction to the persistence of old and new fads is rigorous proof provided by sophisticated methodological procedures, and approvingly quoted an ethicist (Schafer 1982, 723) who said, "If the study of the

---

1. See Majno 1975 and Cope 1958 for detailed histories of surgery.

history of medicine teaches us anything, it is that clinical judgment without the check of scientific controls, is a highly fallible compass."

New surgical techniques, like any other new therapy, require controlled studies to eliminate the effect of bias, but controlled studies are rarely done before new techniques are used in patients. This often means that surgeons, without first employing less invasive techniques, use surgical procedures—such as the past use of colectomy for epilepsy, hysterectomy for hysteria, sympathectomy for hypertension, tonsillectomy for colds, and jejunostomy for duodenal ulcer—that have not been tested in controlled studies for effectiveness.

Because of these factors, surgical procedures are probably more likely to be placebos than is drug treatment, which is subject to more rigorous criteria of controlled study.

Conclusion

Interest in the placebo effect continually waxes and wanes in medical history, decreasing during periods of breakthroughs in medical knowledge and treatment, and increasing in periods when expectations are unfulfilled. Current interest in the placebo effect is probably related to a renewed interest in mind-body concepts, behavioral medicine, and alternative treatment.

Medical treatment, because of the increased use of controlled clinical trials, is less prone overall to placebo effects than are surgical and psychological treatments and many types of unorthodox treatment. Physicians are more skeptical than heretofore about evaluating the efficacy of treatment on the basis of anecdotal reports and uncontrolled studies and generally have more faith in controlled clinical trials. Some of the factors contributing to these attitudes are the FDA's requirement that carefully controlled clinical trials be done before approval and marketing of new drugs, and the subsequent publication of these studies, and other studies with large samples, in peer-reviewed journals; the requirement that studies be well controlled in order to qualify for publication in most professional and academic journals; and the convincing nature of many controlled clinical trials that resolved controversies about the usefulness of vitamin C for colds, the usefulness of megavitamins for prophylaxis against many conditions, and the usefulness of aspirin for decreasing the likelihood of strokes.

The lesser number of problems with placebo effects in medicine may also be related to the fact that it is easier to do controlled studies of drugs than to do controlled studies of surgery and psychotherapy. Placebo effects may still be a problem, however, because of subtle methodological deficiencies in most studies. Some of these methodological lapses include breaking of the double-blind code, the use of inert placebos rather than active placebo controls that have the ability to mimic all, or at least most, of the side effects of the drug being evaluated, and extensive use of uncorrected *post hoc* or group subanalyses.

Surgery is more prone to placebo effects because surgical treatments are not subject to FDA requirements for proof of efficacy and evaluation of side effects. In addition, controlled trials in surgery—which may involve the use of invasive procedures, such as sham surgery as a control for transplants—are technically more difficult to devise and ethically more difficult to justify than controlled trials in medicine. Large-scale examples of surgical interventions that have raised serious questions about overuse, effectiveness, safety, and benefit are cesarean sections, hysterectomies, spinal fusions, transplants, and bypass surgery and other surgery for cardiac problems.

In psychiatry, psychopharmacology is less prone to placebo effects because drugs are subject to controlled clinical trials. Major problems continue, however, as is evident in the literature about many methodological liberties marring most published controlled clinical trials. Psychotherapy, whether provided by psychiatrists, psychologists, social workers, nurse therapists, clerics, or other professionals, is the treatment most subject to placebo effects. Even more placebo prone are the myriad treatments encompassed by alternative medicine, faith healing, and quackery.

An unexpected recent development is the new ethical, emotional, and clinical respect afforded placebos. In fact, belief in the power of placebos has become exaggerated owing to a "bandwagon effect," and the heretofore lowly and unethical placebo now has more of a placebo effect than ever before.

chapter five

Psychiatry and Other Psychotherapies

Psychiatry is the medical specialty that deals with the diagnosis, treatment, and prevention of mental and emotional disorders. Whereas psychiatrists are concerned with the diagnosis and treatment of both organic central nervous system and psychological disorders, other professional groups are primarily but not exclusively involved in the evaluation and treatment of psychological and social distress and disorders. These nonpsychiatrists are predominantly psychologists, social workers, clerics, and nurses, but they may also be members of other, smaller professional groups, and many are nonprofessional individuals with heterogeneous backgrounds.

This chapter examines the relationship of the placebo effect to psychiatric and psychological treatment. One would reasonably expect that psychiatrists and psychologists would be sensitive to and aware of nonspecific psychological factors and of placebo effects associated with treatment. However, psychiatry lags behind medicine and surgery in devising specific and effective nonplacebo treatments, and the need to be concerned about the placebo effect is apparent in the history and present status of psychiatry. The history of psychological treatment traverses the centuries, and the recent literature on the psychotherapies is enormous. We can cite only selected aspects of this history.[1] Our main focus is on examining the possibility that psychotherapy is the major placebo of the late twentieth century.

Psychiatry's Placebo Heritage

The treatment of mental illness before the modern era parallels that of physical illness. The therapies that were used included magic, religion, prayer, incantation, dream divination, myth, philosophy, balancing the four humors, pre-

1. The reader is referred to histories of medicine and psychiatry such as Zilboorg and Henry 1941; Bromberg 1954, 1975; Hunter and Macalpine 1963; Goshen 1967; Rosen 1968; Caldwell 1970, 1978; Ellenberger 1970; Ackerknecht 1971; Roccatagliata 1986; Colp 1989; and several pharmacology texts.

venting a uterus from wandering, faith, suggestion, persuasion, hypnosis, vene-section, diaphoresis, cathartics, emetics, hydrotherapy, and myriad drugs.[2] Hippocrates emphasized diet, baths, and exercise, and to his credit minimized the use of drugs other than mandrake (scopolamine), hellebore (veratrine), henbane (hyoscyamine), and poppy juice (which was administered for pain).

The most prominent drugs used in the eighteenth century were mandrake,[3] hellebore,[4] henbane,[5] opium,[6] and belladonna. Some physicians, during the seventeenth, eighteenth, and nineteenth centuries, used specific drugs for mental illness: a "decoction of pimpernel with purple flower" for the treatment of madness; the "juice of ground ivy"; mandrake to anoint the head; hellebore, alcohol, opium, and quinine sulphate against melancholy; and in 1845 cannabis and chloral hydrate as a depressant. Although none were effective or specific for the treatment of mental illness, they acted as soporifics to dull the senses and make life bearable. Some were inert if used in low dosages, if the active moieties were incorrectly prepared or stored, or if ersatz preparations were dispensed, and all were toxic or lethal at higher dosages.

2. See Caldwell (1970, 1978) for a brief outline of the history of psychopharmacology in Western medicine.

3. Mandragora, also known as European mandrake, contains several alkaloids including hyocine, scopolamine, and mandragorine and has properties similar to those of these alkaloids and stramonium, hyoscyamus, belladonna, and atropine. It has antispasmodic effects and was used for sedation, narcosis, and aphrodisia, and as an inadequate anesthetic. American mandrake, also known as mayapple, is a podophyllin with drastic watery-purging properties.

4. Hellebore, containing mixed alkaloids, is a violent gastrointestinal poison with hydragogic (watery purgation), emmenagogic (menstruation-inducing), cathartic, and antihypertensive properties. The American green hellebore has cardiac, hypotensive, and sedative properties. The white or European hellebore (veratrum album), similar but not identical to green hellebore, has hypotensive properties. Both green and white hellebores are also used as insecticides. Black hellebore *(Helleborus niger)*, or Christmas (or New York) rose, was used as an arterial tonic, diuretic, and cathartic, and there are white *(Veratrum album or V. viride)*, false *(V. adonis)*, and fetid (stinking) hellebores. It would take more study to untangle which of the many hellebores were used at which times and places and for what purposes. It is clear, however, that for mental problems and probably for all other disorders, hellebore was another widely used placebo.

5. Henbane, or hyoscyamus, also known as stinking nightshade, insane root, poison tobacco, and hog bean, contains powerful alkaloids such as hyoscyamus, hyoscine, and scopolamine. (*Hyoscyamus* is the ancient Greek and Latin name formed from two Greek words meaning "hog" and "bean"; this is a reference to its poisonous effect on hogs.)

6. Opium no doubt was used to treat mental illness, and was extensively used to treat depression up to the 1930s. (The limitations of its effective use are described above.)

Hysteria

The history of hysteria is typical of psychiatry's placebo heritage. Hysteria was first described and named by Hippocrates, who believed it to be a women's illness caused by a wandering uterus and recommended marriage and intercourse as cures. Both the concept and the treatment, with minor modifications, lasted more than two thousand years. Edward Jordon, in 1603, wrote the first book in English that labeled hysteria as a disease caused by the uterus (Colp 1989). In the seventeenth century, Thomas Sydenham, the reviver of Hippocratic ethical attitudes and methods of rational clinical observation and experience, more correctly characterized hysteria as having multifaceted nonpsychotic symptoms and occurring in males, but attributed its cause to abnormal animal spirits and recommended treatment with purges and venesection, followed by iron and exercise. Willis, a contemporary of Sydenham, also noted for his careful clinical observation, reported that dissection did not confirm movement of the uterus in hysterical women, but recommended a decoction of pimpernel for madness.

Scholars in the Middle Ages theorized that mental illness was caused by the devil. To corroborate the diagnosis, they examined the patients—especially female patients, who were turned upside down when they were examined—for evidence of nevi or blemishes on any part of the body (Rosen 1968; Kramer and Sprenger 1971).

Placebo Treatments

Many bizarre techniques were used in ancient times and in the nineteenth century to cure mental illness, among them the surprise bath (throwing unwary patients into the sea, or suddenly dropping them through a trap door as they crossed a picturesque bridge over a gently flowing stream); submersion of subjects in water for as long as possible without drowning (at times, drowning indicated innocence and coming to the surface indicated guilt, since the mad were accused of witchcraft); the use of mechanical machines causing vigorous swinging, spinning, and rocking for insomnia, insanity, and unruly patients; and the twirling of patients in a human centrifuge, horizontal and vertical for different indications, leading to ecchymosis of the eyes.

Other treatments in the early 1800s included administration of the juice of ground ivy to tranquilize patients, of granulated tin to reduce hypomania, and of quinine for melancholia (Caldwell 1970, 1978). Other placebo treatments, culled from Anne E. Caldwell's (1970, 1978) history of psychiatric drug therapy, include the introduction of cannabis and hashish in 1845, chloroform and ether inhalations in 1847, hyoscyamine in 1875, cocaine in 1880, sleep therapy in 1897 and 1920, amobarbital (Amytal) narcosis in 1929, carbon dioxide inhalation (first used for psychoses in 1920; later used by Meduna for neurosis in 1947), histamine desensitization in 1938, histamine with insulin for schizophrenia in 1938, and phenbenzamine (an antihistamine) for various mental disorders.

Treatments for Manic-Depressive Disorder and Schizophrenia

More than fifty different treatments, each reported as leading to recovery and improvement, were used to treat manic-depressive disorder, now known as bipolar disorder, before 1950. Among them were testicular vein blood serum, epivector serum, own-blood injections, lysate of the hypophysis, refrigeration, aurora-tone films, puppets, and diencephalic radiation (Bellak 1952). All treatments for bipolar disorder were placebos until the advent of lithium, which went unnoticed when first described in 1949, was recognized in the 1960s, and was ultimately approved by the FDA for treatment of this disorder in 1970. Other drugs currently used for bipolar disorder are valproate (Depakane) and carbamazepine.

The history of placebo treatment for schizophrenia is even more dramatic (Bellak 1948). A telling characterization of the pathology in schizophrenia repetitively reported year after year and by each new generation "would make the schizophrenic patient a sorry physical specimen indeed: his liver, brain, kidney, and circulatory functions are impaired; he is deficient in practically every vitamin; his hormones are out of balance, and his enzymes are askew" (Horwitt 1956, 429). Other reports cited other abnormalities—an abnormal bean sprout test (the beans grew crooked in schizophrenic urine, blood, and cerebrospinal fluid) (Shapiro 1956), the Lehmann-Facius cerebrospinal serological test, the mauve factor in urine, deviant-smelling sweat, abnormal ceruloplasmin levels, too much taraxein in the brain, pink spots in the urine, an abnormal Funkenstein test, and myriad chemical abnormalities extensively reported by the Himwiches and other biologically oriented psychiatrists in the 1950s and 1960s.

All had their day as the latest fad. Today the situation is somewhat different because of the dramatic increase in basic science, knowledge of the brain, and revolutionary medical technology which has resulted in an explosion of biological research in schizophrenia and psychiatry in general. Many of the recent studies, however, violate basic methodological principles and fail to specify and test stated hypotheses, to clearly report and identify retrospective analyses and results, and so on, thus contributing to erroneous conclusions. In addition, reports contradict each other or are not replicated by other studies, inevitably contributing to the conclusion that not much currently is known about the cause of schizophrenia (Rosen 1968; Carpenter et al. 1993).

The physical, mechanical, drug, and psychological therapies used in treatment of manic-depressive disorder and schizophrenia constantly change depending on current fads; the treatments described above are but a sampling of those that have been used. Their use is strongly influenced by the prevailing social, cultural, and economic circumstances—for example, there is one credulity for the upper classes and another for the lower classes (Ellenberger 1970).

Chemical Therapies and Psychopharmacological Treatments

By the nineteenth century some minimally useful treatments had been introduced: bromides (1857), which were used for epilepsy, sedation, hypnosis, and various nervous disorders (but unfortunately caused telltale side effects: nasal pustules and severe brominism); chloral hydrate, the first drug to be used in psychiatry (1869); and paraldehyde (1882), which was largely replaced by barbital (1903), phenobarbital (1912), amobarbital (Amytal) (1929), and subsequently, hundreds of other barbiturates. These treatments, however, were nonspecific and were minimally useful in psychiatry. Specific biological treatments began to appear, very slowly and occasionally, in the twentieth century.

Treatments for General Paresis

Syphilis was the sexual scourge for more than four hundred years, with a lifetime prevalence estimate of 5 to 20 percent in Europe and the United States by the beginning of the twentieth century. By 1914, 3 million people had syphilis in Great Britain (Austin et al. 1992). Its course is unpredictable, it is often debilitating, and it can result in neurosyphilis and early death. The numerous fanciful treatments for general paresis used during the early twentieth century were as impotent as most other medical treatments of the time: treatment was directed primarily at treating the syphilitic chancre with calomel, mercuric chloride, ointments, mercury soaps, arsphenamine (Salvarsan) with bismuth or mercury, and tuberculin.

Another treatment was fever therapy. Malarial therapy, although time-consuming, expensive, and hazardous, was rapidly accepted, many enthusiastic reports were then published, and thousands of patients were treated into the early 1950s, when it was replaced by treatment with penicillin. Austin et al. reviewed the history of malarial treatment and the methodologically primitive published papers on the topic, which were the norm at the time, and concluded that "what is most odd about the whole history is that no one knows, even today, whether malariotherapy was truly efficacious in the treatment of neurosyphilis" (1992, 518). In another report on malarial treatment (1995), Braslow, to account for the fact that medical records showed that malarial fever therapy patients improved, suggested that if physicians have a therapy they believe efficacious, they will be more optimistic. The therapy, he noted, altered physician–patient relationships in a positive way.

Insulin Coma, Metrazol Convulsive Treatment, and Electroconvulsive Treatment

Insulin coma treatment for schizophrenia was introduced by Manfred Sakel in 1933. It ultimately became the *ne plus ultra* treatment for schizophrenia. However, by 1958 it was judged to be a highly dangerous procedure and a complex placebo treatment. Most hospitals soon discontinued its use (Boardman et al. 1956; Ackner et al. 1957; Boling et al. 1957; Fink et al. 1958; Shapiro 1960b).

Ladislav von Meduna in 1934 induced convulsions using camphor, and later pentylenetetrazol (Cardiazol and Metrazol) was used as a treatment for schizophrenia. These therapies were replaced by electroconvulsive treatment, a simpler and safer method of inducing convulsions (Kalinowsky 1970).

Electroconvulsive treatment (ECT) was introduced by Ugo Cerletti and Lucio Bini in 1938. Although ECT was used for most psychiatric conditions for many years after its introduction, over time physicians became aware that it was ineffective for schizophrenia. It was associated with placebo effects, notably because of the finding that there was no difference between unconsciousness during a convulsion and unconsciousness induced by nitrous oxide (Bond and Morris 1954; Brill et al. 1957). By the 1960s, however, ECT was found to be an effective treatment for depression, which now represents the primary indication for ECT.

Psychosurgery

The next notable placebo treatment was prefrontal lobotomy. Examining the history of the use of psychosurgery demonstrates once again how a monstrous treatment, theoretically grounded, developed and used by intelligent and reasonable individuals and evaluated as worthy of the Nobel Prize, can be sanctioned for use in more than fifty thousand patients for more than twenty years and be far worse than a simple placebo. It indicates once again how the desperate need for effective therapies can spawn not only an ineffective therapy—in effect, a placebo treatment—but also a treatment that, like phlebotomy, can covertly cause appalling side effects, all of which could have been avoided by controlled study of a hundred subjects. The data on modern methods of psychosurgery indicate that when the lesions are limited, as in anterior cingulectomies, postoperative complications have been minimal (Henn 1989), and the treatment may be helpful for some patients with chronic intractable depression and obsessional states.

Stimulants

Stimulants were the first useful, effective, and widely used drugs in psychiatry. The most effective were the amphetamines. They were used initially for narcolepsies and then were used extensively to relieve depression, fatigue, sleepiness, obesity, and hyperactivity. It was recognized that amphetamines could be abused, resulting in the development of tolerance, addiction, withdrawal symptoms, and occasional brief but flamboyant paranoid psychoses. As a result, they were labeled controlled drugs, requiring special prescriptions in some states.

Antipsychotic Drugs, or Major Tranquilizers

Rauwolfia serpentina, introduced in Indian psychiatry in 1931, and chlorpromazine, introduced in psychiatry in 1952, contributed to a psychopharmacological revolution. Chlorpromazine was the first effective neuroleptic drug (Deniker 1970; Mitchell 1993).

Many other phenothiazine antipsychotics were developed subsequently, their ability to reduce florid psychotic symptoms confirmed by hundreds of well-controlled studies. At the same time, many drug treatments that initially were heralded as panaceas and used extensively for the treatment of schizophrenia eventually fell into disuse after they proved to be ineffective and it became apparent that they were only temporarily fashionable placebos: these include megavitamins or megadoses of nicotinic acid (vitamin B_3 or niacin), niacinamide, vitamin C, vitamin E, pyridoxine, and drugs such as Deaner (an analogue of choline), the antiepileptic diphenylhydantoin (Dilantin), azacyclonal (Frenquel) for hallucinations, and tetrabenazine (Nitoman).

Antidepressants

Melancholy, or depression as it is called today, long known to pre-Hippocratic physicians, was treated for more than two thousand years with various drugs intended to reduce excessive black bile in patients with melancholic temperaments. Attempts to treat depression with drugs were futile until 1937, when the monoamine oxidase (MAO) inhibitor iproniazid (Marsilid), initially noted to energize chronically fatigued tuberculosis patients, was used to treat depressed psychiatric patients. Although this drug was highly effective in the treatment of about four hundred thousand patients, reports of jaundice began to appear. It was never substantiated that this reaction was due to iproniazid, but the drug was withdrawn from the market (Kline 1970). Other MAO inhibitor antidepressant drugs were introduced soon thereafter: phenelzine (Nardil), tranylcypromine (Parnate), isocarboxazid (Marplan), and nialamide (Niamid). All are still used, except Niamid, which was withdrawn from the market after it was shown to be ineffective even at a dosage of 200 mg/day.

At about the same time, Kuhn (1958) described a drug with a configuration similar to but slightly different from that of chlorpromazine as having antidepressant rather than antipsychotic properties. The drug was imipramine (Tofranil), the first tricyclic antidepressant. Many other tricyclics were marketed subsequently, all similarly effective but each with a different pattern of side effects. Thus the antidepressant era was initiated. It was heralded in thousands of publications, resulting in millions of effectively treated patients and saving billions of dollars by reducing the morbidity of depression. The recent introduction of serotonin reuptake blockers, such as fluoxetine (Prozac), added another category of antidepressant with different and generally better-tolerated side effects. All three categories of antidepressant drugs are equally effective and similar for the postulated depressive subcategories (Davis et al. 1989, 1993).

Hundreds of studies support the effectiveness of antidepressant drugs for the treatment of depression in a range of 45 to 80 percent. All antidepressants have about equal efficacy, differing only in the pattern of side effects. However, placebo effectiveness in depression is also high, ranging from 30 to 50 percent (Brown 1988): placebos are 59 percent as effective as antidepressants (as calculated on the basis of ninety-three studies), 62 percent as effective as lithium (thirteen studies), 58 percent as effective as nonpharmacological treatment of insomnia (thirteen studies), and 54 to 56 percent as effective as injected morphine and common analgesics (twenty-two studies) (Evans 1985).

A serious reservation about the validity of these and other controlled studies of drugs is that inert placebos were used instead of active placebos that mimic the side effects of the experimental drug being evaluated (Blumenthal et al. 1974). This flawed methodology often enables clinicians and patients to discern whether the experimental drug or the placebo control drug is being used, thus breaking the blind. This then renders the study single-blind or entirely nonblind, allowing for serious clinician and patient bias (Shapiro 1978). A growing literature demonstrates that if active placebo controls are used in studies of antidepressants and other drugs, the active drug is only slightly, if at all, better than placebo.[7]

Antianxiety-Sedative-Hypnotic Drugs, or Minor Tranquilizers

The placebo effect has always been an important component of drug treatment of psychological problems, especially anxiety. The recent history of psychochemotherapy indicates that mephenesin, meprobamate, and many other antianxiety drugs that were formerly thought to be effective are now considered placebos. In addition, many effective antianxiety drugs were prescribed both knowingly and unknowingly at placebo dosages—for example, 5 mg of chlordiazepoxide (Librium); 2 mg of diazepam (Valium); 5 mg of prochlorperazine (Compazine) for neurotic and hypochondriacal patients; 2 mg of trifluoperazine (Stelazine) for psychotic patients; and Triavil (2 mg of perphenazine and 10 mg of amitriptyline) and Limbitrol (5 mg of chlordiazepoxide and 10 mg of amitriptyline) for depressed patients.

Mephenesin (Tolserol) was introduced as a muscle relaxant in 1947 and as the first antianxiety drug in 1949–50. It was later shown to be no different than placebo (Hampson et al. 1954). It was replaced by meprobamate (Miltown, Equanil) in 1955. Meprobamate became an immediate success and remained popular until controlled clinical comparisons indicated that it was not superior to barbiturates and placebo. The side effects of meprobamate were similar to those of the barbiturates: sedation, tolerance, addiction, and withdrawal effects, and in some patients could result in suicide (Shapiro 1964e, 1976; Greenblatt and Shader 1971).

The financial success of meprobamate contributed to the introduction of a plethora of antianxiety drugs, none of which was better than barbiturates and placebo, and all of which had similar side effects (Shapiro 1964e, 1976).[8] Much

---

7. See Greenberg and Fisher 1989; Greenberg et al. 1992; and chapter 9 for a detailed discussion of this problem.

8. For example, hydroxyzine hydrochloride (Atarax), promoxolane (Dimethylane), glutethimide (Doriden), emylcamate and hydroxyphenamate (Listica), ectylurea (Levanil), methyprylon (Noludar), benactyzine hydrochloride (Phobex and Suavital), ethylchlorvynol (Placidyl), oxanamide (Quiactin), buclizine hydrochloride (Softran), captodiamine (Suvren), mephenoxalone (Trepidone), chlormezanone (Trancopal), phenaglycodol (Ultran), ethinamate (Valmid), hydroxyzine hydrochloride (Vistaril), and promethazine (Phenergan). This period also saw the use of irrational drug combinations, such as Dexamyl (the stimulant dextroamphetamine combined with the barbiturate amybarbitol), Triavil (10 mg of the antidepressant amitryptyline [Elavil] combined with 2 mg of the antipsychotic perphenazine [Trilafon]), and Librax (5 mg of chlordiazepozide [Librium] and 2.5 mg of clidinium bromide)—all usually prescribed in placebo dosages.

creativity went into giving them proprietary names with antianxiety connotations. The enthusiasm for these drugs was rapidly replaced by the fad for benzodiazepine antianxiety drugs: chlordiazepoxide (Librium) in 1960, diazepam (Valium) in 1963, and dozens of others. Alprazolam (Xanax) and triazolam (Halcion) are the current favorites.

Psychotropic drugs are being prescribed increasingly often by nonpsychiatrists. In a survey in 1980–81, primary care physicians wrote 66 percent of the psychotropic prescriptions, psychiatrists only 17 percent, and other medical specialists 17 percent (Beardsley et al. 1988). A more recent survey indicated a substantial increase in the cost of prescriptions for psychotropic medications in the United States: in 1985, $1.45 billion was spent on outpatient psychotropic medications, compared to $513 million in 1977. About 60 percent of the total was spent on antianxiety and sedative-hypnotic medications, approximately 18 percent on antipsychotic medications, 17 percent on antidepressants, and 5 percent on combination psychotropic medications (Zorc et al. 1991). The expenditures for drugs in all categories skyrocketed in the 1990s. These drugs are often prescribed by nonpsychiatrists and non-psychopharmacologically oriented psychiatrists at placebo dosages, such as 5 mg of chlordiazepoxide or 2 mg of diazepam. The distinction between antianxiety, sedative, and hypnotic effects is unclear and is largely associated with the dosage.

Chloral hydrate, bromides, paraldehyde, barbiturates, nonbarbiturate sedatives, and benzodiazepines all induce essentially the same effects: placebo effects at a low dosage; antianxiety effects at a slightly higher dosage; sedation and hypnosis at a still higher dosage; and anesthesia, coma, and death at the highest dosages. A more proper designation for these drugs might be antianxiety-sedative-hypnotic drugs, since all have similar dosage-related effects (Shapiro 1976; Gorman and Davis 1989).

Controlled studies indicate that benzodiazepines may be effective for patients with acute anxiety, but that the initial dosage is effective only for about one week, after which tolerance develops, requiring an increase in the dosage and the danger of sedative side effects and addiction (Shapiro et al. 1983; Kahn et al. 1986; Lipman 1989).

Faddish beliefs in therapies that come and go are common in the history of medical, psychiatric, and psychological treatment (Deutsch 1949). They are stimulated by economic, political, religious, philosophical, and other societal changes, and often by discoveries of new substances, physical phenomena, technology, and scientific theories. Therapies initially are deemed veritable panaceas by patients and enthusiastic healers who describe impressive results. With time, the results falter, skeptical healers report flagging therapeutic efficacy, and new therapies take the place of the older ones.

This recurrent theme is a reflection of the magnitude of the placebo effect, which since the 1950s has been clearly illustrated by comparison of controlled studies of therapy with uncontrolled studies. In a review of seventy-two studies of treatment published in selected American and British psychiatric journals between 1951 and 1956, uncontrolled studies reported that 83 percent of the treatments were successful and 17 percent were failures; by contrast, (somewhat or variably) controlled studies reported that 75 percent of the treatments were failures and 25 percent were successes (Foulds 1958). Similarly, in a review of fifty-seven studies of treatment published during 1957, unacceptably controlled studies reported 91 percent of treatments as successes and only 9 percent as failures, whereas acceptably controlled studies reported 54 percent as successes and 46 percent as failures (Fox 1961). Regarding the use of glutamic acid in brain-damaged children, fourteen uncontrolled studies reported success and none reported failure, while 68 percent of controlled studies reported failure and 32 percent reported success (Astin and Ross 1960). The percentages of successes for the controlled studies probably were overly generous, since only minimal criteria were required and none of the studies was double blind.

Psychological Treatments

A brief summary of the history of psychotherapy is not possible because of the length, myriad manifestations, and diffuseness of that history, and the failure to authenticate any of the multitudinous psychotherapeutic theories, systems, or treatments. This discussion, therefore, focuses on selected highlights and generalizations, primarily to examine psychotherapy as possible placebo.[9]

A study of the placebo effect provides an approach to the question of what is specific and what is nonspecific in psychotherapy. This concept is not popular among psychotherapists, many of whom believe that psychotherapy is a modern treatment based on scientific principles and view the placebo effect as a suggestion-related response to a drug. Psychiatrists holding these attitudes believe that the placebo effect is not a factor in—or the entire basis for—the existence, popularity, and effectiveness of the majority of the numerous methods of psychotherapy now in use. We believe strongly that there is much to be learned about a treatment if it is examined in relation to basic principles applicable to all treat-

---

9. The literature about psychotherapy and efficacy is immense, consisting of thousands of papers and books. Comprehensive discussion of the many facets of psychotherapy research can be found in the references cited in this section, their bibliographies, and the national psychotherapy databases.

ments and also to psychotherapy by considering its relationship to the placebo effect (Shapiro 1971; Shapiro and Morris 1978; Shapiro and Shapiro 1984b).

The History of Psychotherapy

Contrary to popular belief, psychotherapy did not begin with Freud. Even before Freud, mental patients were treated not only with methods similar to those used to treat medical illness but also with methods that strongly resemble current psychotherapies. A comprehensive study of the development of psychotherapy, including many primary sources and original historic documentation, abundantly documents parallels between modern psychotherapeutic methods and primitive, Greco-Roman, and subsequent healing methods, and religious methods, right up to our current period (Janet 1909, 1924, 1925; Ellenberger 1970; Roccatagliata 1986). The patterns and details of this history have been subject to cryptomnesia in every generation.[10] The history shows an unwitting repetition of old, abandoned psychotherapeutic ideas, which are heralded as new discoveries and insights, their recurrent periods of popularity and rejection being determined by social and economic factors affecting society, patients, and healers. Henri E. Ellenberger (1970) traced the origin of dynamic psychotherapy, labeled as a recent breakthrough and elevated to a scientific method of treatment, to a long line of ancestors and forerunners. Medical, philosophical, and healing ideas in the past had "a surprisingly high degree of insight into what are usually considered the most recent discoveries" (3). The ebb and flow of these ideas and practices are influenced, as persuasively described by Ellenberger, by socioeconomic and religious factors, political background, cultural trends, the personality of pioneers, and changes in class ascendancy, as well as changes in general knowledge, discontinuity of tenacious traditions, and new paradigms.

Histories of psychotherapy frequently highlight the influence of Friedrich A. Mesmer, Valentine Greatrakes, hypnotism, Christian Science, and Freud.[11] All, however, had many antecedents (Janet 1909, 1924, 1925; Podmore 1963; El-

10. Cryptomnesia about previous psychotherapy research and literature can be illustrated by a major three-day conference of the American Psychopathological Association in 1983 (Williams and Spitzer 1984). Four papers summarized the results of psychotherapy of anxiety, depression, schizophrenia, and conduct disorder. Of the 325 references in these papers, 91.4 percent had been published in the preceding ten years, 7.7 percent between 1963 and 1973, and only 3 before 1963; the oldest cited reference was from 1953.

11. See the three-volume assessment and comparison of methods of psychotherapy edited by W. B. Parker (1908–9).

lenberger 1970; Roccatagliata 1986). Psychotherapy was a burgeoning enterprise at the turn of the century, with published descriptions of many techniques—persuasive, suggestive, re-educative, cognitive, and other—similar to those used today.

Psychoanalysis

Psychoanalysis, ignored for many years, was frequently derogated after its introduction in 1894. For example, Morris Fishbein, the long-time editor of *JAMA,* entitled a chapter of his *New Medical Follies* (1927) "Psychoanalysis: A Cultist Movement?" According to Fishbein, psychoanalysis slowly became the plaything of artists, littérateurs, and critics, and Torrey (1992) commented on its absorption by liberal intellectuals, social reformers, anthropologists, educators, and writers; Grünbaum (1993) noted that it influenced literary criticism, esthetics, history, biography, religion, and all of society. It attracted the interest of the upper classes and was characterized by Ellenberger (1970) as a therapy for wealthy persons who were concerned about amorous problems. Others may have been attracted by the sexual license that psychoanalysis implied, the free play of fantasy in psychoanalysis, and the extensive, well-written works by Freud (who won the Goethe Prize for Literature) and other psychoanalysts.

Many creative psychoanalysts migrated to the United States from Germany in the 1930s, increasing both the number of psychoanalytic practitioners in the United States and the number of their publications (usually favorably reviewed). They began to influence the younger generation of psychiatrists and psychologists after World War II. Psychoanalytic philosophy soon began to permeate much of American life—child rearing, education, psychology, anthropology, history, sociology, social work, art, literature, drama, cinema. Percival Bailey (1965) concluded that psychoanalysis had an "overwhelmingly hypertrophied and distorted influence . . . in the United States" and did "great damage to psychiatry as well as to our civilization in general." Martin Gross (1978) characterized it as a new faith and dogma, having all the earmarks of a new religion, transmogrifying the United States into a "psychological society."

Freudian psychoanalysis dominated the training of psychiatrists and medical students at most U.S. medical schools in the 1950s. The chairs of most departments of psychiatry were psychoanalysts or psychoanalytically oriented, as were most members of the faculty (Garfield 1980). The prestige treatment was a classical psychoanalysis; if this was not possible, patients did the best they could with a psychodynamically oriented therapy. And psychiatrists treated everything—hyperthyroidism, hypertension, asthma, migraine, ulcers, ulcerative colitis, rheumatoid arthritis, myasthenia gravis, Tourette syndrome, schizophrenia, manic depression, and much more—with analytic therapy.

Psychiatrists had a monopoly on treatment in the 1950s and 1960s. Psychologists, also influenced by psychoanalytic theory, were limited mainly to administering projective tests such as the Rorschach Ink Blot Test ("What do the inkblots resemble?"), the Thematic Apperception Test ("Tell a story about the pictures"), and intelligence tests. Patients both in and out of the hospital were often tested, and the results were viewed with the respect and awe otherwise reserved for a pathologist's postmortem. A few doctoral programs in clinical psychology offered therapeutic training, but these were in nonanalytic techniques such as Rogerian (client-centered) therapy. There were a few other therapies here and there—such as psychoanalytic offshoots, eclectic, nondirective, rational, and hypnotic therapies, and some behavioral therapies—but they had less prestige and were not taught at major training centers. Psychologists were not accepted for training at most psychoanalytic centers, and it took many years before specific centers were established to train psychologists as psychoanalysts.

The pervasive influence of Freudian psychoanalysis is illustrated by the common use of many Freudian concepts, words, and terms. For example, the word *unconscious* is commonly used to explain slips of the tongue, forgetting, mistakes, mispronunciation, misattribution, tardiness, or punctuality; to interpret dreams; and to explain a host of peccadillos. However, the Freudian unconscious is defined as mental life not subject to recall, unretrievable, and completely unknowable—except, during intensive and prolonged psychoanalysis, to psychoanalysts who have been trained to understand the language of the unconscious (Fenichel 1954; Salter 1952; Grünbaum 1993). The analyst's selective interpretation of resistance, repression, transference, dreams, fantasies, slips of the tongue, and free association, repetitively given to the patient during the psychoanalysis, may cause the patient to intellectually accept the interpretation of his or her unconscious, but the patient never actually remembers having had the unconscious wish or thought. The Freudian unconscious is different from the preconscious, which is retrievable by the patient. It also does not include concepts and studies about the unconscious by psychologists (Loftus and Klinger 1992) dealing with topics such as selective attention, subliminal perception, dichotic listening, perceptual processing, retinal image stabilization, binocular rivalry, backward masking, or other cognitive issues.

Unconscious interpretations and other psychoanalytic formulations may be correct, however, only if there is evidence to support their reliability and validity. But such data are not available. For example, the reliability of psychoanalytic interpretations and formulations has never been demonstrated, and there is some indication of negative findings reported by psychoanalysts themselves.[12] Similarly for validity:[13] two uncontrolled reports, by psychoanalysts, about the effectiveness of psychoanalysis were disappointing.[14] There has never been a controlled study of psychoanalytic treatment (Nagel 1959; Scriven 1959; Fisher and Greenberg 1977; Luborsky and Spence 1978; Grünbaum 1986, 1993; Strupp 1994; and many others), and accumulated data from clinical observation and studies of therapy support the notion that no one therapy is better than another (Frank 1973; Luborsky and Spence 1978; Bergin and Lambert 1978; Fisher and Greenberg 1989).[15]

Many psychoanalysts acknowledge the importance of nonspecific factors in therapy. Indeed, some refer to such factors as suggestion (construed as transference). Very few, however, take the logical plunge of referring to them as the placebo effect. Questioned about the placebo effect, psychoanalysts did not agree with the statement that the placebo effect was a part of all treatment, and they excluded psychotherapy from the definition of the placebo (Shapiro and Streuning 1973a, 1973b).

12. Preliminary results of an ambitious study of the reliability of psychoanalytic interpretations were presented at a meeting in New York City in the 1970s. Partial results were subsequently published by Dahl (1983). After listening to selected sessions of a tape-recorded psychoanalysis, six to eight psychoanalysts judged the evidence supporting postulated unconscious wishes and clinical generalizations and made predictions, as did the psychoanalyst conducting treatment. The number of items supporting the hypotheses differed markedly for each of the participants, who also overvalued their proposed evidence supporting their hypotheses compared to the ideas of other judges. On only one occasion did the reviewing psychoanalysts agree, and their conclusions differed from that of the treating psychoanalyst.

13. For example, at a psychoanalytic seminar on the changes of technique since Freud given at the New York Psychoanalytic Institute in 1959, Freud's analytic technique was described as much simpler than the analytic technique then in use. Freud's therapy was very brief and less advanced; Freud was more informal and more active and talked much more than current therapists. Yet, Freud's results were very good. As a young analyst at the time, I (AKS) found this puzzling, but my question about what it implied about the importance of technique was rebuffed by the training psychoanalyst.

14. See discussions by Salter (1952) and Gross (1978) of the reports about the results of treatment by Knight (1941), and the American Psychoanalytic Association's *Central Fact-Gathering Committee: Summary and Final Report* (American Psychoanalytic Association 1958).

15. For reference to many other authors who discuss the inadequate reliability and validity of psychoanalytic formulations, including the absence of evidence demonstrating effectiveness and the likelihood of little difference among psychoanalytic and other types of therapy, see especially Salter 1952; Gross 1978; and Grünbaum 1984, 1986. See also the discussion of Grünbaum in *Behavioral and Brain Sciences* (1986) and in his more recent book of collected papers (1993).

After the influence of psychoanalysis peaked in the 1950s and early 1960s, it began to decline owing to many interacting contributing factors. Not unimportant are the accumulation of the aforementioned methodological shortcomings and disappointing clinical therapeutic effects, and the absence of controlled studies—an absence that is more striking when seen in light of the stringent FDA requirements for the approval of new drugs, which established precedents for the types of procedures and evidence considered adequate to demonstrate the reliability and validity of study data and the effectiveness of the agent under study. The remarkable progress in medicine, psychiatry, and psychology may have stimulated greater interest and faith in the scientific method.

An indirect indication of the decline of psychoanalysis is the fall from grace of previously omnipotent, largely psychoanalytically formulated projective tests, as negative data about their usefulness were accumulated repeatedly by data-oriented psychologists over a period of years. The development of sophisticated instrumentation, the acquisition of new knowledge about the functioning of the brain, and the promise of important and dramatic scientific discoveries provide the possibility of answering questions that hitherto could only be speculated about, and probably contributed to a shift in interest away from psychological psychiatry and toward biological psychiatry. Another factor is the discouraging theoretical instability resulting from the existence of dozens of different psychoanalytic institutes, orientations, and schools, and the mutual rejection by the orthodox psychoanalytic institutes, as well as the internecine struggles of the advocates of many other psychoanalytic approaches.

Other important factors contributing to the decline of psychoanalysis include the expense of psychoanalytic training, competition from clinical psychologists and social workers (whose fees are generally lower than those of psychoanalysts), a progressive decrease in insurance reimbursement for a treatment that necessitates three to five visits a week, and the growth of managed care facilities. Psychiatry itself is experiencing a dramatic decrease in the percentage of U.S. medical students applying for residencies, dropping 41 percent from 745 in 1988 to 438 in 1994, according to the *Psychiatric News* (Anonymous 1994b), and there has been a similar erosion in the number of psychiatrists applying for psychoanalytic training.

Despite these factors, and many others described in greater detail in other references, most practicing psychoanalysts have maintained that psychoanalysis is a science, whereas many nonpsychoanalysts challenge its scientific foundations (Grünbaum 1993). It is unlikely that this argument—like other irreconcilable controversies, such as those of creationism versus evolution, religion versus atheism, and belief in inherited biological versus psychological determinants of human behavior—can ever be resolved.

This brief, highly selective, and focused examination of psychoanalysis as this century's most infamous placebo treatment requires several caveats. Does psychoanalytic treatment help? There is little doubt that it does, certainly for particular patients. But are its effects any better than those of the many other contending therapies? Probably not. Unfortunately, the only way of resolving the issue would be to conduct controlled studies, which would be so difficult to do that it is unlikely that it will ever be done. One possible method is to contrast disparate psychoanalytic orientations—such as orthodox Freudian treatment versus Jungian treatment, in patients motivated for treatment with either approach, as has been done in studies of Adlerian versus Rogerian client-centered therapy (Shlien et al. 1962); psychoanalytically oriented therapy versus behavior therapy (Sloane et al. 1975); experienced psychoanalytically oriented therapists versus popular but nontherapist faculty members at a college (Strupp and Hadley 1979); and cognitive therapy versus interpersonal psychodynamic therapy (Elkin et al. 1989).

Nothing that has been said should reflect on psychoanalysts' commitment to helping their patients and concern about their welfare. The only problem is that such commitment and concern characterize all innovative healers, clinicians, and physicians who, with the best intentions, and on the basis of insight and clinical experience, develop or strongly espouse therapies that in retrospect are seen to be placebo treatments.

Placebo-Related Themes in the History of Psychotherapy

The literature on psychotherapy extends back to antiquity; it expanded rapidly at the end of the nineteenth century and has grown explosively since the 1950s.[16] It is more extensive than the literature on psychoanalysis and is beyond one person's ability to completely read or master. Only snippets of the history and literature on psychotherapy are noted here; the reader is referred to the histories and studies cited, as well as to others that are not cited but are readily available. Many of the placebo-related factors described for psychoanalysis apply equally to the psychotherapies, and vice versa. This section examines selected features of psychotherapy that can be attributed to placebo effects.

Psychotherapeutic methods constantly replace one another. Older therapies are often unknowingly repackaged as innovative and are then believed to be

16. See the references cited in the previous section on psychoanalysis.

more effective than their progenitors and other current psychotherapies. Pierre Janet, among many others, reflected on this theme. According to Janet: "When, for the first time, they [psychotherapists] come across the phenomena of suggestion [placebo effects], they believe that they have made a discovery, and they are satisfied that they are going to exhibit something which is both peculiar and unfamiliar" (1925, 215).

Schools of Psychotherapy

Schools exist in medicine (and in all other human endeavors) when there is an absence of knowledge, and disappear after facts and controlled studies accumulate and lead to coherent theories. The breakup of psychoanalysis into dozens of schools is exceeded only by a mushrooming of the psychotherapies. The number of distinct psychotherapies was estimated to be 200 in 1977 (Wolberg 1977) and more than 250 in 1980 (Herink 1980; Parloff 1980). It probably would have been 500 in 1995; the total number of different psychotherapies that have been described in history probably exceeds 1,000.

The number of practitioners has increased as well. The spectrum includes psychiatrists, psychologists, social workers, counselors, paraprofessionals, and an ill-defined assortment of other mental health professionals and nonprofessionals, holding degrees such as M.D., D.O., Ph.D., Ed.D., Psy.D., M.S.W., B.A.; some have only a high-school diploma, others have assorted certificates testifying to competence, and some have no diploma at all. The number of psychiatrists in the United States increased from about 7,000 in 1965 to about 42,000 in 1994, an increase of 600 percent. More patients are treated by about 50,000 clinical psychologists, who are exceeded by more than 100,000 social workers and more than 50,000 other mental health professionals, all competing with an uncounted number of assorted and ill-defined lay and quack therapists (Fink 1994). Psychotherapy is big business, with more than 250,000 psychotherapists in the United States; almost 80 million visits to psychotherapists, accounting for $4.2 billion in fees (Sledge 1994); and 2.5 million children receiving treatment at an annual cost of $1.5 billion (Weisz et al. 1992). With the estimate that fewer than 100,000 psychotherapists will be needed in the coming health reform era (Fink 1994), psychotherapy is in crisis.

The proliferation of psychotherapeutic schools suggests that the treatments provided by all types of psychotherapists may work to some extent, not because of the theories or therapeutic procedures but because of underlying, unspecified or not clearly determined nonspecific effects—or what we now subsume under the rubric of placebo effects.

One Therapy for Many Disorders

Many psychoanalytic and psychotherapeutic schools treat different psychiatric disorders with the same underlying theoretical framework or therapeutic approach. The disorders include most psychiatric disorders (e.g., anxiety, hysteria, phobias, obsessions, compulsions, minor and major depression, personality problems, psychoses, and addictions), and many somatic symptoms and disorders. Each school, working from its own theoretical framework, postulates an etiology for many or all of these disorders and derives a therapy, which then is used to treat them. For example, orthodox followers of Freud focus on Freud's theories of the unconscious; Carl Jung's followers focus on archetypes in the collective unconscious; Alfred Adler's, on inferiority; Karen Horney's, on situation and character neurosis; Harry Stack Sullivan's, on interpersonal relationships; Carl Rogers's, on client-centered therapy; and Aaron Beck's, on cognitive therapy. Whenever one therapy is used to treat many different disorders, it is likely that therapeutic effects are due to the placebo effect.

The largely nonspecific treatment for emotional illness is underscored by the remarkable proliferation of psychotherapeutic schools, orientations, and types of treatment. The literature is replete with thousands of clinical and anecdotal testimonials, uncontrolled, retrospective reports, and poorly controlled studies. Most of the studies that attempt to use controls are seriously flawed. The studies use waiting-list controls (assignment of patients to a waiting list, a practice that may result in deterioration of patients), inadequate, nonmatching placebos (brief visits at longer intervals, administered by less-interested therapists), and extensive analysis of nonhypothesized or retrospective variables that maximize the occurrence of irrelevant, nonreplicable findings and leave the findings open to serious question. Adding to the problem is the failure of adequately controlled studies to detect significant therapeutic differences between specific therapies and their controls. As a result, clinical and research psychiatrists, psychologists, psychoanalysts, and others have extensively discussed the nonspecific effects of psychotherapy, and most leading clinical researchers have concluded that nonspecific effects strongly outweigh specific effects.[17] With more than 600 stud-

17. Current views about the preeminent importance of nonspecific factors in psychotherapy are acknowledged by many psychoanalysts and most prominent analytic, dynamic, eclectic, and behaviorally oriented psychotherapist researchers. Study of these factors has become a major area of research, and the references in this area are so numerous that they would fill several pages. We refer the reader to previous references about psychoanalysis and to a sampling of an enormous psychotherapy literature: Janet 1925; Murphy 1951; Eysenck 1952, 1961, 1965, 1966; Rosenthal and Frank 1956; Tibbets and Hawkings

ies of psychotherapy today (Herink 1980), and 230 studies of techniques for therapy with children (Kazdin 1988), many controlled to one extent or another, there is no conclusion as to what specifically works in psychotherapy. An inescapable speculation is that psychotherapy has become this century's major placebo.

Denial That a Placebo Is a Placebo

Another problem is that many (e.g., APA Commission on Psychotherapies 1982; some discussants in Prioleau et al. 1983; Parloff 1986) but not all psychotherapeutic researchers reject the use of placebos and the term *placebo* to designate controls in studies of psychotherapy (the exceptions include Rosenthal and Frank 1956; Shapiro 1971; other discussants in Prioleau et al. 1983; Critelli and Neumann 1984; Grünbaum 1984, 1985, 1986, 1993; Critelli 1985).[18] This rejection is reflected in Morris Parloff's (1986, 86) interesting and thoughtful paper, which builds on previous papers about the placebo and concludes that "the advocates of placebo control research are encouraged to go forth and sine qua non no more." While the arguments for these views are appropriate for some research strategies and are compelling given some assumptions, they ignore historic, heuristic, and methodological factors essential for unflawed clinical trials. These issues are discussed fully in chapter 6; here we briefly discuss some of the recurrent errors in the literature.

The placebo frequently is mentioned as an inappropriate control because it is defined as inert, involves deception, is unethical, and/or is a deterrent to treatment, and because it is appropriate for the study of drugs but not psychotherapy because the placebo itself is a psychological therapy. An appropriate control is described frequently as a procedure or therapy that includes some of the psy-

---

1956; Frank et al. 1957; Imber et al. 1957; Smith and Wittson 1957; Shapiro 1960b, 1971, 1984; Frank 1961, 1973; Torrey 1972, 1992; Luborsky et al. 1975; Sloane et al. 1975; Gross 1978; Shapiro and Morris 1978; Shepherd 1979; Rachman and Wilson 1980; Garfield 1980, 1983, 1984; Smith et al. 1980; APA Commission on Psychotherapies 1982; D. A. Shapiro and D. Shapiro 1982; *Behavioral and Brain Sciences* 1983; Prioleau et al. 1983; Critelli and Neumann 1984; Shapiro and Shapiro 1984b; Williams and Spitzer 1984; Parloff 1986.

18. Controls for use in studies of behavior therapy have been discussed extensively by behaviorists. Particularly thoughtful are comprehensive papers about the importance of using creditable placebos, developing controls with positive expectations about therapy, and standardizing demand characteristics and other factors in studies. However, it is curious to us that the blinding of therapists and others is not considered to be important (Kazdin and Wilcoxon 1976; Jacobson and Baucom 1977; Kirsch 1985; and other references above).

chological factors associated with the psychotherapy to be evaluated, but not the postulated specific or essential factors.

As discussed in chapter 2, for most of its semantic history the placebo was not defined as inert. The original definition that appeared in 1785 referred to "a commonplace method or medicine." By about 1820, when medication became more important, this definition had been replaced by a definition that, with minor variations, described the term *placebo* as "an epithet given to any medicine adopted more to please than to benefit the patient." The next change came in 1947, when Dorland defined the placebo as "a make-believe medicine." The definition was changed in 1951, possibly as a result of the beginning of the use of inert placebos as controls in studies, to "an inactive substance or preparation." *Placebo* then generally became defined as an inert substance, and later, reference was made to its use as a control in clinical studies. At the same time, with increased study of the placebo effect, the definition of *placebo* in the literature and dictionaries began to resemble the original definition, in that it included both medication (inert or active) and methods (surgery, psychological treatment, and other treatment). In fact, if the placebo is considered inert, there would be no problem with deception or ethics, or with the placebo as a deterrent to treatment, because the prescription of inert substances has been exceedingly infrequent. The overwhelming, predominant, and usual use of placebos has been and still is as a treatment believed to be effective. Moreover, with the development of controlled clinical trials it became apparent that an inert placebo is an inadequate control because it often can be detected, which breaks the double blind (the study thus becoming a single-blind study) and may increase positive findings for the active drug.

Psychotherapists may be as defensive in their rejection of the concept of placebo as are those surgeons who deny using placebos because they do not use medicines; the internists who make the same denial because they use only active medicines, such as vitamin B_{12} injections; and the psychoanalytically oriented psychiatrists who do so because they do not use drugs but use psychological treatment, which they do not define as a placebo. These groups thought that the use of placebos in treatment was unethical, and attributed such use significantly more often to other physicians in their own and other specialties than they did to themselves (Shapiro and Struening 1973a, 1973b; Shapiro et al. 1983).

There is a tendency to use a bewildering melange of terms to describe placebo controls in studies of psychotherapy: for example, minimal treatment, medical management, best available treatment, neutral expectancy, counter demand, component control, attention control, expectation control, and treatment element control. Discussion of many of these myriad control procedures is appropriate and relevant, but the terms also may be used defensively to disassociate psychotherapy from a placebo stigma. Psychology's corollary to the "frenetic efforts at remedicalization of the practice of psychiatry" (Parloff 1986, 82) may be the frantic efforts to destigmatize the placebo implications of psychotherapy by abolishing the placebo from psychology. The generic concept of a placebo control in clinical trials does portray the placebo not as inert or active, limited to one therapy or another, but rather as a credible control for everything except the proposed specific or hypothesized components of the treatment to be evaluated.

Actually, the question of inert versus active placebo is academic, because, as discussed in chapter 2, there is no such thing as an inactive substance: the dose of a drug determines whether it is inert or active. But what psychological factors, and what quantitative differences in these factors, would differentiate between an inert psychotherapeutic placebo, an active psychotherapeutic placebo, and an effective psychological treatment? All of these therapeutic agents can be differentiated only by controlled-study comparison with an established placebo.

There are other problems in using placebos in studies of psychotherapy (Parloff 1982, 1986). It is clear from extensive data in the literature that studies using no-treatment controls, waiting-list controls, inactive or inert placebos, or active placebos or procedures without adequate credibility are almost guaranteed to produce results showing that psychotherapy—in fact, any treatment— is more effective than controls. Moreover, none of these procedures can be double-blinded, and the double-blind method is necessary to control for the effect of bias. A frequently proposed alternative concept to placebo controls is to develop a psychological concoction that incorporates nonspecific psychological elements but not the unique therapeutic factors hypothesized as associated with the psychotherapy being studied. However, the resultant psychological placebo package is likely to be inadequate, because both psychotherapeutic and placebo-related factors are not yet adequately understood, and it would not be possible to specify reliable, valid, and predictable elements associated with the placebo effect (Parloff 1986). In addition, it would be difficult for a psychotherapist to invest in placebo therapy to the same extent as a psychotherapist supplying the real therapy, and bias could not be controlled by blinding the treatments.

Studies of Psychotherapy

A major problem is devising an adequate placebo control for use in studies of psychotherapy. As in any study, it is essential that the placebo control be a credible therapeutic procedure, identical to the therapy to be tested except for the specific theoretical principles of the therapy to be evaluated (e.g., the placebo must be the same with regard to the number and duration of visits, the patients' motivation for the therapy, and the therapists' interest in the treatment, and the study must be adequately double-blinded). No study of psychotherapy has been able to accomplish all of these goals, in part because of the difficulty of finding a psychotherapy placebo that is not used as a specific therapeutic technique in another form of psychotherapy (Shapiro 1984; Parloff 1986).

A way out of this dilemma is to contrast one type of therapy with another, such as orthodox versus Jungian psychoanalysis (Rosenthal and Frank 1956; Shapiro 1984; Parloff 1986). This solves many of the problems of using traditional placebo double-blind methods that are more appropriate for therapies, such as drug therapies, that have agreed-upon specific effects. This approach assumes that the therapists are experienced representatives of their theoretical orientations, that the patients are motivated to be treated by the therapies, that patient assignment is randomized, and that other established methodological safeguards are included. It ensures that therapists will treat patients using the specific principles of their own therapeutic orientation, and controls nonspecific variables such as enthusiasm about treatment, coherence of theoretical framework, and many other variables that are difficult to specify and control. The main research question to be answered is clear-cut: Is one therapy better than the other, or are they both equally effective? If a number of such therapies are compared with each other and one or more therapies consistently produce superior results, this would indicate that the therapy with better results is not a placebo treatment, and it would highlight and encourage further study of that therapy. Alternatively, if there are no differences among the therapies, the inevitable supposition would be that therapeutic benefits are due to the placebo effect, which would encourage more intense study of other factors now referred to as nonspecific. Another possibility, one of many, is that the results may show that one therapy works better with certain types of patients than another does.[19]

Several studies illustrate the potential usefulness of comparing established therapies with each other. One study compared twenty-three patients treated twice weekly for a maximum of twenty sessions by experienced Adlerian psychoanalytic and Rogerian client-centered psychotherapists (Shlien et al. 1962).

19. Short-term studies of targeted symptoms, frequently done by behavior therapists and by students writing dissertations, are easier to do than studies of psychodynamic therapies oriented to personality reorganization, requiring prolonged treatment. The problems of the latter—such as the difficulty of assembling an adequate number of therapists and patients who could commit themselves to prolonged treatment, attrition of the sample over time, the costs of such studies, and other tactical and strategic problems—are formidable.

All of the patients improved, without significant differences between therapies. Jerome Frank and colleagues (1959) compared the treatment of three individual groups of fifty-four outpatients with psychoneurosis and personality disorder who were treated by three second- and third-year psychiatric residents for six months. One group was treated with one-hour weekly individual psychotherapy, another with one and one-half hour weekly group psychotherapy, and the third with half-hour visits every two weeks as a minimal-contact control. Discomfort scores significantly decreased for all three groups, but there were no differences between groups at six-month evaluation, and discomfort scores continued to decrease at subsequent one- and five-year evaluations in each group. Measures of social effectiveness improved for all groups, but at six-month evaluation the improvement was greater for patients in group psychotherapy; there was continued improvement at one- and five-year evaluations for all groups, and there were no significant differences among the three groups when they were evaluated after five years.

One of the best studies of psychotherapy was conducted by R. Bruce Sloane and co-workers (1975, 1984). Ninety-four outpatients with anxiety neurosis and personality disorders were treated by experienced therapists for four months with psychoanalytically oriented or behavior therapy, and the members of a control group were given only an initial assessment, assigned to a waiting list, and called every few weeks. The severity of target symptoms improved significantly for all three groups, but more so for the two treatment groups, which, however, were not significantly different from each other. At follow-up evaluations one and two years later, all three groups showed improvement, but did not differ significantly in the extent of this improvement.

In another study, ninety-one depressed elderly patients were treated for sixteen to twenty sessions with cognitive behavioral and brief psychodynamic therapies. The therapists were doctoral-level psychologists with one year of specialized training in each of the three modalities, eight therapists trained by the therapists who had developed the therapies, and two carefully supervised by authorities in each of the therapies. The three therapies were equally effective (Thompson et al. 1987).

Another important study is the $3.4 million, carefully designed National Institute of Mental Health (NIMH) study comparing 239 mildly to moderately depressed patients, some of whom were treated by trained therapists for four months with weekly cognitive or interpersonal psychotherapy, whereas others were treated with the antidepressant drug imipramine plus clinical management for twenty to thirty minutes; and a placebo group was treated with clinical management for twenty to thirty minutes plus supportive discussions (Elkin et al.

1989). Improvement was similar, not significantly different, for all four groups. It appears that all treatments in which the patients were engaged led to a substantial relief of symptoms, particularly among the less severely ill. There was a modest gradient of efficiency across the several outcome measures and across the four treatments. Imipramine did the best, the two psychotherapies were intermediate in efficiency, and placebo did the worst.[20]

The specificity of cognitive behavioral treatment for panic disorder was compared with a control treatment that used a focused nonprescriptive treatment for panic. Cognitive behavioral treatment included prescribed techniques targeting each component of the panic reaction (e.g., breath retraining, progressive muscle relaxation). The contrasting treatment focused attention on frightening symptoms, life problems, and stress (Shear et al. 1994). Forty-five patients were treated for fifteen weekly sessions by psychotherapists who had two years' experience using cognitive behavioral treatment and were supervised by a more experienced cognitive behavioral therapist, and sessions were rated for adherence to the two treatments. Post-treatment and six-month follow-up evaluations revealed a high rate of panic remission and equally significant improvement in both treatment groups.

20. Several *post hoc,* retrospective, or subgroup analyses were performed on the data of this study. Some, but not all, clearly stated that the analysis is *post hoc* and is useful primarily to generate hypotheses for another hypothesis-oriented study.

A frequently reported and discussed retrospective analysis is that, although the treatments (including placebo) were equally effective for milder depressions, imipramine was the best treatment for moderate depression, resulting in about 70 percent recovery, compared to 40 to 50 percent for the two psychotherapies and 10 to 20 percent for placebo.

In our opinion, the placebo condition was a nonmatching, nonidentical, and inadequate control (Shapiro 1984; Parloff 1986). It is possible that if the placebo treatment had been more adequately matched in terms of providing equal amounts of time during sessions and had included a popular alternative-type therapy, such as pleasant college professors or loquacious and personable actors, with enthusiasm and faith in the treatment by both patient and healer, there would have been no difference between the placebo treatment and the two psychotherapies, even for patients with moderate depression. It is even possible, since improvement was similar for drug and psychotherapeutic treatment for patients with mild depression, that drug treatment would have been better than the psychotherapies if the amount of time per session and nonspecific conditions in the imipramine group had been the same as in the two psychotherapeutic groups or if drug treatment sessions had included a credible-appearing pseudotherapy.

Another *post hoc* analysis of data from this study evaluated whether there were differential effects of the therapies which could have been obscured by general outcome measures. Differential effects, also referred to as mode-specific effects, were not detected for the different therapies (Imber et al. 1990). It was also reported that the severity of depression and the duration of treatment were not significantly different for the two psychotherapies (Shapiro et al. 1994).

The literature indicates an increase in the number of controlled psychotherapy studies that compare different treatments by psychotherapists who are committed to different theoretical orientations. Although these studies have a more limited psychotherapeutic scope and include therapies of shorter duration, behavioral techniques for specific symptoms, and the use of therapists with varying amounts of training and experience, they illustrate the usefulness of contrasting therapies with each other. Most of the studies report little or no difference in the efficacy of the compared therapies.[21]

Many of the small, discrete, controlled studies of behavior therapy and popular lay therapies that pit therapies, or components within therapies, against each other are innovative, creative, and carefully supervised dissertations, and may contribute procedures and techniques that can be used in larger clinical studies. The accumulated results could help differentiate effective from ineffective therapy.[22]

21. Several such studies have come to our attention:

In one of these, the results of cognitive-behavioral therapy and of psychodynamic psychotherapy for 117 depressed patients treated for eight sessions by five clinicians were not significantly different (Shapiro et al. 1994).

In another study, parents of children with conduct problems were treated with discussion with a group of therapists and videotape modeling treatment, individual self-administered videotape modeling treatment, and group discussion treatment without videotape modeling. At post-treatment and at evaluation after one year, there were no significant differences among treatments (Webster-Stratton et al. 1989).

In a third study, fifty-nine depressed religious patients were treated either with cognitive-behavioral therapy with religious content (therapists with religious interests), with cognitive-behavioral therapy without religious content, or with pastoral counseling for eighteen to twenty one-hour sessions over three months. The results of cognitive-behavioral therapy with religious content and of pastoral counseling were significantly better post-treatment but not at three-month and two-year evaluations (Propst et al. 1992).

In a fourth study, thirty children were randomly assigned to treatment with time-limited, time-unlimited, and a minimal-contact control group to evaluate family functioning in children and their parents. The minimal-contact situation resulted in significantly more improvement at post-testing and after four years (Smyrnios and Kirkby 1993).

And finally, cognitive-behavioral intervention for panic disorder administered as bibliotherapy alone produced results that at post-test, three-month, and six-month evaluations did not significantly differ from those of cognitive-behavioral intervention administered as group therapy, although both groups of patients had better results than the waiting-list control group (Lidren et al. 1994).

22. In one study, progressive relaxation/meditation and a quasi-desensitization placebo control equally reduced moderate and severe insomnia, but only when the credibility of the placebo control was increased (Steinmark and Borkovec 1974; Borkovec, Kaloupek, and Slama 1975; Carr-Kaffashan and Woolfolk 1979).

"Box Score" Studies

By 1975 the number of published psychotherapy studies enabled comparisons among some psychotherapies. Lester Luborsky and colleagues (1975) selected ninety-one studies fulfilling minimal criteria for adequate controlled comparisons and graded the studies for methodological adequacy. Therapeutic effects were categorized in "box score" comparisons of therapy pairs as better, the same, or worse. Results were reported for traditional psychotherapy versus client-centered therapy, traditional psychotherapy versus behavior therapy, individual versus group therapy, and time-limited versus time-unlimited therapy. The authors concluded that "everybody has won and all must have prizes," meaning that psychotherapies were not significantly different from each other with regard to effectiveness. Of further interest, drug therapy was superior to psychotherapy, and psychotherapy with drug therapy was better than psychotherapy alone. The results and conclusions were striking, especially because the senior author was a respected and long-term psychotherapy researcher, a committed psychotherapist, and a psychoanalyst.

Box score studies have been extensively and critically discussed in the literature, especially the Luborsky 1975 study. The report, in our opinion, is excessively defensive about various therapeutic orientations (APA Commission on Psychotherapies 1982).[23] One limitation of box score studies is the neglect of interactions among variables and outcome. One list contained seventy-two pa-

---

In another, patients who received either progressive relaxation, stimulus control, or paradoxical intention administered by one therapist showed equal improvement in sleep difficulties and significantly more improvement than waiting-list and placebo control groups (Turner and Ascher 1979).

For anxiety reduction in students, no differences among treatments were reported for Zen meditation and two control groups, antimeditation and no-treatment, in seventy-two subjects (Goldman et al. 1979); and for mantra meditation, antimeditation control, progressive relaxation control, and no-treatment control in eighty undergraduate students (Boswell and Murray 1979).

For student speech anxiety, no differences among treatments were reported for heart rate biofeedback, false feedback, and systematic desensitization (Gatchel et al. 1979), and for manual self-treatment with systematic desensitization, desensitization with meditation replacing progressive relaxation, and meditation alone (Kirsch and Henry 1979).

23. Although the commission report is comprehensive, detailed, and thoughtful, it has, in our opinion, a tendency to find psychotherapy effective, possibly influenced by the fact that nine of the twenty-one members were psychoanalysts. Moreover, although many of the nonspecific and other variables influencing clinical treatment and the evaluation of efficacy are discussed, there is no mention of the placebo effect or of the possibility of psychotherapy being a placebo.

tient, therapist, and therapy variables, which would require about five hundred thousand potential combinations for study (Beutler 1991). With the recognition of the difficulty of demonstrating differences among therapies and the development of more sophisticated methodology in general, studies of psychotherapy became more focused and better controlled methodologically.

Meta-analytic Comparisons

Meta-analysis is a sophisticated statistical methodology that can parsimoniously summarize the results of many studies. Although complicated to use, it has been heralded as the *sine qua non* for future analyses of cumulative—especially clinical—studies (Schmidt 1992; Nowak 1994). With more than six hundred studies of psychotherapy having some sort of control, and with the proliferation of published comparisons among therapies (especially studies by psychologists), meta-analyses are flooding the literature.

The first meta-analysis, by Mary Lee Smith and colleagues (1977), which was updated in 1980, is the most frequently cited meta-analysis of psychotherapy. The study comprised 1,766 outcome comparisons from 475 outcome studies of psychotherapy that used some form of a placebo, waiting-list, or other control; the studies involved twenty-five thousand patients who were treated with seventy-eight different forms of psychotherapy (Smith et al. 1980). Although psychotherapy was found to be superior to placebo, the authors "did not expect that the demonstrable benefits of quite different types of psychotherapy would be so little different," noting that it is the "most startling and intriguing finding" (185). They concluded that different schools of therapies do not produce different types or degrees of benefit. Nonspecific elements that unite different psychotherapies appear to be more important than the specific elements that distinguish them. Counting for little are the methods of psychotherapy, the setting (individual or group), the duration of therapy, the training and experience of therapists, and the types of clients and their problems; and the benefits are often not permanent.

Some of the limitations of the sample, discussed extensively in the literature, are that over 60 percent of the subjects were solicited or were volunteers, about 50 percent of the studies were behavioral studies and about 13 percent were psychodynamic studies, the therapists were largely psychology graduate students or psychiatric residents, and 3 percent of subjects were depressed. The studies were not evaluated for scientific rigor, were of uneven quality, and were usually of brief duration; the diagnoses were diverse, the outcome measures variable, and the sample sizes small; and studies with very few subjects were given equal weight to studies with many subjects.

Other meta-analyses, many reanalyzing selected subsets of the Smith et al. sample, came to conclusions similar to those of the Smith et al. (1980) study—namely, that psychotherapy as a whole, which includes an incredible number of different types of therapy, most of them not typically referred to as psychotherapy, is more effective than nontreatments with which it is compared.[24]

Some of the studies in the Smith et al. (1980) meta-analysis are of brief duration; include student, volunteer, and nonclinical subjects (such as students with questionable clinical symptoms of snake phobia); include no-treatment, waiting-list, and placebo controls without adequate credibility; and use poor methodology. Most are well-done analogue studies, dissertations, and behavioral and other studies on psychological or psychotherapeutic minutiae. Meta-analyses evaluating the effectiveness of psychotherapy exemplify the problem of GIGO (garbage in, garbage out). These and many other limitations of meta-analyses, as well as methods of improving meta-analyses, and the promise of their utility as a method of reviewing accumulated research have been discussed extensively in the literature (*Behavioral and Brain Sciences* 1983).

Even Smith and colleagues' conclusion that psychotherapy is more effective than controls has been criticized as a sampling and methodological artifact. When a reanalysis of the Smith et al. study included only real patients (psychiatric inpatients and outpatients) and excluded subjects solicited to participate in a research study and subjects who were treated in studies comparing psychotherapy with placebo treatment, the effect size for the thirty-two studies that met these criteria was similar for patients treated with placebo and those treated with psychotherapy (Prioleau et al. 1983). (The effect size is a statistical measure of the magnitude of the difference between the experimental and the control group in controlled clinical trials.)

Thirty-six discussants responded to the Prioleau et al. 1983 paper (*Behavioral and Brain Sciences* 1983). The papers by the discussants reflect current controversies about how to study psychotherapy, about the need for controls (including placebo controls), and about types of controls. Also included were personal opinions about the use of meta-analysis and about whether psychotherapy is effec-

24. From a reanalysis of a subset of the Smith et al. sample, which included randomization to treatment or a no-treatment or placebo control, Landman and Dawes (1982) concluded that psychotherapy is effective. A reanalysis of Smith et al. data that included a subsample of "real patients" who sought treatment compared to diverse controls also concluded that psychotherapy was effective (Andrews and Harvey 1981). A more recent meta-analysis of 290 studies similarly concluded that psychotherapy was effective, with published studies being reported as more effective than unpublished studies (Lipsey and Wilson 1993).

tive, is more effective than placebo, or is itself a placebo. The discussions were prepossessing and dramatic, and were so engaging and compelling that the reader tended to agree with the last paper read. Interestingly, one-third of the discussants believed that the effectiveness of psychotherapy was supported by the meta-analysis of Smith et al. and one-third that psychotherapy was ineffective or placebo, while the remainder were noncommittal. It was obvious that the writers held on to their original beliefs. In fact, as is apparent throughout the history of psychotherapy during the past century, opinions and beliefs appear to be minimally influenced by studies, research, data, and logic.

A meta-analysis concluded that brief dynamic therapy was more effective than placement on a waiting list, slightly superior to nonpsychiatric treatment (various types of active placebo control, such as self-help groups, clinical management, drug counseling, low-contact treatment), and about equal to other psychotherapies and medication: that is, the various psychotherapies did not differ in effectiveness (Crits-Christoph 1992).

In a meta-analysis comparing Albert Ellis's rational-emotive therapy (RET) with other therapies (on the basis of twenty-eight studies), RET was found to be superior to placebo and no treatment but equally as effective as variants such as RET bibliotherapy, RET classroom education, RET role-playing exercises with or without homework, rational role reversal with or without rational-emotive imagery, and RET combined with systematic desensitization, client-centered behavior therapy, eclectic dynamic therapy, vocational training, and psychodynamic therapy. As expected, meta-analysis showed RET to be more effective than placebo and no treatment but equally effective in comparison with other types of treatment such as combination therapies and systematic desensitization (Engels et al. 1993).

A meta-analysis of 163 randomized trials compared the outcomes of therapy provided by practitioners of different therapeutic orientations; the types of therapy included family and marital psychotherapies and individual therapies. The analyses were complicated. The essence of the results was that marital and family therapies were mildly positive compared to controls but were not significantly different from each other, nor did they show significant differences when compared with individual therapies, and orientations within therapies were not different from each other, except that humanistic therapies were less effective (Shadish et al. 1993).

A meta-analysis of 143 outcome studies in which two or more treatment groups were compared with a control group led to the conclusion that active treatments were superior to minimal placebo treatments, and that the effects of different treatment methods were not impressively different from each other except that the results of behavioral and cognitive methods were modest whereas the results for dynamic and humanistic treatments were poor (D. A. Shapiro and D. Shapiro 1982). The limitations of meta-analyses cited by D. A. Shapiro and D. Shapiro (1982) include a predominance of behavioral (analogue) treatment, the analyzed studies' use of recruited student volunteers and few clinically referred patients, and the use of the results from dissertations, from published studies (which are more likely to report positive rather than negative findings), and from meta-analytic studies that are unrepresentative of clinical practice situations (thus limiting their generalizability to everyday practice).

A review of four meta-analyses of more than twelve thousand subjects who participated in more than two hundred controlled studies concluded that, overall, children and adolescents benefited from treatment. However, benefit was associated more with the treatment of recruited subjects for focal problems by specially trained therapists with small caseloads, as well as with other features not representative of typical clinical treatment. Clinical studies of referred patients treated in clinics for more general psychopathology did not show significant therapeutic effects (Weisz et al. 1992). Alan E. Kazdin's (1991) review of meta-analytic studies of child and adolescent treatment also concluded that individual treatment techniques have not been found to differ from each other.

This review of meta-analytic studies demonstrates that many psychotherapies are clearly better than no treatment or a variety of different controls. Meta-analysis is an important new analytic method for assessing the results of research but has been criticized for including questionable data (Eysenck 1994, 1995).

Problems in the Evaluation of the Psychotherapies

Psychotherapy manuals or guides intended to ensure treatment integrity within different types of therapies have proliferated in psychotherapy research (Sifneos 1972; Mann 1973; Horowitz 1976; Beck et al. 1979; Davanloo 1980; Luborsky 1984; Klerman et al. 1984; Strupp and Binder 1982; Fawcett et al. 1987). Various factors stimulated this attempt to standardize psychotherapy provided by psychotherapists. It has long been known that published theoretical descriptions of therapies are usually not accurate depictions of how psychotherapists behave in their clinical treatment of patients (Glover 1955; Klein et al. 1969; Lieberman et al. 1973; Luborsky and Spence 1978). Clinical treatment by practitioners and theories about treatment evolve over time, deviating from the original descriptions of new therapies (Parloff 1986). Acknowledgment of these changes is especially apparent in classical Freudian theory and treatment, which in classical texts is usually assumed to be immutable (Grünbaum 1986). The use of various nonspecific therapeutic techniques and procedures, and the behavior of therapists, unwittingly may outweigh the presumed specific principles of a particular therapy. These and other problems may prevent adequate evaluation of different therapies. Another factor is the popularity of standardized forms and manuals for interviewing, collecting data, and evaluating results, which have contributed to the attempt to standardize studies of psychotherapy. In addition, it has become increasingly difficult, if not impossible, to obtain approval and funding for a psychotherapy study without the inclusion of therapy manuals.

While the use of standardized psychotherapeutic manuals is praiseworthy, to an unknown extent they deprive psychotherapists of their spontaneity, sensitivity, flexibility, warmth, genuineness, empathy, ability to resourcefully respond to unpredictable and idiosyncratic situations, and adequate motivation for effective psychotherapy—factors also applicable to the use of noncredible placebos (Parloff 1986). Psychotherapists may feel like dull-witted clods, dispensing fortune-cookie advice, maxims, and predictions. It is possible that manual-based therapies would be so stereotyped, dull, and platitudinous that therapeutic factors would be similar for all of the therapies and lead to nonsignificant differences among them.

A relevant study would be to evaluate the equivalence of manual-based therapies by comparing the similarities, differences, and effectiveness of psychotherapy done by two groups of therapists with similar experience and orientations (e.g., cognitive-behavioral), one group trained in and committed to manual-based psychotherapy, the other to clinical treatment. If two different manual-based therapies are used, it is necessary to clearly define the treatment intervention and to identify actual differences between the treatments in the therapy sessions. It is curious that such studies were not done before therapists plunged into the extensive use of manual-based therapies.

Paradoxically, the embrace and extensive use of fortune-cookie-type therapy by major psychotherapy researchers and governmental granting agencies lends support to the concept of psychotherapy as placebo. Moreover, what if studies of manual-based and clinical therapy were to result in equivalent therapeutic effects? Would this mean that simple, manual-based training (not requiring advanced medical and psychological degrees) should replace years of intensive and expensive clinical training? Would psychotherapy then be reimbursed by insurance at current levels? Would such results provide further support for the concept of psychotherapy as placebo?

With some creative imagination and sufficient motivation, more relevant, suitable, credible, and ethical placebo therapies should not be difficult to construct. These might include some of the fashionable therapies that frequently erupt onto the therapeutic landscape—therapies provided by loquacious, persuasive, and popular television advice givers and passionate faith healers, as well as Christian Science healing, laying on of hands, meditation, primal scream therapy, orgone therapy, Rolfing, Dianetics, and other holistic and alternative treatments described previously. The only problem is, are we willing to take the chance?

The limitations of controlled studies are discussed extensively in the literature (APA Commission on Psychotherapies 1982), which includes the criticism that most of the studies were short-term and that there were no comparative studies of the more open-ended or long-term psychotherapy usually believed to be therapeutically necessary by dynamic psychotherapists. However, on the basis of the previously reviewed studies, almost all psychotherapy researchers, including researchers with psychoanalytic, psychodynamic, and other theoretical and clinical psychotherapeutic orientations, have concluded that nonspecific factors clearly outweigh potential specific factors, that not all of the specific factors have been identified, and that the specific effectiveness of psychotherapy has not been supported by controlled studies.[25] The onus, therefore, is now on those upholding the alternative hypothesis that a particular method of psychotherapy is specifically effective and not a psychological theriac or placebo. In response to this challenge, recent studies have improved methodologically.

Recent Studies of Psychotherapy

The number of methodologically improved studies of psychotherapy has increased dramatically over the past decade.[26] The reasons include the general de-

25. For example, see the support for this conclusion among major psychoanalytically oriented psychotherapeutic researchers, such as Luborsky et al. (1975); Parloff (1986); Strupp (1994). See also Grünbaum 1986.

Relevant to the general topic of whether psychotherapy is effective is an article published in *Consumer Reports* (Anonymous 1995) giving the results of a readers' survey using a self-report questionnaire methodology. *Consumer Reports* sent to 184,000 randomly selected subscribers questionnaires that included questions about their experience with mental health services. The results showed that the people surveyed were generally favorable about their psychotherapeutic treatment, and their responses were unrelated to the type of treatment or addition of medication. The sample of people contacted in such surveys, however, has been criticized for being unrepresentative of the general U.S. population or the typical psychotherapy patient. In addition, self-report surveys, it has been said, "are no substitute for controlled clinical trials when it comes to drawing causal inferences" (Hollon 1996, 1025). Although the *Consumer Reports* report was generally favorable toward psychotherapy, it still leaves us with the troublesome question, is psychotherapy effective?

26. This increase in the literature on psychotherapy has been paralleled by an increase in medical, scientific, and psychological publications generally (175,000 papers each day in

velopment of and emphasis on sophisticated research methodology in medicine, psychiatry, and psychology (the research being required for grant support), and the availability of computers that efficiently manage many routine tasks and more readily permit sophisticated statistical analysis. Studies include more hypotheses or predictive designs, improved diagnostic criteria for patient samples, larger sample sizes, more carefully defined methods of psychotherapy, better descriptions of methods and procedures, more reliable and valid independent and dependent measures and scales, more attention to appropriate control samples, more sophisticated statistical planning and analysis of results, improved methods of summarizing the results of many studies (i.e., meta-analysis), and better research design in general. There is some evidence to suggest that patients in various diagnostic groups, with different symptoms and levels of severity, may respond better to one type of psychotherapy (used alone, or in combination with drugs) than to another, or to drugs alone. Many more studies are focusing on meaningful factors such as patients' therapy preference, their goals, their expectations (faith, hope, motivation, etc.) about therapy, and important aspects of the relationship between patient and therapist (mutual background, respect, interest, liking, warmth, attractiveness). These factors auger well for the quality and the meaningfulness of future research on psychotherapy.

However, major methodological problems plague studies of psychotherapy. These studies are much more expensive, take much longer to do, and are more difficult to design and conduct than are drug studies. Only a few of the methodological problems will be noted here.

First, the diagnostic criteria in the *Diagnostic and Statistical Manual of Mental Disorders–IV* (DSM-IV) are problematic, inexorably destined to expand and contract every five years with the appearance of data from isolated and unsystematic research; as a result, comparing studies becomes difficult. A similar problem occurs with changes in interview schedules and scales.

Second, and even more important, is researchers' failure to adhere to several fundamental principles of research. The most important of these principles is that one must clearly state the specific hypotheses to be tested, the specific independent and dependent variables that will be used to confirm or reject hy-

---

1994 in the medical literature alone), making it impossible to do a complete review. There are now hundreds of papers published in dozens of publications, including specialized psychotherapy journals, handbooks, edited books, published symposia, and individually authored books. The reader is referred to the many references that are readily available. In this section, we restrict our attention to features that are related to the study of psychotherapy as placebo.

potheses, and the statistical procedures that will be used in analyses. These features of a study should be clearly described in published papers, any deviations from the design detailed, and all retrospective analyses, including appropriate adjustments for multiple statistical analyses, clearly specified. Many published studies do not include such deviations from the design. In fact, most studies tend to report or highlight a few significant relationships (out of dozens that happen to be significant), usually those that support the author's bias. This is known as "milking the data," and as in the process of milking a cow, there is always a little more—but not very good—milk that comes with the last squeeze of the udder. Data milking, or retrospective analysis, an irresistible indulgence for researchers, usually yields unreplicable findings and is useful only for generating hypotheses for future study.

Does Psychotherapy Help?

Most, if not all, researchers have concluded that psychotherapy has beneficial therapeutic effects. By comparison with previous therapies having psychological effects, say these researchers, current psychotherapies are less mystical and more firmly anchored to current psychological and neurological principles and explanations about the cause and treatment of disease. However, though today's theories and treatment may be more rational and may conform to what is known today, the theories and treatment of yesteryear also were founded on the best scientific principles of their time.

History is filled with testimonials about the usefulness of psychological ministration in many forms—whether magical, mystical, religious, metaphysical, fraudulent, medical, or psychological—as long as it is credible as a therapy to the supplicants. Cures are testified to by Galen in the first century; by Maimonides, writing in the twelfth century about the use of senseless remedies; by Paracelsus, writing in the fifteenth century about miracles produced by real or false faith in saints or their images; and by Pietro Pomponazzi, writing in the sixteenth century about marvelous cures resulting from confidence and imagination about real or unreal religious relics (saintly bones). Other claims included those attributing impressive powers to Valentine Greatrakes, in the seventeenth century; those made by Benjamin Franklin, in the eighteenth century, about "Franklinism" (static electricity and electric shock treatment); those of Armand Trousseau, in the nineteenth century, about using the new drugs while they work; and those recounting cures at Lourdes, and cures produced by faith in gods and saints, by pills, and by hypnosis. Added to these testimonials is the extensive history of healing by hundreds of thousands of witch doctors, herbalists, and religious, quack, faith, psychic, and other unorthodox healers, as well as by physicians who administered untold number of placebos to billions of sufferers throughout history.

Healing superstitions and fads may be even more extensive than is described here. Most are lost in medical history, but in light of the deluge of patent medicines and other cures that are advertised, it is easy to see that their numbers keep increasing. Television and other media first advertise the new cures and later expose them as fraudulent or ineffective treatments. Quackery and faith healing continue to grow despite better education and scientific advances, and scholars despair that they will ever be eradicated (Young 1992; Hilts 1995).

Whereas some of the apparently positive results of these treatments are due to nonspecific effects such as the natural course, spontaneous remission, and waxing and waning of most symptoms and disorders; the occasional treatment of "disorders" that do not exist; and lying, deception, and skullduggery, most scholars acknowledge that potent therapeutic factors exist within all healing methods. These factors are commonly referred to as the placebo effect because their cause is not yet known. It remains to be determined whether psychotherapy is merely another example in the long history of the placebo effect. We believe, as do many others, that the question of whether psychotherapy is an effective, nonplacebo therapy can be answered only by pragmatic controlled studies. Much more will have to be done to demonstrate its therapeutic power and effectiveness.

Future Psychotherapies

What scenarios can be posed for the future of psychotherapy? One possibility is that future research will provide evidence that certain psychotherapeutic procedures are effective for specific symptoms or disorders. With more than 250 different types of psychotherapy and hundreds of DSM-IV diagnoses, it may be necessary to establish a new governmental agency, a "Food, Drug, and Psychotherapy Administration," to evaluate the evidence regarding the effectiveness and possible adverse effects of various psychotherapies, and to publish a *Psychotherapist's Desk Reference* to fully describe the therapies' ingredients, effects on the body and brain, cautions, contraindications, and adverse effects.

A second possible scenario is the development of computerized models of brain function similar to those already being developed by neuroscientists, identifying the normal number and type of neurons and axons in different areas of the brain; normal types and concentrations of neurotransmitters, enzymes, and other substances; and appropriate neurophysiological relationships. With non-invasive imaging techniques, psychopathology could be detected; and it might be possible to correct it by increasing inadequate brain areas, decreasing excessive areas, extirpating totally abnormal brain tissue, transplanting normal healthy brain tissue, or performing other neurochemicophysiological modifications of abnormally functioning brains.

A final possibility is that, despite extensive study, the efficacy of psychotherapy will not be supported. Psychological treatments would then continue their wobbling course, new methods continually easing out older ones, shaped by an evolving culture and zeitgeist.

The factors that characterize psychotherapy—repackaging, myriad schools, the use of one therapy for many disorders, the use of many therapies for one disorder, the predominance of nonspecific effects, and the absence of proof of specific effectiveness—suggest that psychotherapy, like theriac, is

> a general cure-all that could be used in every possible case because there had been put into it by the hundred all the active agents that were known. The patient was made to swallow it all in the hope that the disease, whatever it might be, could find in this mixture what it demanded. The therapeutic methods that I have just described seem to me identical with a sort of psychological theriac, that calls forth indiscriminately all the psychic phenomena, that appeals to all the mental operations in every patient whoever he may be, in the hope that each of them will be able to find what he needs in this mixture. This happens occasionally and psychological theriacs have certainly had some successes. But one should not be surprised if they do not always succeed, or that such treatments are considered as lotteries by official science. (Janet 1925, 122–23)

chapter six

The History of Clinical Trials

Three important developments ultimately decreased the power of the placebo effect. The first was the discovery of the scientific method, and the second was the advent of clinical trials. The third, and most important, was the advent of *controlled* clinical trials using placebo controls and the double-blind method to evaluate therapeutics. Formal experimental methods did not exist before the nineteenth century, and the few fledgling experiments that were done had little systematic impact on medical practice. Without methodological safeguards, treatment was determined by elaborate theories, mysticism, superstition, and tradition. In this chapter, we discuss the development of clinical trials;[1] in chapter 7 we discuss the use of placebo controls and the development and use of the double-blind method.

The Ancient and Medieval Periods

There is no evidence of the use of clinical trials in ancient medicine. Despite the belief that medical practice in ancient Egypt was tremendously advanced, the situation was in reality one of confusion and chaos. "Once and for all beware: next to nothing is known about the effectiveness of ancient drugs; and even when the drug itself is known, experimental studies are almost nil" (Majno 1975, 108). Likewise, there is no evidence that the ancient Assyrians or Babylonians conducted clinical trials (Jayne 1962).

Although the disciples of Asclepius relied on the innate properties of healing, which were clearly less harmful than the elaborate pharmacopoeias of other ancient civilizations, Greek medicine was "a failure as a science" (Majno 1975, 178). Galen, the most famous Greco-Roman physician, wrote twenty-two volumes, of which two-thirds still exist. Because he was held in profound reverence by his colleagues, medicine did not advance under his tutelage beyond Hippo-

---

1. Our history of controlled clinical trials relies on Bull (1959, 1970) and the references cited in the text.

cratic medicine. No attempt was made to test the efficacy of his materia medica. His reliance on pure theory to explain everything was responsible, according to Fielding Garrison (1929), for the failure of medicine to advance for nearly fourteen centuries after his death. Despite this, Galen's statement that "he cures
most in whom the people have the most confidence" reveals an awareness of the
placebo effect.

Ambroise Paré conducted one of the first clinical experiments. He applied
onions to one-half of the face of a German guard who had been burned, and
applied medicines commonly in use to the other half. He reported that the side
treated with onions was free of blisters and excoriation, whereas the other side
was troubled with both (Anonymous 1960a). In another instance, more by
serendipity than by true experimentation, he found the use of salve to be more
effective than the use of burning oil to treat gunshot wounds. Unlike other
physicians of the time, he readily discarded ineffective remedies and was critical
of remedies that were highly esteemed by others. Thus, he criticized the use of
Egyptian mummy and unicorn horn as therapeutic agents despite their widespread use by physicians. He demonstrated that bezoar stone was ineffective
against poison by giving mercuric chloride, and immediately afterward bezoar
stone, to a palace cook condemned to death, who then died in agony. These
studies are early examples of clinical trials involving the use of a control in the
treatment of a single patient.

Such critical thinking was uncommon. Superstition, herb doctoring, and
quackery were the rule in medical treatment, and physicians were content to rely
on astrology to determine when to perform bloodletting or when to purge.

The Seventeenth Century

The growth of the scientific method in physics, chemistry, and biology in the
seventeenth century was not reflected generally in medicine. Most medical ideas
were speculative and most medical hypotheses were untested, and physicians
continued to rely on a priori reasoning (Bull 1959). Some challenged established
practices, calling for "experimental" methods to evaluate treatment. One skep-
tic was Robert Boyle, who suggested that naturalists could be of use by testing
whether advocated cures had any medicinal virtue. Sir Kenneth Digby proposed
using the experimental method in his discourse on the "powder of sympathy."
Although unaware that he was proposing an experiment using the single-blind
method on a single patient, he was, in fact, doing just that. Digby is described as
a Renaissance man—versatile, intellectual, practical, and critical (King 1966).

His explanation of how sympathetic powder could heal wounds was based on a complex and reasoned rationale and reliance on the scientific theories of the day, rather than on mysticism. A shift in the basis for demonstrating the effectiveness of treatment is seen in Digby's report of a man with a potentially gangrenous sword wound of the hand who was treated with sympathetic powder. Unknown to the patient, blood from the wound which had dried on a garter was dipped into a vitriol solution, and the patient suddenly felt better. Digby later removed the garter from the solution, and the patient again felt pain. After the garter was returned to the solution, the pain disappeared, and the patient recovered five or six days later. Changes in the patient's pain were explained by reference to current concepts about sympathetic powder.

The Eighteenth Century

Experimentation was still a rarity in the eighteenth century. The meticulous observation of patients by physicians—seen in William Withering's work on the specific use of foxglove (digitalis) for heart disease and Thomas Sydenham's advocacy of cinchona bark for fevers of malarial origin—contributed to greater understanding of the nature of disease and the need to differentiate symptoms from disorders but did little to advance experimental methods.

Here and there, rudimentary experiments were undertaken. C. Maitland inoculated six Newgate convicts against smallpox, and all of them survived. The results were later criticized because a prior history of smallpox could not be ruled out (Bull 1959). Joseph Lister's experiments, at the end of the century, provided a more adequate demonstration of the value of inoculation against smallpox.

Reference was made in chapter 3 to an innovative experiment proposed by Bishop Berkeley to demonstrate the effectiveness of his tar-water treatment. He suggested comparing tar-water to a standard treatment of the time, keeping other factors constant. If this comparison had been carried out, it would have been one of the first comparative experiments.

James Lind, a Scottish physician to the Royal Naval Hospital, noted that scurvy was ravaging the naval fleet. Lind's study of scurvy in 1747 was the first controlled nonblind investigation of a clinical treatment. During a ten-week voyage, Lind reported 350 cases of scurvy and proposed a comparative trial of several different cures. Two men were given a quart of cider a day, two were given an elixir of vitriol, two were given oranges and lemons, and two were given an electuary (a medicine that melts in the mouth) (Lind 1753). Although Lind reported that the addition of citrus fruits was the most effective remedy for scurvy, he failed to accept his own findings and recommended instead fresh air and a changed diet. Perhaps the weight of tradition proved too strong and influenced his judgment.

Withering used foxglove to treat heart disease and was instrumental in approximating the correct dosage of the drug. He made elementary comparisons of the patient's condition before and after treatment, as well as charting the rate of relapse when treatment was discontinued. John Bull (1959) regarded Withering's use of the historical technique (comparing treatments over time) as appropriate for such a problem. He clarified which patients would benefit from digitalis and criticized fellow physicians for their massive abuse of that drug.

Other studies included experiments with vaccination. Edward Jenner published the results of a trial of smallpox vaccination in twenty-three individuals in 1798 (Garrison 1929). Although an important advance in the use of inoculation, the design was flawed and the trial inconclusive. The results related only to artificial inoculation and not to the naturally occurring disease. In 1800 an American physician, Benjamin Waterhouse, was the first to demonstrate the value of inoculation in preventing smallpox by vaccinating nineteen boys, twelve of whom were subsequently inoculated with smallpox, and inoculating two boys with smallpox who had not been previously vaccinated. The two boys who had not been vaccinated developed the disease.

Belief in folk medicine and methods nevertheless continued to dominate medical practice, with one belief replacing another. Methods such as electricity, Mesmerism, and tractors, although adopted by many mystics, were reviewed skeptically by others, who believed them to be charlatanism and quackery and urged that they be subjected to experimental review. The report of the Royal Academy of Medicine in Paris, which subjected magnetism to experimentation, found these methods to be of no use (DuBois 1837).

Other experiments, including those of Benjamin Franklin, used static electricity. Franklin described his electric shock treatment for paralyzed patients in a letter to John Pringle, president of the Royal Society in 1757 (Franklin 1757). Franklin placed the patient on an electric stool and sent shocks through the affected limb or limbs, repeating the procedure three times each day. The treatment did not result in permanent cure of the palsies, leading Franklin to comment that the spirits of the patients were improved "by the hope of success enabling them to exert more strength in moving their limbs" (Franklin 1757, 347).

Particularly noteworthy for the time is the experimental design that John Haygarth used to evaluate the usefulness of metallic rods ("tractors") advocated by Elisha Perkins. The stroking of afflicted parts of the body with metallic rods of dissimilar alloys was used to relieve numerous painful ailments (Quen 1963).

Perkins, a well-trained physician (a rarity at that time), aroused controversy, as did his treatment. Haygarth, skeptical about the effectiveness of Perkins's tractors, designed one of the earliest, and possibly the first, placebo-controlled single-blind studies. Wooden tractors shaped and painted to resemble the metallic ones used by Perkins were applied to five patients with rheumatism. One day Haygarth would use the wooden tractors, the next the metallic. Only he knew which tractors were being used; the patient was blind to the choice. The results were the same with both. The curative factors, he believed, were the patient's and physician's imagination and faith. The physician's fame, he believed, was an additional factor that contributed to the patient's faith: that is, the more important the physician, the more likely it was that the treatment would be effective (Haygarth 1801). Haygarth's experiment was an early example of the use of the experimental method, although it had little effect on medical practice at the time.

The Nineteenth Century

The Prayer-Gauge Debate (Means 1876) and "The Prayer Test" (Brush 1974) dramatically illustrate the growing controversy between proponents of authority and those advocating scientific experiment. Although the prayer test debate was about whether religious prayer worked (does God answer prayers?) and how the efficacy of prayer could be tested (by reliance on the authority of the Bible, or by experiment?), the issue is strikingly similar to the authority-versus-experiment controversy in medicine. The debate erupted in July 1872, when "The Prayer for the Sick: Hints towards a Serious Attempt to Estimate Its Value" was published in the *London Contemporary Review*. "Prof. John Tyndall [its author] fathered it with an Introduction, while disavowing authorship." He recommended testing the effectiveness of prayer in the same way that a proposed remedy for a disease or a scientific theory is tested. He proposed that a hospital treating a disease with known mortality rates "be made . . . the object of special prayer by the whole body of the faithful . . . for not less than three to five years" (Brush 1974, 561). Proof of the power of prayer would be obtained by comparing the mortality rate for the prayed-for patients to that of a control group suffering from the same disease in other hospitals during the same period of time, for whom prayer had not been offered.

Rejoinders flooded the *London Contemporary Review,* the *Fortnightly Review,* the *Spectator,* and the great newspapers of London for many months thereafter. Francis Galton, a cousin of Darwin, responded to the controversy one month later. He had collected data for several years about the effect of prayer and presented tables indicating that royalty, usually the object of public prayers, die earlier than lawyers, gentry, and military officers, that clerics, a prayerful class, do not live longer than lawyers and physicians, that missionaries tend to die at a younger age, and that the numbers of stillbirths in praying and nonpraying groups were identical. The believers in prayer contemptuously questioned the motives, integrity, logic, and intelligence of the nonbelievers. The test was criticized for suggesting the use of a control group of patients for whom one does not deliberately pray, compared to a group of sick patients prayed for, in order to evaluate the worth of prayers; and for showing a misunderstanding of the purpose of prayer. Praying for one group and not for the control group was considered unethical. Intuition was thought to be more cogent than observation and statistically based conclusions. The reliance on and belief in experimentation rather than authority was limited to a small group of scientifically oriented individuals who appeared to be more numerous than they actually were because of their proclivity to write about and articulate their ideas. Those in the majority, although they did not write about it, embraced older, authoritarian, nonscientific ideas.

Skepticism about quack treatments continued to grow. Some physicians objected to the development of increasingly elaborate pharmacopoeias and to the treatment of the same illness with many different therapies. Nothing was known about the effectiveness of most medications, and clearly, methods of evaluation were needed. Some physicians advocated using statistics. As early as 1800, William Cobbett questioned the value of bleeding and purging for yellow fever and suggested using statistical methods to demonstrate their ineffectiveness. Pierre C. A. Louis (1834) discussed the need to "count," which he called the Numerical Method (Bull 1959). With this method he showed that whether or not a person was bled did not affect outcome. Ian Hacking (1988) cited a study published by Jean Civiale in 1838, comparing the mortality rates associated with a traditional method of operating on gallstones (in which 1,141 of 5,615 patients died) to those of a new operation in which only 6 of 307 patients died.[2] Henry G. Sutton (1865) recognized that greater knowledge of the natural course of disease was needed before one could attribute cure to a particular remedy. In the following year, John H. Bennett (1866) astutely commented that physicians were

2. We are indebted to Dr. Harry M. Marks, of the History of Medicine Department at Johns Hopkins University, for bringing to our attention papers on the history of randomization (Hacking 1988), cooperative clinical trials (Marks 1987), the regulation of and reporting on new drugs by the FDA (Hutt 1983), the pioneering work of Sollmann, and the earliest example of a clinical double-blind study (of which we had been unaware), which was initiated by the AMA's Council on Pharmacy and Chemistry in 1911 (Hewlett 1913).

quick to remember their successes and slow to remember failures. He advised that statistics be used to control for the lack of objectivity, that all recorded cases be numbered and analyzed, and that particular note be made of factors such as sex, age, severity, mortality, and duration of illness.

Arithmetical Observationists

Ulrich Trohler (1978) traced the development of mathematical methods in medical therapeutics in Great Britain from 1750 to 1830. He attributed the beginning of this development to a number of British physicians in the second half of the eighteenth century who recognized the need to verify the effectiveness of remedies by expressing the results of comparative trials by simple "medical arithmetic." They departed from the then-current acknowledged methods of authoritative reporting, oracular aphorisms, and mere opinions of individuals, and stressed the primacy of facts expressed in numerical analysis over speculative theories. They were referred to as arithmetical observationists, who advocated the science of medical arithmetic and the numerical method. The method was accepted by scientifically oriented physicians, particularly in the army, the navy, and the Department of Ordinance.

Trohler described the social background of the arithmetical observationists. They were "quite clearly," with some exceptions, Scots—provincial and insignificant or marginal men who had attended less-prestigious schools and had done postgraduate apprenticeships. They differed from physicians with more established lineages, who had attended the best schools and belonged to the landed gentry and the privileged social class. Because of their inferior backgrounds, they were excluded from the centers of influence and power and thus had difficulty in developing a successful private practice. One method of obtaining prestige and success which was open to the more upwardly mobile, ambitious, and gifted of them was to absorb and reflect emerging new ideas. The "arithmetical observationists" are described as dissenters, interested in change and having an altruistic spirit of reform: they favored reform of medical care for the poor, of traditional treatments of disease, of medicine in general, of the way the profession was organized, and of the confused state of medical scholarship; and the elimination of quacks, proprietary secret remedies, and nostrums. Because dissenters were excluded from established centers of influence and power, they were encouraged to make a distinctive contribution to the nation's education and scientific, industrial, and commercial progress, and to become a meritocracy strongly espousing numerical and other scientific methods for evaluation in clinical medicine. Their scientific work distinguished them from the majority of practitioners. Included in their ranks were Lind, Pringle, Haygarth, Thomas Percival, and other prominent physicians. Their work led to improved studies of the relationship of weather to disease, scurvy, smallpox, amputation, lithotomy, and fevers, and was a strong influence on future generations of physicians. Trohler concluded that the habits of observation, of careful, regular, and comprehensive recording, and of systematic interpretation by means of simple arithmetic were important developments in the history of medical science in the eighteenth century. The social roots of the arithmetical observationists contributed to the correlation of disease with living conditions and ultimately to the scientific analysis of the relationship of social conditions to disease. Arithmetic observation began to be called "statistics" in 1830.

The advance in statistical techniques impelled the development of the experimental method, but whether statistics or the experimental method took precedence is difficult to say. Edwin G. Boring (1954) believed that the initial relationship between the two developments was coordinate, not causal.

Randomization

Hacking (1988), in a comprehensive history of randomization, an important method of selecting patients, attributed the first use of randomization to Charles S. Pierce and Joseph Jastrow (1885), who described the method in their studies to differentiate between very slightly different weights. However, the method was essentially ignored. A separate development came from the popularity of spiritism, mediums, telepathy, and parapsychology, which began in New York in 1848 and soon swept the world. This fad attracted the attention of scientists, who, though initially skeptical, began to study the phenomena. Their studies stimulated the development and use of probability and controls. John E. Coover (1917) is noted for the first use of the terms *controlled, control experiments,* and *randomization.* Randomization was not used in experiments until many years later. Although the concept was initially described by Sir Ronald Fisher in 1926, it did not became commonplace until after the publication of his important book *The Design of Experiments* (1935).

Despite advances in methodology, physicians in the nineteenth century continued to be primarily clinicians and to rely on clinical intuition. Oliver Wendell Holmes strongly advocated greater scientific rigor on the part of the medical profession (1891). He chastised physicians for lack of observation, for failure to weigh evidence, for the disregard of failures and spontaneous improvement, for failing to heed the *"post hoc ergo propter hoc"* fallacy, and for their inability to learn by experience (Bull 1959).

Some clinical studies did attempt to evaluate the effectiveness of treatment. The method of historical comparison, evaluating the difference in outcome between treated and untreated cases, was used to document the advantages of antiseptics and vaccines. Lister, in 1870, experimenting with the use of antiseptics in amputations, compared old amputation cases in which the amputations had been done without antiseptics to new cases in which antiseptics had been used. Only small numbers of patients were involved, numbers that Lister felt were too small for statistical comparison, thus arousing some question about his findings. In addition, the reliability of the criteria used to select the old cases was criticized. Because Lister's methodology was inadequate, his results were open to bitter controversy and delayed the introduction of a beneficial technique. This underscores the importance of using adequate methodology.

Louis Pasteur, known as the founder of bacteriology and a pioneer in preventive inoculation, used a more sophisticated design to test his antitoxin (Bull 1959). The sample consisted of twenty-five sheep protected by inoculation and infected with the virus, twenty-five sheep infected but not inoculated, and ten sheep neither inoculated nor infected. Equal dosages of the virus were given, and injections were alternated between protected and unprotected sheep. All of the infected and uninoculated sheep died, while the inoculated sheep survived. Because of the excellent design, the results of this controlled experiment could not be disputed, and this led to immediate application of immunization.

The number of experimental studies increased slowly. Controlled trials of the diphtheria vaccine were conducted during the late 1800s. In Johannes Fibinger's adequately controlled study in Denmark in 1898, patients with diphtheria were alternated, one patient treated and the next patient untreated. The two groups, treated and untreated, were compared on the basis of age, symptoms, severity, and other factors. Although the experiment demonstrated that the mortality rate was less among the treated cases, the patients in the samples studied had mild symptoms that lowered the final mortality rates, thus lessening the impact of the results (Bull 1959).

The nineteenth century, building on the rapid changes and advances of the eighteenth century, is characterized as "an era of stupendous progress in medicine" (King 1963, 221). Rapid progress came from many sources, such as new knowledge about chemistry and cells; new sciences such as bacteriology, pharmacology, genetics, and the study of evolution; the use of asepsis, antisepsis, and anesthesia in surgery; improved microscopy; the discovery of viruses, x-rays, and radioactivity; increased use of statistics, historical controls, and controlled trials; and the emphasis on science and experimentation personified by the work of Francis Bacon, Claude Bernard, Louis Pasteur, Robert Koch, and Rudolph Virchow, to name a few. There was a rapid development of new therapies brought about by these developments, which in turn stimulated interest in methods to evaluate the efficacy of therapy in the twentieth century.

The Twentieth Century

Although before the twentieth century individual clinicians recognized how important it was to carefully observe patients, record all cases, describe the methods of treatment, and specify demography, length of treatment, severity of illness, natural course of illness, and so on, controlled clinical trials were still rare. By the beginning of the twentieth century, however, the medical community began to institute changes.

Federal Regulations

The Food and Drug Act, passed in 1906, placed drugs under federal control. The main emphasis at the time was on measures to ensure the purity of foods. Enforcement, investigations, and reports of violations, fraud, and dishonest advertising were conducted by the Food and Drug Administration, the Post Office Department, and the Federal Trade Commission. Amendments to the act—such as the 1938 requirement that drug manufacturers conduct tests to ensure safety before marketing, the 1962 amendment requiring sponsors of a new drug to submit substantial evidence of efficacy, the 1966 legislation to control drug abuse, and so on—were enacted slowly. (See Hutt 1983 for a detailed history of FDA regulation up to 1973; subsequent changes in FDA regulations are described in chapter 7.)

The Campaign against Nostrums and Quackery

There was growing concern over unrestricted claims about the effectiveness and safety of numerous nostrums, patent and proprietary medicines, and quackery, which became a floodtide at the end of the nineteenth century in the United States. James H. Young (1961, 1967) comprehensively described the history of quackery in Britain from the eighteenth century to the 1960s. In 1905 a series of articles about the nostrum evil and quackery, entitled "Great American Fraud," appeared in *Collier's* (Adams 1905) and was reprinted and sold by the American Medical Association.

At about the same time, the AMA established a Council on Pharmacy and Chemistry to determine which products were acceptable to advertise in the *Jour-*

nal of the American Medical Association (JAMA), and soon thereafter set up a Propaganda Department to combat quackery. Its director was Arthur J. Cramp, whom Young (1967) described as dignified, reserved, modest, sensitive, cautious, thorough, perfectionistic, courageous, honest, moral, and dedicated to a lifelong fight against quackery and secret proprietary preparations advertised to laypeople. Cramp's writing is characterized as vivid, eloquent, effective, and manifesting a fine sense of style. The AMA later published a weekly series of similar articles in *JAMA,* which were then published as pamphlets for physicians and the public. These articles and reviews of hundreds of then-prevalent treatments were published by Cramp in *Nostrums and Quackery,* a 500-page volume, in 1911; this work was expanded to 700 pages with the 1913 second edition, and to 800 pages in 1921; finally, after ill health forced Cramp to retire in 1935, a 232-page volume, *Nostrums and Quackery and Pseudo-Medicine* (volume 3) was published in 1936. The 1936 work is a lucid, encyclopedic discussion of nostrums and quackery in America. Cramp even studied a baldness cure advertised by the Professor Sholder Institute, which claimed success in treating Theodore Roosevelt and Harry Houdini for their hair problems. This claim was made after the death of Roosevelt and Houdini (Young 1967). Cramp submitted hairs from a fox-fur coat to Sholder, who replied that microscopic analysis revealed seriously undernourished roots and grave danger of continuous and increasing hair loss unless the condition was treated. Cramp then serially submitted hairs from a wolf, hairs from a girl with long, luxurious hair, short strands of twine dyed black, and twine dyed brown. Sholder sent the same letter after each submission. The study could be classified as a single-blind study of an individual healer.

Both Cramp (1921) and Young (1961, 1967) provided insightful analyses of the reasons for the perennial and universal success of quackery, which also apply to the placebo effect of treatment. Ironically, although the treatments used by physicians at the time were essentially ineffective, there was no discussion of this, nor were physicians' treatments classified as largely placebo. This is another example of the ability of healers to detect placebo treatments used by others more easily than those they used themselves (Shapiro and Struening 1973a, 1973b). Shortly thereafter, as described later in this chapter, the AMA instituted a program to evaluate questionably effective remedies.

Changes in Medical Education

Another important development, reflecting changes in the medical zeitgeist and resulting in important changes in medical education and practice, was the Flexner report (Flexner 1910). It was stimulated by the Carnegie Foundation for the

Advancement of Teaching (Barzansky and Gevitz 1992). The report advocated changing medical training and giving medical students a postgraduate medical education centered in a university hospital taught by a full-time faculty; it emphasized a research and scientific orientation. It had a profound influence on the subsequent course of medical education in the United States and resulted in the closing of the majority of the "doctor mills" within the next twenty years (Barzansky and Gevitz 1992).

Despite these auspicious beginnings and the subsequent implementation of legal restraints by the FDA, Cramp later wrote in disappointment that "credulity is bred less by a lack of brains than by a dearth of knowledge. We are all credulous when we wander in fields that are strange to us. Knowledge, rather than intelligence, is the best antidote for credulity. . . . In the field of medicine human credulity learns little from experience" (1936, vii). "In from 80 to 85 percent of all cases of human ailments, it is probable that the individual will get well whether he does something for his indisposition or does nothing for it. The healing power of nature—vis medicatrix natura—fortunately for biologic perpetuity, works that way. The seller of medicaments then, obviously starts with at least an eighty percent chance in his favor" (vii). Despite this and other meaningful assaults on quackery, Young, as late as the mid-1960s, concluded that "quackery is not only not vanquished; never in previous history has medical quackery been such a big business as it is now" (1967, 247); and quackery has not abated since then.

Also influential in combating quackery were the many essays by Morris Fishbein (1925, 1927, 1932), the long-time editor of *JAMA,* who unrelentingly described the fads and foibles of healing cults and medical follies.

The twentieth-century changes in medical education and the intrinsic scientific basis of medicine slowly but inexorably contributed to sensitivity about the placebo effect and the development of methodology to control its unbridled effect.

Sollmann and the Committee on Therapeutic Research

The Council on Pharmacy and Chemistry of the AMA established a Committee on Therapeutic Research in 1912 and provided funds "to focus attention of experimental and clinical investigators on some of the urgent but neglected problems of practical therapeutics, and help bridge the chasm between science and its application" (Sollmann 1916, 1439; for additional history, see Marks 1987). Torald Sollmann, professor and chair of the Department of Pharmacology at the Medical School of Western Reserve University, was appointed chair of the committee. A major figure in pharmacology, Sollmann was referred to as "Mr. Pharmacology" and "the dean of pharmacology" (Riker 1992; Marks 1992b) and wrote many editions of an influential text on pharmacology. He was an astute and perceptive pharmacologist who was acutely aware of the need for controlled clinical experimentation. He guided and strongly influenced the policies and activities of the committee for many years, together with other distinguished leaders in chemistry, pharmacology, and clinical medicine who were affiliated with the foremost medical colleges and hospitals. The views of these leaders, reflecting the evolving changes in clinical research, strongly influenced subsequent developments in medicine. The council published important volumes throughout the years: *Useful Drugs* (Council on Pharmacy and Chemistry 1930b), dealing with nonproprietary drugs, and *New and Non-Official Remedies* (Council on Pharmacy and Chemistry 1930a), dealing with proprietary substances (Gold 1930). The council's orientation is reflected in Sollmann's 1912 paper on experimental therapeutics, in which the "paucity of exact, quantitative, critical records as to the effect of drugs on the human individual, either in health or disease" is cited, as well as "the need of experimental therapeutics—the carefully planned, accurately executed, and intelligently digested study of the effects of drugs in human patients"; Sollmann asserted that it was "essential that clinical experimentation should follow the canons of other scientific experimentation" (243).

Four years after the creation of the Committee on Therapeutic Research, Sollmann (1916) summarized the committee's work evaluating controversial and suspect commercial remedies. Comprehensive pharmacological studies usually preceded clinical studies of the effectiveness and toxicity of the examined remedies.[3] The results are noteworthy; more was accomplished in four years than would probably be possible today in ten years. The report reads like a *Consumer Reports* evaluation of questionable claims and advertisements for soaps, and as expected, cherished beliefs about the effectiveness of most of the examined remedies were not confirmed.

The period 1912 to 1930, influenced by Sollmann and the publications of the Committee on Therapeutic Research in *JAMA* and summary volumes, revealed

---

3. Studies were done comparing natural and synthetic salicylates, the duration of digitalis action, the effect of iodides on the circulation, organic iodin preparations, salicylate toxicity, the interaction of ferments, the action of bromids, hexamethylenamine, digestive ferments, cardiac stimulants, pancreatic preparations, opium alkaloids, the synergism of the activity of hydrochloric acid, the stability of digitalis infusions, the toxicity of different samples of chloroform, the distribution of hypophosphites in all body fluids and tissues, epinephrine in pituitary extracts, uric acid solvents, and strontium salicylate (Sollman 1916).

increased sensitivity about how to conduct clinical trials, including references to the "blind test" and the publication of an early—and probably the first—clinical study using what is now called the double-blind procedure. Unfortunately, the work of Sollmann and the committee had little effect on subsequent research.

The inclusion of the terms *placebo effect* and *double-blind method* as references in the computer files of the National Library of Medicine in 1990 is perhaps a symbolic indication of a belated triumph over the several-thousand-year hegemony of the placebo effect.

chapter seven

The History of the Double-Blind Procedure

This chapter examines the most important and notable developments in the history of clinical trials: the use of placebo controls and the double-blind method. In early experiments, control groups were usually passive comparison groups. Either individual patients were given an active drug and a placebo at different times, or they were alternately given an active agent and no treatment, or historical controls were used (the experimental group was compared with a group previously treated with another medication, or an untreated group for which the outcome was known). The next development was the use of control substances. The earliest technique used was the single-blind procedure. In this paradigm the physician or investigator knows that control substances are being used and knows which patients are receiving them, but the patient does not know. The control substance is usually an inert placebo. While this design theoretically would control for the influence of the patient's hopes or expectations and other variables on the treatment outcome, it would not control for the influence of the physician's bias or behavior on the patient (Rivers 1908).

Very slowly, controls gained acceptance. Most of the early studies were isolated experiments and had limited impact on the therapeutic community.

Early Studies Using Controls and Blinding

The first recorded use of an inert material as a control was in W.H.R. Rivers's (1908) laboratory study of the influence of alcohol and other drugs on fatigue. Controls are necessary to account for the sensory stimulation caused by the experiment, and Rivers advocated using an inert substance (not referred to as a placebo) as a control for the active agent. The inert material was designed to taste and appear indistinguishable from the experimental drug. The subjects, who included the experimenter (Rivers), had no knowledge of the substances they received. Many methodological variables were considered, including the need for baseline measurement, the need to keep all conditions of life constant, and the need to control for many factors: the effects of knowing the character of the dose, sensory stimulation, suggestion, excitement, interest, and practice. For example, writing of his own experience as an experimental subject, Rivers recalled:

> I felt at once stimulated by the fact of having taken the substance, the action of which I was trying to test, and it was obvious that I had no means of telling whether any effect which might be produced was due to this interest or to the physiological action of the drug. In all future experiment I, therefore, determined to endeavor to disguise the days on which the drug was being taken and all the new work to be described in this lecture has been carried out with the use of control mixtures which have usually been wholly indistinguishable from those containing the active substances. The subject of an experiment has taken every day at some time in its course a dose of a mixture, and has been wholly unaware whether he has taken the substance which is the motive of the experiment or some inactive imitation of it . . . and it has only been at the end of the experiment that I have been made acquainted with the exact nature of their contents. (Rivers 1908, 18)

This study demonstrates an early understanding of the placebo effect and probably was the first use of the double-blind procedure. Although important historically and methodologically, to the best of our knowledge it was never widely cited.

Rivers's erudition and prescience appeared again in his posthumously published book *Medicine, Magic, and Religion* (1927), written for the most part before 1920. He said, "The action of suggestion can never be excluded in any form of medical treatment, whether it be explicitly designed to act upon the mind or whether ostensibly, it is purely physical in character" (137). "If we confine our attention to our own culture, it is only within the last fifty or sixty years that there has been any clear recognition of the vast importance of the mental factor in the production and treatment of disease, and even now this knowledge is far from being fully recognized either by the medical profession or the laity" (123).

H. L. Hollingsworth (1912) referred extensively to Rivers's influence on his experiment on the influence of caffeine and alcohol on mental and motor efficiency. Like Rivers's study, Hollingsworth's was double blind. An inactive substance (sugar or milk) was disguised to appear and taste the same as the active drugs, and was administered in the same manner and at the same time as the caffeine and alcohol. Neither the subjects nor the assistants making the measurements knew which was being administered. Other notable early controlled studies included those of Albion W. Hewlett (1913), David I. Macht and colleagues (1916), and Adolf Bingel (1918).

Torald Sollmann (1917) revealed increased interest in and sophistication about methodological safeguards in clinical trials. Moreover, he referred for the first time to the use of an identical inactive preparation as a control (not yet referring to it as a placebo) and to the use of the "comparative method or the 'blind test.'" In his paper "The Crucial Test of Therapeutic Evidence," Sollmann cited *post hoc* reasoning as "apt to creep in unawares, unless one takes great precautions . . . and that clinical experiments must be surrounded with extra painstaking precautions" (1917, 198). He rejected enthusiastic but unsubstantiated testimonials, letters, clinical reports, and impressions submitted by commercial firms as evidence of the effectiveness of a remedy. He recommended adequate controls (untreated patients who were ill) for the natural course of an illness, samples large enough to permit statistical comparisons, and alternating patients who receive the test preparation and another inactive preparation, and he noted that the active and inactive preparations should resemble each other physically and taste the same. To avoid the pitfalls of clinical observation, he urged that researchers use the "comparative method or the 'blind test' . . . as the only method that makes the results purely objective, really independent of the bias of the observer and the patient. It is the only method, therefore, which determines" whether a drug is effective (Sollmann 1917, 199).

We do not know what were the scientific and methodological influences on Sollmann. The use of the term *comparative method,* which is linked with the term *blind test,* may be related to Claude Bernard's 1867 recommendation of the use of the "comparative observation" or "comparative experiment" to "reason about what we have observed, compare the facts and judge them by other facts used as controls" (Bernard 1927, 128).

Subsequently, in the 1920s, the Council on Pharmacy relied on reviews by experts, rather than on controlled studies, to evaluate drugs (Marks 1987). Moreover, it appears that until the early 1930s the reviews had little effect in terms of hastening the use of the "blind" test or method and advancing the need for better experimental methodology to evaluate the effect of treatment.

The evolution of Sollmann's concepts can be seen in his paper "The Evaluation of Therapeutic Remedies in the Hospital" (1930), which may reflect changes generally taking place in medicine. Sollmann again recommended the use of the "blind test," for the first time used the term *placebo* to refer to a control in studies, linked the placebo to the "blind test," and dropped the use of the term *comparative method.* He commented in the paper: "Apparent results must be checked by the 'blind test,' i.e., another remedy, or a placebo, without the knowledge of the observer, if possible. The placebo, if expectant treatment is permissible, also furnishes the comparative check of the natural course of the disease; comparison with another remedy helps toward a just perspective" (1280).

A somewhat parallel development occurred in Great Britain with the passage of the Therapeutic Substance Act in 1925. Its purpose was "to provide for the regulation of the manufacture, sale, and importation of therapeutic substances, the purity or potency of which cannot be tested by chemical means. . . . The duties of . . . carrying out control tests are entrusted to the National Institute of Medical Research" (Hampshire 1933, 275). The Medical Research Council appointed a Therapeutic Trials Committee in 1931 "to advise and assist them in arranging for properly controlled clinical tests of new products that seem likely, on experimental grounds, to have value in the treatment of disease. Its object was to supply clinical reports on new therapeutic agents which manufacturers were preparing to place on the market" and to arrange "appropriate clinical trials . . . in suitable cases" (Anonymous 1931, 304). Lilienfeld (1982) cited this report as one of the first publications to use the term *clinical trials* (Anonymous 1931; Hampshire 1933). Reports by the committee were essentially reviews of various drugs, however, and as far as we know the committee conducted no controlled studies.

In the 1920s and 1930s, investigators slowly began to use controls but not blinding. Several studies used nonblind controls for the active treatment, and many used large samples and multiple outcome measures. These include the studies of Von Sholly and Park (1921), Ferguson et al. (1927), Leighton and McKinlay (1930), Finland (1930), the Medical Research Council's Therapeutic Trials Committee (1934), Wyckoff et al. (1930), Amberson et al. (1931), Diehl (1933, 1935), and Hoagland et al. (1950). Donald W. Cowan et al. (1942) referred to the tablets used in their study as a placebo. However, this was not the first use of the term: Harry A. Gold had used placebos since 1932, and published his study on the xanthines in 1937 (Gold et al. 1937).

The blind procedure and placebo controls were uncommon in studies in the early 1930s. This may have been due partly to attitudes about the use of placebos at the time. According to Gold (1968), "The commonly accepted belief was that placebos were given to deceive patients. . . . Doctors were criticized for using a dummy pill." Walter Modell (1967) noted that he "never heard the word placebo mentioned. . . . People didn't speak of placebos at all, a kind of word you avoided. . . . It was not common to refer to the placebo effect in 1930. . . . Doctors wouldn't admit using placebos. . . . [and] gave vitamins instead, or something bitter, like tincture of valerian. . . . No one ever [called these substances] placebos except for Gold. [Gold was] the only one I ever heard refer to

the placebo effect. . . . Others called it suggestion." Nathaniel Kwit (1969) and
McKeen Cattell (1969) made similar comments: placebos were considered to be
inert and were not openly used by physicians, and if you wanted to give something for its psychological or suggestive effect you gave an ineffective substance
such as tincture of strychnine or valerian. Both had been unaware of the blind
procedure before Gold used it in his ether and xanthine studies. These initial
studies using the blind test and placebo controls were important historically because after them Gold used the methods in all of his studies. This was not true
of the controlled and blinded studies conducted by investigators before him,
which were usually isolated experiments.

The Evolution of Double-Blind Studies

A study by Ella M. Hediger and Gold (1935) compared the deterioration and
complications caused by the use of ether supplied in expensive twenty-seven-
to fifty-five-pound drums with those caused by ether supplied in small, inex-
pensive quarter-pound tins. The significance of the study, according to the authors, was that "general appraisals were made entirely free of possible prejudices
and preconceived notions regarding the relative value of different types of ether,
since those who made them had no knowledge of the source of the ether" (2246).
The authors made only a casual reference, without other explanation, to the fact
that the study was conducted with the "blind test." This study, like those of aspirin and diphtheria, compared two active agents, without comparison to placebo. A placebo control was not necessary because both active agents were known
to be effective. But inevitably, these studies comparing two active drugs were
followed by studies comparing an active drug to placebo.

   An early placebo study was undertaken in the 1930s, stimulated not only by
a growing interest in the use of placebo controls but also by growing skepticism
about the treatment of angina pectoris. Somewhat similar studies were carried
out to test drugs used in the treatment of angina: in New York, Gold et al. (1937)
began a study of xanthines compared to placebo, while a single-blind London
study treated ninety patients with thirteen drugs commonly used for angina.
None was reported to be more effective than placebo (Evans and Hoyle 1933).

   According to Gold (1968), "In the 1920s and 1930s the placebo was something you gave the patient to take and swallow . . . and not something that had
something in it such as quinine or strychnine. . . . A doctor who used placebos
was considered a quack. . . . The reputation of a placebo was so bad that doctors in general had no use for either its name or its use." Modell, a student of
Gold, who worked with him in pharmacology, remarked, "Placebos were used

very often in Gold's clinic, but not elsewhere; [placebos were] in the formulary at Beth Israel Hospital, designated as #35 white or pink tablets" (1967). According to Cattell (1969), "placebos were not given as such because there was so much ineffective medicine being used. . . . Vitamins were the most popular placebos, but were given for their placebo effects. . . . Placebo effects were often more important than the pharmacological action. . . . The doses were so small that they didn't do anything half the time."

Kwit (1969), a co-investigator, co-author, and member of the Gold group, described the evolution of the xanthine study. Since 1895, xanthines (aminophylline and theobromine) had been thought to be effective for the relief of angina pectoris. By 1932 most patients with cardiac pain had been treated with xanthines at some time during their illness. Gold was skeptical about xanthines' effectiveness and designed a study to compare the effectiveness of xanthines to that of inert (lactose) placebo in one hundred patients with anginal pain. The study began in 1932 as a single blind study. As the study progressed (after about two or three years), according to Kwit (1969) and Gold (1968),[1] they realized that the physicians administering the drug were asking the patients "leading questions" about its effect on the severity of pain and thus could be biasing the results. A review of the charts revealed that patients were giving contradictory answers to the physicians' questions, making it essential to blind the physicians. The authors emphasized the need for objectivity: "The method we employed for determining cause and effect was more objective and relatively free of personal judgments. The procedure was based on this general formulation; namely, if the relief of pain during the use of xanthine is due to the specific action of the drug, the patient should be able to distinguish its effects, and to do so repeatedly, from the effects of a placebo given under similar conditions and in such form as to preclude its detection by the patient through any means other than the relief of pain" (Gold et al. 1937, 2175). In the summary they stated, "The data were obtained in a manner relatively free of bias by the use of the 'blind test'" (2178). However, it is not clear at what point in the study the physician was blinded and how consistently this was done, since the authors used the phrase "the questioner usually refrained from informing himself as to the agent that had been used," when they described the physicians' role in appraising the patients (2175). Kwit (1969) described their thinking: "Toward the end of the study we realized that the doctor must not know what he gives, the patient must not know what he receives, and the questioner must not know what was given. The study

---

1. Information not available in the 1937 paper is derived from tape-recorded interviews (Modell 1967; Gold 1967a, 1968, 1969; Kwit 1969).

started out single blind, it then became partially, and finally fully blind. . . . By the time we finished the paper, we had already established what we meant by the double-blind test, and that the only proper way of evaluating anything was with a double-blind." (The term *double blind* was not used in the paper, however.) "We realized the importance of the method but didn't realize its importance historically. We just knew that we had devised what we thought was a fool proof way of testing a drug and the only way of testing a drug." Needless to say, the use of xanthines for cardiac pain decreased after this and other studies. After the 1937 xanthine study, all clinical studies from the Gold laboratory used double-blind methodology.

Although the xanthine study was not entirely double blind, it is nevertheless important historically. It was the first clinical treatment study to use a placebo as a control in a double-blind study. Gold's (1968) comments about the congruence of the two methods (placebo control and double-blind procedure) are of interest. Gold believed that by calling the control substance a placebo, they gave the term legitimacy. Before then, the term had a pejorative meaning: a placebo was a pill used to deceive a patient. Gold said during this interview, "the placebo and the double-blind were companions after the 1937 study."

Another interesting feature of the study was the use of medications similar in size, shape, color, and taste, to ensure that the placebo was indistinguishable from the active medication. Early in the study, either cascara or lactose was used as a placebo. Patients detected differences between the placebo and the active drug and wanted the active drug. The investigators recognized that this introduced a subjective bias on the patient's part, and that it was, therefore, essential to use identical agents. Drug manufacturers were asked to provide an identical matching placebo for the study. More so than in previous papers, the authors listed factors that could influence the response to treatment: spontaneous changes, changes in weather, occupation, work, domestic affairs, diet, eating habits, amount of rest, bowel function, and amount of emotional strain; reassurance, the confidence aroused in the treatment, the encouragement afforded by any new procedure, a change of physicians, and other unknown factors.

Gold, the primary author, was a pharmacologist who was trained to do animal research in the laboratory. He became interested in treating patients with drugs, stressing the importance of doing "the same experiments in humans as done in the laboratory on animals." The 1937 study convinced him that human clinical trials required better and different types of controls than were traditionally used in the laboratory. Apparent in the well-written paper on the xanthines is the five-year struggle by the authors to perfect their methodology, and the evolution of their thinking about how to derive reliable, meaningful, scientific data from clinical trials. Their failure to recognize the importance of their contribution to experimental methodology or to recognize that they had broken new ground was in keeping with the general scientific zeitgeist. The new methodology generated little interest among their colleagues and had little influence on other investigators. It was not discussed in the literature, nor was it used in clinical studies for many years afterward. Some physicians, however, were influenced. They heard of Gold's interest in controls and placebos and wanted a chance to work with him (Gold 1968). Their contact with Gold planted a seed that led to the prominence of controls and placebos, interest in the placebo effect, and the evolution of the double-blind procedure.

The 1937 study by Gold et al. incorporated many new features. Its pioneering use of a placebo as a control gave legitimacy to the placebo, which heretofore had been viewed derisively as a substance in the form of a drug given by unethical clinicians to satisfy or fool a patient (Gold 1968). It used matching placebo and active drugs to ensure that they were indistinguishable from one another, and administered them in the same way. The authors recognized and stated that clinical experience is only observation and does not fulfill the essential standards of scientific evidence. According to Modell (1967), "Gold believed that you can't study drug effects in man without the double-blind. There may be other previous double-blind studies, but Gold was the one who implanted it, who stuck the standard in the ground." Gold, according to Kwit (1969), believed that "the importance of the study was how it evolved." In later studies, the Gold team recommended increasingly sophisticated statistical analyses and randomization.

Gold established the Cornell Conferences on Therapy (1946). He was active in research and teaching and continued to develop and communicate his ideas to students and staff at Cornell, probably with considerable discussion and interaction. The staff included Eugene F. DuBois, McKeen Cattell, Harold Wolff, Stewart Wolf, Walter Modell, Theodore Greiner, and others. They too were aware of placebo effects and the need for controlled studies. The conferences on therapy were very popular and well attended. The proceedings were published in the *New York State Journal of Medicine,* in *JAMA,* and in collected volumes. The conference titled "The Use of Placebos in Therapy" (Gold 1946), the first such conference that we know of, was cited for many years after its publication. Judging by the participants' discussions, knowledge about the placebo effect was increasing.

During the 1946 conference Gold explicitly stated that the power of the placebo (the placebo effect) had to be accounted for and controlled in clinical evaluation studies in order to establish the therapeutic efficacy of any new agent.

Further, the importance of the placebo in the investigation of drug action in humans could not be overestimated. His interest lay not in studying the variables that contribute to the placebo effect but in the use of the placebo as a control for study of medication. Only by using the blind test, he stated, is it possible to ascertain the amount of improvement due to the specific action of the drug and the amount due to the psychotherapeutic action of just administering a medicine.

The conferences stimulated a growing appreciation of the placebo effect. Discussions focused on many issues: indications for the use of placebos in treatment and research; the effects of placebos; the use of pure and impure placebos; the ethics of using placebos; and the doctor–patient relationship, conditioning, attitudes, and other psychological variables associated with positive and negative placebo reactions.

The comments at the conference by Oskar Diethelm, chair of the Department of Psychiatry at Cornell for many years, illustrated the paradoxical and belated interest by psychiatrists in the placebo effect: he recognized the importance of knowing how patient variables influence placebo effects, and he emphasized the importance of belief, the symbolic value of the drug, and the personality and unconscious factors in the physician which may influence his or her reliability when evaluating the effect of the drug (Diethelm 1946). Diethelm (1967) later commented that he would not allow placebos to be used at the Payne Whitney Psychiatric Clinic at Cornell while he was chair. Although almost all of the treatments then in use were impure or active placebos, the Payne Whitney staff was not interested in studying the placebo effect or the methodology of evaluating treatment, even though they had been exposed to innovative ideas about the placebo by internists and pharmacologists at Cornell. This negative attitude was common among psychiatrists, including not only academic psychiatrists but also, especially, clinicians, psychotherapists, and psychoanalysts. It was so pervasive that virtually no papers on the placebo were published by psychiatrists and psychologists until many years after there had been interest in and study of the placebo phenomenon among nonpsychiatrists.

The importance of Gold's specific contribution to clinical pharmacology was recognized in 1947, when he was appointed the first professor of clinical pharmacology at Cornell University Medical College (Gold 1967a). Pharmacology, before his work, had involved testing the effect of pharmaceuticals in animals, whereas Gold, quoting Alexander Pope's statement "The proper study of mankind is man," advocated studying their effects in humans. Thus began a new field, clinical pharmacology (Gold 1952). According to Gold (1967a), the application of scientific methods, specifically the use of controls, double-blind design, and statistical analysis of data, was a major factor advancing this development.

An interesting double-blind study (although not referred to as such) of the cardiac glycoside strophanthin for preoperative treatment of 421 patients without congestive heart failure began in 1944 and was published in Finland in 1948 (Elovainio and Ostling 1948). Patients were randomly assigned to group A or group B. The code for the injection vials labeled A or B was not broken until the end of the study. Gustaf Ostling, in response to our inquiry about whether the authors had prior knowledge of the double-blind method, replied: "My double-blind strophanthin study was neither based on personal communications from other workers nor from ideas obtained in the literature" (Ostling 1970). The physicians were blinded because he knew that "all surgeons in the hospital believed firmly in the strophanthin prophylaxis and we thought it unwise to inform them that one of two sets only contained saline." It was his impression that the paper's influence was insignificant because it was published in a journal with a very restricted circulation.

The evolution of the double-blind procedure in the 1940s was stimulated by a slow increase in comparative studies, the use of placebos in single-blind studies, and an influential controlled study of the use of streptomycin to treat pulmonary tuberculosis (Medical Research Council 1948). The Medical Research Council stressed the importance of conducting a rigorously planned investigation with concurrent controls to validly establish the clinical effectiveness of a new chemotherapeutic agent in tuberculosis. To this end, the study (Sir Austin Bradford Hill was one of its planners) incorporated methodological advances such as establishing criteria for patient selection, the use of random numbers in each sex group to determine patient assignment, and blind radiological evaluation. Because patients ($N = 107$) were assigned to either streptomycin and bed rest or bed rest alone, without placebo control for streptomycin, the treatment was not blind. Hill indicated to us in 1970 that a blind placebo control for streptomycin would have been desirable but that at the time of the study it had been decided not to use a placebo control, since streptomycin-treated patients received up to four daily injections for six months, and it would have been inappropriate to treat bed-rest patients with frequent and prolonged placebo injections. The final outcome of treatment, however, was determined independently by two radiologists and a clinician, who were blind to patient assignment. By using a control group, the investigators demonstrated significant radiological and clinical improvement, and showed that patients treated with streptomycin showed decreased mortality by comparison with patients treated with bed rest.

Other blind studies done under Gold's direction included studies by Herman

Bakst et al. (1948), Seymour Rinzler et al. (1950), and Modell et al. (1945), and the Greiner et al. study in 1950, in which the blind test was more accurately named the double-blind test. Greiner and Gold were responsible for the design, analysis, and publication of the last-named study. The other authors participated primarily in the clinical aspects of the study. The authors called the method the "double-blind test" to underscore the blinding of all participants and highlighted the importance of the method in the title: "A Method for Evaluation of the Effects of Drugs on Cardiac Pain in Patients with Angina of Effort." They used a crossover double-blind design and identical tablets to compare khellin and placebo. The patients' logs of pain experienced were reviewed by a physician, who "decided on changes in dosage and dispensed the supply of tablets with directions for their use" (Greiner et al. 1950, 144). Although the physician knew what the patients had been taking, he did not participate in the treatment or evaluation of the results. Another physician recorded the evaluation of the patient "made by skilled questioning under the 'double-blind test' in which neither doctor nor patient knew at the time whether the evaluation related to the placebo or khellin" (146). According to the authors, this method was essentially similar to the method used in their 1937 xanthine study, and offered the greatest freedom from distortion by innumerable factors affecting patients' statements. The results indicated no difference in effectiveness between khellin and placebo, and khellin was not used subsequently for the treatment of anginal pain.

This paper (Greiner et al. 1950) provides many creative insights about the placebo effect and the methodology of clinical trials. The authors noted the effect on treatment of "spontaneous variations in the severity of the anginal state, and the several factors of suggestion, such as taking a new medication, and the physician's personality and enthusiasm for the new agent" (152). They commented on the importance of making the active drug and placebo control identical, stating, "the physician's enthusiasm is inadmissible in a scientific experiment for the purpose of seeking out the specific pharmacologic merits of an agent in the control of the angina of effort" (153). They suggested that the influence of suggestion "can be neutralized by the use of an appropriate placebo in a 'double-blind test' in which the identity of the drug and placebo remain unknown to the patient and physician until the analysis of the data is completed" (153). As in the xanthine study, in order to maintain the double blind the allocation code was not revealed until after the analysis—an important procedure seldom included in studies. Moreover, as in a 1948 study (Bakst et al. 1948), they advocated the use of statistical tests to analyze the results.

This paper contained the most forceful recommendation and comprehensive explanation about the necessity of using the double-blind procedure in clinical trials. It is probably the most important and influential paper in the history of the double-blind procedure. Nevertheless, according to Greiner (1969), Gold had his detractors. As far as Greiner knew, at that time there was no one else in New York City using the double-blind method, although people were aware of the technique.

The 1954 Cornell conference on therapy explored methods for clinical evaluation of new drugs in human subjects. Gold cited the serious bottleneck to therapeutic progress caused by the absence of controlled clinical trials and the lack of sufficiently well trained physicians, suitable clinical facilities, and adequate methods to clinically evaluate all the new available drugs. He advocated a comparison between

> an allegedly potent agent and a blank of such physical properties as to render a distinction between the two impossible except through some pharmacologic potency which may exist. On the other hand, the two compounds may both be potent and we then have to determine a difference in potency. In this type of drug evaluation there are two indispensable elements: one is the notion of a comparison of one thing with another, the other is the factor of the double-blind procedure which calls for an investigation in which neither the patient nor the doctor is aware of the identity of the two agents until the results are in and analyzed. This is imperative to avoid the influence of subconscious bias. The failure to use the double-blind test and the placebo in the attempt to evaluate a new drug is responsible for a large proportion of erroneous conclusions in clinical testings. . . . I am not sure why it is that the use of a placebo is considered by many physicians objectionable in a method of clinical evaluation and why there seems to be so much resistance to the idea that the experimenting doctor and the patient should remain in the dark about the identity of the agent until the comparison is finished. (1954, 724)

This statement by Gold culminated twenty years of pioneering study of methods with which to reliably and validly evaluate the effectiveness of new drugs. In it, the "blind test" (previously written with quotation marks) is more appropriately referred to as the double-blind procedure (without quotation marks). An essential requirement for a clinical study is that *all* of the ingredients of the drugs being compared be identical, so that the *only* distinction is the specific pharmacological or psychological effect. This then requires that the compared drugs be physically identical, that patients experience their administration as identical, that clinicians administer them identically, and that the results and the statistical analysis be completed before the identity of the compared drugs is revealed. The reasons for doing a study comparing one active drug or two active drugs with a placebo are clarified.

All of the clinical studies conducted by Gold and his colleagues beginning about halfway through the 1937 xanthine study used the same format: a physician, otherwise not associated with the study, reviewed daily reports completed by patients and the records of the clinicians, determined the dosage, and gave the medication to patients; an active drug was compared with a placebo identical to it in color, form, shape, smell, and taste; patients and physicians evaluating the clinical course were unaware of which patient received the active drug and which the placebo; and the results or statistical analysis were done blindly before the code for drug allocation was revealed. Technically, it is possible that the physicians deciding on dosage and dispensing the drug were not blind to drug allocation and unknowingly could have influenced the results, although their role is described as casual and uninvolved.

The procedure evolved over time, and today in studies of drug efficacy all physicians are blind to drug allocation. However, identical placebos are not always used. Although the placebo control is described in most studies as an "identical matching placebo," the studies do not specify that the experimental drug and placebo be identically matched with regard to form, shape, color, and taste. The need for the placebo control to mimic the adverse effects of the active agent so that true double-blindness is maintained was not considered at the time. Although well known today, it is still rarely taken into account in studies. In Gold's procedure the allocation code was not revealed until after the results had been tabulated or statistically analyzed. We know of no other studies that used this method of blind data analysis to control for unintended bias on the part of investigators and statisticians. These stipulations fulfill Gold's criteria that all elements or variables in a clinical trial be identical except for the pharmacological or specific therapeutic effects of the drug under study.

By the 1950s the controlled clinical trial was accepted by some in the research community; however, wider acceptance did not come easily or quickly. The number of controlled trials in one hundred papers published in five leading American medical periodicals between January and June of 1950 was reviewed in 1951 (Ross 1951). Of these, 27 percent were well controlled (an increase over past periods), 45 percent did not use controls, and 18 percent used inadequate controls, which indicates that the use of controls was not yet required for publication, nor was the double-blind method.

Cattell, chair of the Department of Pharmacology at Cornell, who advocated the use of controls, was critical of investigators who failed to do so, noting, "It is an unfortunate fact that a considerable proportion of papers in the current literature neglect this elementary principle" (1950). Cattell (1969) credited Harry Gold as the greatest contributor to the development of controlled clinical trials, an opinion supported by Gold's consistent advocacy and use of controlled studies during the previous fifteen years and the publication of his definitive khellin study in 1950.

Other members of the Gold group subsequently added to, elaborated on, and refined the double-blind procedure and the conduct of clinical trials:

Janet Travell (1953, 135) comprehensively discussed many aspects of controlled clinical trials. The "blind test" is referred to as the double-blind method, and the assessment by evaluators as "by the blindfold members of the team."

Greiner et al. (1957), describing the results of a double-blind study of laxative use, recommended the use of randomization and more sophisticated statistics, discussed the rights of patients, and provided sensitive insights about the complexities of clinical trials. In this and other papers Greiner discussed the potential for unmasking of the double blind as a result of untoward side reactions of the active drug, which suggests the need to use placebo controls with expected side reactions (1959); the use of the controlled clinical trial in the earliest screening of drugs (Greiner et al. 1959); the value and interaction of clinical intuition and scientific verification (1961); the role of hypothesis in studies (1962b); the ethics of drug research on patients (1962a); and the subjective bias of the clinician (1962c).

Modell and Raymond W. Houde further refined the methods of conducting clinical trials in their classic paper "Factors Influencing Clinical Evaluation of Drugs with Special Reference to the Double-Blind Technique" (1958). The AMA Council on Drugs signified the paper's importance by authorizing its publication in *JAMA*. The AMA at the same time approved the use of the double-blind method, controlled comparisons, randomization, statistics, and other procedures recommended for use in clinical trials. Paul Leber, director of the Division of Neuropsychopharmacology at the FDA, traced "most of the formulations about trial design to Modell and Houde" and referred to the paper as "the definitive paper in the modern development of controlled trials . . . the one we usually give credit to as being the paper that really describes to the medical community what you have to do in studies" (Leber 1992). Modell referred to the "blind test" in this paper (Modell and Houde 1958) as "the double-blind technique . . . double-blind control" and as "blindfolds" for subjects and evaluators which are removed if the drug reveals its effect. Modell published important papers on methodology for many years (Modell 1955a, 1955b, 1962, 1976; Modell and Garrett 1960; Modell and Lansing 1967).

Although the foregoing historical review indicates that the first double-blind study was not done by Gold, nor was he the first to use the term *blind,* his contributions set in place the essential, universally accepted guidelines for controlled clinical studies and the use of the double-blind procedure which have lasted to the present time.

The Origin of the Terms "Blind Test" and "Double-Blind Method"

Our interest in the origin of the term *blind test* was piqued during our historical research. Although probably not a scientific name, it is a creative and perfect description of the method.

I (AKS) had the good fortune to interview Gold and many of his associates.[2] Several of those interviewed (Cattell, Kwit, Modell, Wolf) described the years from about 1925 to 1935 as a time in which methodological concerns were in the air, although there was no recognition of this in the literature of the period. The evolution of the double-blind methodology is in some ways reflected by the phrase used to describe it.

The first use of the term *blind* was by William Stanley Jevons (1874, 43), who referred to "blind or test experiments." The phrase was not used, however, in accordance with the mid-twentieth-century understanding of a blind or controlled experiment (Boring 1954). For example, in a study to determine the amount of arsenic or magnetism in a substance, an initial study was conducted to ensure that arsenic or magnetism was not present in the chemical reagents or measurement apparatus. Jevons's use of the term, not referred to subsequently, was not likely to have influenced concepts about blind testing. Neither Rivers (1908) nor Hollingsworth (1912) used the term *blind test* to describe their method. For some reason, the studies by Jevons (1874), Rivers (1908), and Hollingsworth (1912) were unknown to the researchers we spoke to and to au-

2. Those interviewed were Harry Gold; Nathaniel Kwit, student colleague, collaborator, coauthor, and friend of Gold; McKeen Cattell, of the Department of Physiology and chair of the Department of Pharmacology at Cornell from 1956 to 1983; Walter Modell, director of Clinical Pharmacology, Cornell University Medical College; Stewart Wolf, who was at Cornell as an intern in 1938, was later professor in the Department of Medicine until 1952, and subsequently was head of the department at the University of Oklahoma Medical School; Ted Greiner, research fellow in the Department of Pharmacology, coauthor and colleague of Gold from 1948 to 1956, later a psychiatrist; Oskar Diethelm, chair of the Department of Psychiatry; Harry M. Marks; and Muriel Gold Morris, a psychiatrist in New York City, who is Gold's daughter. Riker reminisces about the relationship of Cattell and Gold in a 1989 interview (Minick and Haimowitz 1989).

thors discussing controlled studies (Solomon 1949; Boring 1954). We came across
the studies fortuitously in our historical search of the literature. They were unlikely, because of their relative obscurity, to have influenced the subsequent development of the double blind method.

A blind study of natural and synthetic sodium salicylate was initiated by the
Committee on Therapeutic Research under the direction of Sollmann in 1911
and published in 1913 (Hewlett 1913). The term *blind* was not used in the research report and was not used in any of Sollmann's papers until 1917, when he
recommended the "comparative method or the blind test." One year later, Bingel (1918) used the phrase *blind method* to describe the methodology used in a
study of the effect of two antitoxins on diphtheria. No other mention of the
blind method was made until Sollmann recommended the use of the "blind test"
in a paper discussing the evaluation of remedies in hospitals (1930, 1280). Although Gold (1930) referred to "the comparative study and evaluation," his
first reference to the blind test ("The study was made with the blind test") was
made in the ether study by Hediger and Gold (1935, 2245). This was the second
study using the term. The term *blind test* was used again in the more definitive
xanthine-versus-placebo study (Gold et al. 1937). Single-blind studies were more
frequent, and although seven double-blind studies were published, only three
used the term *blind test* (Bingel 1918; Hediger and Gold 1935; Gold et al. 1937).
Subsequently, only the Gold group used the phrase "blind test" (always in quotation marks) in their papers and in all of their clinical studies (they had done
most of the blind studies), until 1950. In the 1950 khellin study, they referred to
the procedure for the first time as the "double-blind test" (Greiner et al. 1950).
The phrase then evolved into its more appropriate and current form, without
quotation marks, as the *double-blind method or test* (Travell 1953; Greiner et al.
1959), the *double-blind technique or control* (Modell and Houde 1958), and *double-
blind designs* (Gold 1967a). The method has also been referred to in the literature
as the double-blind procedure, or simply as the double blind.

The available history suggests that the use of the double-blind technique was
independently arrived at by six individuals—Rivers and Hollingsworth, Sollmann, Bingel, Diehl, and Gold—who did not seem to be aware of the use of the
term by others and did not refer to each other. The use of quotation marks
around the phrase "blind test" suggests that it was being defined in a new or unusual way. However, the specific use of the same, somewhat unusual phrase, always in quotation marks, suggests that one of these researchers coined the term,
which then was quoted by others. Unless other historical details become available, the phrase *blind test* should be attributed to someone unknown or to Sollmann, who first used the term in 1917.

The associates of Gold who were interviewed at Cornell were unaware of any use either of the term *blind test* or of the method itself prior to its use in Gold's work. They believed that Gold had coined the phrase, had done the first blind study, was entirely responsible for the idea, and had not been influenced by anyone else (Modell 1967; Cattell 1969; Kwit 1969; Riker 1992). They all mentioned that interest in controlled clinical trials was in the air at the time, as was evident from the literature. Gold (1968) was unaware of the Rivers, Hollingsworth, Hewlett, and Bingel studies, or of any previous use of the term *blind test*. It seems reasonable to assume that Gold knew of Sollmann's ideas and the work of the Committee on Research—particularly because Robert Hatcher, chair of the Department of Pharmacology at Cornell University Medical College, was an original member of the committee and a friend of Sollmann and is likely to have influenced Gold. Cattell, however, described Hatcher as a laboratory pharmacologist who was not interested in methods of clinical trials and had no influence on Gold. Perhaps Gold was unaware of the previous ideas and studies because they had been published while he was a college student. Some support for this is apparent in Gold's paper (1930), in which he discussed scientific methods of conducting clinical trials without referring to blind methodology. It is more difficult to accept, however, that he was unaware of Sollmann's article on the blind test published in 1930. However, none of the individuals interviewed about the history of blind methodology—including Cattell, Modell, Kwit, Wolf, Riker, and others in the United States; Hill, Bull, and Laurence in England; and Pichot in France—knew of any of these studies. Moreover, they are not cited in the literature as far as we know.

Also relevant is Gold's use of the quoted phrase "blind test" in his 1935 ether study (Hediger and Gold 1935). This use of the term, exactly as it had been used previously, casually and without explanation, suggests that the term had been used by others. These subtle issues concerning the origin of the term might have been resolved had Gold been asked about them. Unfortunately, unaware of the issues when we interviewed him in the late 1960s, we failed to ask.

The Gold xanthine study began in 1932 and was published in 1937. Gold, Kwit, and Harold Otto, after their clinical work at the hospital, would meet to discuss the progress of the study. About halfway through the study, according to Kwit (1969), they "realized that blinding only the patient was not enough, that we could influence the patient's judgment by being more involved with and asking more 'leading questions' of patients on xanthine than those on placebo." They realized that it was necessary to eliminate the possibility that they were inducing more placebo effects in patients receiving xanthine, and that knowing which patients were on active medication and which were on placebo might influence their judgments about the response to treatment. The decision was made to have one physician administer medication but not be involved in judgments about the response to treatment, and to have other physicians rate improvement but be unaware of which medication patients were receiving. They called this procedure the "blind test."

As Kwit reminisced about the history, he seemed perplexed about how they decided to use such a strikingly descriptive term as *blind test*. He muttered, "Where did the idea come from?" After a minute or so, he exclaimed, "I know where we got it! It came from the 'Take the Blindfold Test' advertising campaign for Old Gold cigarettes. In this campaign, smokers were asked to compare Old Gold cigarettes with another brand while blindfolded—in other words, blind about which brand they were smoking. Our design was similar, except that patients were not blindfolded, so we called it the blind test" (Kwit 1969). This may be the first time that an advance in research methodology was creatively stimulated by an advertising slogan.

The Placebo and the Double Blind Become Companions

Interest in the placebo effect and the double-blind procedure increased in the late 1950s, resulting in an avalanche of meetings, symposia, papers, and books, and the elaboration of the methodology of clinical trials. Initially the emphasis was on the use of the double-blind procedure to minimize or provide a control for the placebo effect in clinical studies. Concern with the placebo effect itself was minimal. However, the focus shifted from methodology to the study of the placebo effect in the early 1950s. The study of the placebo effect and the development of the double-blind method took separate paths but continued to influence each other.

Stewart Wolf carried out important placebo studies in the 1950s. In his classic experiments on a patient named Tom, he demonstrated how placebos could reverse the pharmacological action of drugs and cause end organ changes (Wolf and Wolff 1947; Wolf 1950). Wolf noted that every medication given to Tom caused a physostigmine effect, which led him to use placebos in subsequent studies because the placebo effect could outweigh the ordinary effect of drugs. This was the first demonstration of the observable, measurable effect of placebos. Other papers provided documentation attesting that placebos could induce toxic effects (Wolf and Pinsky 1954) and that placebo effects were variable for individuals over time (Wolf et al. 1957). Many other papers were published on various aspects of the placebo effect and are summarized in Wolf's classic paper "The Pharmacology of Placebos" (1959b). Although Wolf did not use the double-blind procedure in these and other studies, his work had an important impact on the use of placebos and ultimately contributed to the expanded use of the double-blind method.

In 1955, Henry K. Beecher, an anesthesiologist at Harvard, reported that placebos have a high degree of therapeutic effectiveness in treating subjective responses. This effect was seen with a wide variety of symptoms, including wound pain, the pain of angina pectoris, headache, and nausea, indicating that placebo effects may have a fundamental mechanism in common and should be studied more closely. The importance that Beecher attributed to this phenomenon is reflected in the title of his important and very frequently cited paper "The Powerful Placebo" (Beecher 1955). This, and many other studies by Beecher and others which are summarized in his book *Measurement of Subjective Responses: Quantitative Effects of Drugs* (1959b), profoundly expanded knowledge of and stimulated study of the placebo effect and had a worldwide effect on the use of the double-blind method and the development of clinical trials.

Further awareness of these issues is evident in articles in *JAMA* on the use of statistics (Council on Pharmacy and Chemistry 1930a, 1930b) and on the placebo effect and the double-blind method (Hailman 1953); in the influential paper by Modell and Houde (1958) authorized by the Council on Drugs; in a report in the *Lancet* (Anonymous 1954) on the placebo effect; and even in the title of a novel, *The Double Blind* (Wilson 1960).

Papers on the placebo effect, the double-blind method, and controlled clinical trials increased noticeably after 1955; notable among these are papers by Walter Modell and Louis Lasagna, both pharmacologists, and the papers by many physicians in other specialties that are cited throughout this book. Interest continued to accelerate, as documented in the citation of 986 papers on the placebo effect in the English language from 1900 to 1978, most published since the 1950s (Turner et al. 1980).

The Double-Blind Method and Clinical Trials in Europe

The detailed history of the double-blind procedure in this chapter has focused largely on the development of the methodology in the United States. Controlled clinical trials and double-blind methodology developed and were used later in other countries (Modell 1962). There is a need for a more detailed study than we have attempted of the history of controlled clinical trials in Europe—particularly England, Sweden, France, and Germany.

Interest in the double-blind method and placebo controls was slow to develop in Great Britain. A symposium reviewing the progress in the past fifty years of medicine in the *British Medical Journal* (British Medical Association 1950) did not mention or cite the blind procedure or clinical trials and discussed statistical methods only briefly. In interviews, Hill (1970), Bull (1970), and Laurence (1970) agreed with this assessment. They were aware neither of the first double-blind study done by Rivers in 1908, although Rivers was English, nor of Gold's work or the literature on the double-blind method in the United States.

Bull, head of the Industrial Injuries and Burns Research Unit in Birmingham, published a very comprehensive review of the history of clinical trials (Bull 1959). Alive to the application of statistical methods in medicine, he selected the history of clinical trials as the subject for a thesis required by the Cambridge University medical school. Bull's thesis was completed in 1950 and approved in 1951, and a shortened version was published in 1959 (Bull 1959). The early history of clinical trials briefly sketched here is largely based on his work; for a more complete review of clinical trials over the past four thousand years, the reader is referred to his paper. Bull (1970) attributed his interest in clinical trials to several sources: his degree in experimental psychology and physiology from Cambridge, the influence of Sir Ronald Fisher's *Statistical Methods for Research Workers* (1926), and his experience with experiment-oriented teachers in medical school. The comprehensive and detailed history extended from about 2000 B.C. to about 1951. In this thesis, he noted that, although the principles of clinical trials were implied in the classical writings of Hippocrates, Celsus, Avicenna, Roger Bacon, Francis Bacon, and others, "there are very few records of tests of therapy until the last two centuries" (Bull 1959, 242). He speculated about the reasons for their absence: the reverence for authority, the relationship of physician and patient (ethical considerations, authoritarian attitudes on the part of the physician, and the inconvenience of time-consuming trials in a busy practice), the paucity of records (the recording and printing of scientific evidence is a recent development), the lack of facilities for investigations (inadequate hospitals, inaccurate diagnosis and assessment, insufficient numbers of similar cases for study), the belief in polypharmacy (which perpetuated ignorance), and most important, the lack of active remedies during this period. The situation began to change in the nineteenth century with the development of organic chemistry, biochemistry, bacteriology, and a more critical appraisal of treatment. Bull noted that "the years since 1935 [to 1950] have possibly seen more clinical trials than occurred in the whole of previous medical history," so much so that it is "not feasible to review even briefly all these therapeutic studies" (238).

Although Bull's review extended to 1950, it did not mention the placebo effect, although an awareness of the placebo effect is implied, nor did it refer to the double-blind method or its use in clinical trials, the double-blind studies by

Gold, or many of the controlled trials published in the United States. Bull (1970) explained that the term *placebo effect* was not used in England until some time after the publication of Beecher's work in the 1950s "and that the double-blind was only overtly discussed in the American literature . . . it being in its infancy in the research community at the time." Although aware of the procedure, he thought that it was "mostly used in fields other than clinical trials . . . more applicable to observer error in psychological experimentation." According to Bull, the development of clinical trials was stimulated after World War II by the need to evaluate many new compounds that had been formulated, and by the experience of many scientists and physicians assigned to study important problems associated with the conduct of the war, such as antimalarial prophylaxis, structure for shelters, diet, exposure to cold, casualty statistics, and blood transfusion. These studies had practical utility, and their results were considered very important. The techniques used to study these problems were brought back to the hospitals and medical facilities by these physicians after the war and influenced the subsequent conduct of clinical trials.

Sir Austin Bradford Hill was one of the great figures in the development of controlled clinical trials in Great Britain (Laurence 1970). He is often referred to as the "father of clinical trials" and was one of the pioneers in the use of statistical methods for clinical trials. Hill, seriously ill with tuberculosis for five years after World War I, could not attend medical school. Instead, he became an epidemiologist, worked in public health, and later became professor of medical statistics at the London School of Hygiene and Tropical Medicine and honorary director of the Medical Research Council's Statistical Research Unit. His interest in clinical trials was stimulated by his involvement in the Medical Research Council's Streptomycin in Tuberculosis Trials Committee (Medical Research Council 1948, 1950).

The history of the treatment of tuberculosis was similar to that of many other diseases, a record of many fruitless treatments, including such ineffective remedies as gold therapy, introduced in 1924 and still being used in 1944 (Hart 1946). Shortly after streptomycin was developed, Hill and his colleagues on the committee designed a sophisticated clinical trial to compare the results of treatment with streptomycin and the results of treatment with bed rest, which had been a standard treatment for tuberculosis for thirty years. Several factors might have contributed to Hill's interest in this study and in the design of this and other studies: his experience as a patient with tuberculosis provided clinical sensitivity to the design of studies, his epidemiological and public health background contributed a broad scope to his ideas, and his statistical background led to the use of controls and statistics. Hill was asked why placebo controls, blind treatment, and blind clinical evaluation were not used (Hill 1970). He responded that, although aware of the desirability of these methods, he felt that it would have been too great a hardship for sick tuberculosis patients to endure intramuscular placebo injections every six hours for four months. This methodological shortcoming was offset by assessing mortality and having the x-ray films read and radiological changes assessed by more than one person who was blind regarding the treatment groups to which the patient belonged (Hill 1952). The methodology used in this study set a new standard for clinical trials.

Hill also participated in the Medical Research Council's controlled antihistaminic trials for the common cold (Medical Research Special Committee 1950). The trials included a comparison of placebo with chlorocyclizine hydrochloride (Histantin) ($N = 16$), promethazine hydrochloride (Phenergan) ($N = 20$), and thonzylamine (Neohetrame or Anahist) ($N = 1,156$). Although this study was not described as a blind study, subjects and investigators were unaware of the random assignment to treatment with active drug or placebo control. The innovations used in the study were strict randomization, the use of an active placebo containing a small dose of phenobarbital to mimic the sedation effects of the antihistaminics in the first two studies, and the use of quinine to obscure the taste of the placebo in the third study. The results clearly showed that antihistaminics did not have any value for the common cold.

Hill knew and accepted the concept of blinding in the late 1940s. He said, "The blind was in but not referred to as the blind or the double-blind until later". He did not remember being influenced by anyone about the concept: "the idea was obvious." He was not aware of Gold's work or of the literature on blinding and had read very little about the placebo effect in England or the United States (Hill 1970).

When asked what factors contributed to the development of clinical trials in England, he identified three: (1) the streptomycin study, because it demonstrated efficiency of design, using few patients, careful clinical observation, objective evaluations, and statistics; (2) the proliferation of new drugs such as the sulfonamides, analgesics, corticoids, and others, whereas previously there had been few drugs to evaluate; and (3) the enormous amount of operational research done by physicians during World War II (Hill 1970). During wartime, many questions—the conditions under which soldiers and sailors could live, what kind of tank would increase survival, and so on—had been investigated using experimental designs. Such exposures to methods of experimental design contributed to the use of these methods in evaluating clinical problems.

Hill more specifically recommended that clinical judgments be made "without any possibility of bias. . . . In other words the assessment must whenever possible be 'blind'" (Hill 1952, 118). Later, the method was commonly referred to as the double blind (Hill 1970). The first step in clinical trial design, Hill noted, is random allocation; the second is assessment of therapeutic efficacy in such a way that the physician or rater is kept ignorant, or blind, about the group or treatment the patient was assigned to (Hill 1952). Hill emphasized randomization, replication, unbiased observation, and the use but not the tyranny of statistics, and discussed many other facets of controlled clinical trials. This emphasis amplified and extended Gold's focus on the double-blind method, calling attention to the placebo effect and other aspects of clinical trials.

The history of clinical trials in England recounted by both Hill and Bull suggests that the double-blind method was developed independently in England and the United States, although there may have been inapparent mutual influences. In England as in the United States—although according to Hill (1970) "the double-blind would go against the grain of most doctors"—double-blind methodology and controlled clinical trials were increasingly accepted and used after the 1950s.

There are interesting differences in the history of clinical trials in the United States and Great Britain before the middle of the 1950s. It is striking how authors in both countries did not refer to each other's work in published papers. The controlled studies by Gold and many other Americans were not referred to in the English literature, and the papers by Hill and others in England were not referred to in the American literature. The development of clinical trials in the United States initially focused on the double-blind method and the placebo effect, whereas in England the focus was on randomization, statistics, the use of an active placebo (e.g., phenobarbital in the study on the common cold), and other clinical design characteristics. Perhaps the difference in initial focus was related to British and American researchers' lack of information about other researchers' work (as reflected in the sparsity of references to other authors and studies in papers published before 1950), and to British and American chauvinistic proclivities.

The use of controlled clinical trials occurred much later in France. According to Paul Pichot (1970), professor of psychiatry at the Salpêtrière in Paris, medical opinion about the need for controlled studies changed in France in about 1965. Even as late as 1970, he recounted, there were very few controlled studies, since most French physicians knew nothing about statistics and were unable to use statistical methods. Indeed, most French physicians felt that it was unnatural to do such studies. However, once they had presented at an international meeting, they recognized that no one would take heed of their findings unless they used statistics. According to Pichot, the development of research methods was propelled by research on cancer (especially research on the relationship of smoking and cancer), research on heart disease, and rising medical costs. Placebos, he noted, were referred to as *johe,* a pill made from bread. Since 70 percent of the drugs dispensed to patients were considered placebos, this became a political issue and stimulated research.

Pichot's impressions were confirmed in a review by J. D. Guelfi and colleagues (1983) of 120 controlled psychotropic drug trials. Guelfi showed that placebos were rarely used in France before 1978. In fact, most French investigators were still suspicious about the practicality and ethics of using placebos. An indication that things were changing, however, is Kissel and Barrucand's *Placebos and Placebo Effect in Medicine* (1964), and later Pichot's edited volume *Psychological Measurement in Psychopharmacology* (1974).

According to Modell (1962), Pichot (1970), and our knowledge of the literature, the use of controlled studies came even later in most other European countries (except for Sweden, influenced by medical trends in Britain; and Germany, where Haas et al.'s paper "Das Placebo Problem" appeared in 1959) and elsewhere.

The Double Blind and Clinical Trials in Psychiatry and Psychology

The introduction of many new drugs to treat mental illness in the 1950s led to the development of clinical research methods in psychiatry and gave rise to the discipline of psychopharmacology. Two studies in psychiatry using double-blind methods were published in 1954 (the Weyburn chronic nucleotide project was reported in Clancy et al. 1954; the mephenesin project, in Hampson et al. 1954).

We learned about the background of the 1954 study by Clancy, Hoffer, Lucy, Osmond, Smythies, and Stefaniuk from Hoffer (1970b) and from correspondence in 1970 with Hoffer, Clancy, Osmond, and Fisher. The Mental Health Division of the Canadian Department of Health and Welfare had asked Hoffer and his group at the Saskatchewan Hospital to conduct a study of mixed nucleotides (adenylic acid, cytidylic acid, guanylic acid, and uridylic acid), which had been reported in an uncontrolled study as effective for the treatment of chronic schizophrenia. Funds for the study were provided, and James W. Fisher, a statistician from the Mental Health Division, in collaboration with other department colleagues, was responsible for the design and statistical analysis. The study was begun in late 1952 or early 1953. The design specified the testing of a priori hypotheses, random selection of patients, and random assignment of forty patients to daily treatment with identical-seeming intramuscular injections of nucleotide or placebo. Patients and evaluators were blind to allocation. However, in this otherwise well-designed study, drug allocation became apparent because the nucleotide injection was a thick liquid that caused pain, irritation, and occasionally pyrexia (Clancy et al. 1954; Osmond 1970). No significant improvement was reported for treatment with nucleotides. According to all informants, Fisher was mainly responsible for interesting the group in using blind evaluation, despite the participants' initial reservations. Fisher was "not aware of previously published double-blind studies being conducted in Canada. I was a protagonist of this approach in clinical trials . . . owing . . . to previous knowledge of placebo reactions, Beecher's work, and the need for devices to reduce errors in statistically designed studies" (Fisher 1970).

Hoffer (1970), on the basis of the 1953 publication of a very brief description of a study in the *Saskatchewan Psychiatric Journal* (McIlmoyl 1953), claimed precedence for conducting the first double-blind study in psychiatry. However, the report focused on some staff attitudes to the study, incidentally described the design, and did not present the results of the study. The definitive study, which in our opinion deserves priority, appeared in 1954 (Clancy et al. 1954).

Interestingly, the term *double blind* was not used in the nucleotide study. Hoffer (1970b) explained the omission: "Although we did not talk about placebo or double-blind procedures, you will notice that these were in fact what we were using." In a letter, James Fisher (1970) quoted Hoffer's written comments to him: "that we had not invented the idea, that in fact I [Hoffer] had not considered it such a substantial contribution, but that it had been advised that we follow it, and that you (Fisher) [the consultant on the study] had been the person mainly responsible for getting us interested in it."

Ironically, although Hoffer was eager to establish his priority for the first use of the double-blind procedure in psychiatry, he essentially rejected the use of the procedure afterward (Hoffer 1967; see response by Auerbach 1967; Sprott 1968).

We corresponded with Hampson, Rosenthal, and Frank, the researchers who conducted the mephenesin study (Hampson et al. 1954). John L. Hampson, who had a background in neurophysiology and biological research, was chief resident in psychiatry at the Johns Hopkins University School of Medicine and later became professor of psychiatry at the University of Washington (Hampson 1970). He became interested in mephenesin (Tolserol), a drug widely used in the early 1950s to treat many different psychiatric conditions, especially muscular tension and anxiety. He proposed a study of the effect of mephenesin on a mixed group of psychiatric outpatients to Jerome Frank, professor of psychiatry, and David Rosenthal, a psychologist at the Phipps Clinic who later became chief of the Laboratory of Psychology at the National Institutes of Health (Frank 1970; Rosenthal 1970). The study was well designed, well described, and well executed, especially when compared to studies done in the early 1950s. The study was started at the end of 1952 or early in 1953, submitted for publication in July 1954, and published in October 1954. It used a double-blind design, although the term *double blind* does not appear in the published paper. Both Hampson and Rosenthal, however, stated that they had been familiar with the concept of the double blind at the time. Frank and Hampson attributed the methodology and the double-blind design to Rosenthal, who said, "I don't know why we did not use the term double-blind, especially since it seems so obvious now. My psychological background in research has always emphasized that the investigators be blind so it was no big deal for me" (Rosenthal 1970).

The overall finding of the study was that patients had reduced symptoms on both placebo and mephenesin, which prompted the authors to discuss the placebo effect. The use of mephenesin rapidly declined, but mephenesin was replaced by its derivative, meprobamate (Miltown), which became the first massively used placebo drug for the treatment of anxiety.

Frank credited Rosenthal for stimulating him to think about the placebo effect of psychotherapy discussed in their classic paper "Psychotherapy and the Placebo Effect" (Rosenthal and Frank 1956). Frank subsequently published widely on the placebo effect of psychotherapy, writing numerous papers and three editions of an influential book, *Persuasion and Healing* (1961, 1973; Frank and Frank 1991).

With regard to the matter of priority for the first use of the double-blind method in psychiatry: although both papers were published in 1954, the Clancy et al. paper was published in July 1954—earlier than the Hampson et al. paper, which was published in October 1954. Both papers describe the double-blind procedure casually, without special comment or citation of previous literature, and do not refer to the procedure by its name. The use of the procedure was initiated by a statistician in the Clancy study and by a psychologist in the Hampson study, not by the psychiatrists associated with the studies.

Controlled studies, placebo controls, and double-blind methodology were infrequent in psychiatry and psychology during the 1950s. Clinical psychiatry and psychology were dominated by psychoanalytic philosophy and relied on anecdotal or case history reports to demonstrate the efficacy of psychoanalytic and psychotherapeutic treatment. The use of placebos in psychoanalytic treatment and research was summarily rejected, and the placebo effect was explained as transference.

The Influence of Psychopharmacology

Psychiatric drug treatment before the twentieth century was not specifically psychoactive. Treatment of mental disorders—essentially depletion with cathartics, diaphoretics, emetics, bloodletting, and dehydration, and the use of drugs such as mandrake, hellebore, belladonna, hyoscyamine, opium, alcohol, and cannabis—was largely similar to the treatment of other medical conditions. Also used were cocaine, chloroform, chloral hydrate, paraldehyde, bromides, barbiturates, and sleep therapy. Introduced in the 1930s were insulin coma therapy, camphor and then Metrazol shock therapy, insulin coma combined with ECT, carbon dioxide inhalation, antihistamines, histamine desensitization, continuous sleep treatment, narcotherapy, amphetamine (Benzedrine, or prophylhexedrine), methamphetamine shock, phenacemide (Phenurone), adrenalin desensitization, atropine toxicity treatment, hydrotherapy, continuous tub, cold pack, and prefrontal lobotomy; some of these were still in use until about 1960. The paucity of effective treatments in psychiatry before 1959 is illustrated in the treatment sections of commonly used psychiatric texts.[3]

It is likely that most of the treatments referred to in the three major psychiatric texts were ineffective and often harmful, and that their therapeutic benefits can be ascribed to the placebo effect. The few exceptions were ECT for depression; possibly lobotomy for obsessive-compulsive disorder; amphetamines for attention deficit hyperactivity disorder, narcolepsy, and short-term treatment of depression; and lithium for manic-depressive disorder.

Up to about 1953, the prospects for biological research were not auspicious. Clinicians had few effective somatic treatments. Researchers did not have promising new drugs for study. Psychoanalysis and insight-oriented or psycho-

---

3. *Modern Clinical Psychiatry,* by Noyes (1948), describes only twelve treatments then in common use: insulin shock treatment, combined insulin-convulsive therapy, Metrazol convulsive therapy, electric convulsive therapy, prefrontal lobotomy, Meyerian psychobiology, Freudian psychoanalysis, hypnoanalysis, narcoanalysis, hypnosis, supportive psychotherapy, and mental catharsis. Kalinowsky and Hoch, in *Shock Treatments, Psychosurgery, and Other Somatic Treatments* (1952), highlighted the effectiveness of the treatments on which their text focused: shock, psychosurgery, and insulin coma therapy. An indication that similar treatments were being used in Great Britain is provided by the Sargant and Slater text *An Introduction to Physical Methods of Treatment in Psychiatry* (1956). Somatic treatment had not changed very much by 1959, except for the addition of several nonbarbiturate sedatives, rauwolfia, and chlorpromazine, as indicated in *The American Handbook of Psychiatry,* volumes 1 and 2, by Arieti (1959). None of these books discusses the placebo effect or the double-blind procedure.

dynamic psychotherapy became the predominant orientation in the 1950s, with competition from social or community psychiatry toward the end of the 1950s. Biological psychiatry was in the doldrums. This therapeutic vacuum might have contributed to the enthusiasm for the study and use of psychoanalytic and other psychological and social methods of treatment.

The introduction of chlorpromazine and rauwolfia at about the same time had a dramatic effect on biologically oriented psychiatrists. As a medical student before and after the introduction of chlorpromazine, I (AKS) observed, as did others, the transformation of large hospital wards from literal madhouses to reasonable domiciliary wards. This change stimulated optimism and unleashed creative energy and led to the new discipline of psychopharmacology.

Although the term *psychopharmacology* was used by Macht et al. (1920) and in psychiatry by Thorner (1935) (see Caldwell 1970 for a history of psychopharmacology), it was not used in American psychiatry until after introduction of chlorpromazine (Thorazine) in 1952 (Caldwell 1970) and rauwolfia (reserpine) in 1954 (Miner 1955; Kline 1956). A year later, meprobamate (Miltown) was marketed; it rapidly became the first antianxiety panacea, and the first of many antianxiety drugs to be subsequently evaluated as a fashionable placebo (Shapiro 1976).

Others soon followed. By 1956, forty antipsychotic and antianxiety drugs, seven stimulants, and eighteen hallucinogens had come and gone (Caldwell 1970). The number of psychotropic drugs continued to increase dramatically, as indicated in the 1967 listing of 690 psychotropic drugs by the Psychopharmacology Research Branch of the National Institute of Mental Health (Usdin and Efron 1967); this list had swelled to 1,555 references by 1972 (Usdin and Efron 1972). Some of the major drugs in use by 1964 are described by Shapiro (1964e, 1964g).

A flurry of publications explored many different facets of the new drugs. Although the double-blind procedure was recommended by many researchers in the 1950s (Hailman 1953; Lasagna et al. 1954; Lasagna 1955; Beecher 1955, 1957; Palmer 1955; Fischer and Dlin 1956; Pfeiffer 1957; Mason-Browne et al. 1957; Rosenthal 1966), others had little interest in or appreciation of the placebo effect and the use of the double-blind procedure to control it.[4]

---

4. The books demonstrating indifference to the placebo effect and the double-blind procedure usually are collections of papers presented at symposia. For example, neither the placebo effect nor the double-blind procedure is discussed in *Psychiatric Research Reports of the American Psychiatric Association: An Evaluation of the Newer Psychopharmacologic Agents and Their Role in the Current Psychiatric Practice* (APA 1956); *Chlorpromazine and Mental Health* (1955); *Psychotherapeutic Drugs* (Welsh 1958); *Psychopharmacology* (Kline 1956); *Psychopharmacology Frontiers* (Kline 1959); *Psychochemotherapy: The Physician's Manual* (Remmen et al. 1962).

Interest in the placebo effect and use of the double blind in clinical trials finally began a dramatic increase in about 1959, when interest in the methodology of evaluating treatment and the conduct of clinical trials was stimulated by symposia and new drug studies. Investigators soon became cognizant of the placebo effect and the necessity of using the double-blind procedure. Many studies of the placebo effect were done, and many presented data demonstrating the need for the use of the double-blind procedure. Most investigators actively involved in studying the new psychopharmacological drugs readily accepted the concept of the double blind, recommended its use, and used it in their studies. This is demonstrated in the flurry of papers, symposia, and books that began in the late 1950s (the books include Kline 1956, 1959; Beecher 1959b; Featherstone and Simon 1959; Reznikoff and Toomey 1959; Waife and Shapiro 1959; Uhr and Miller 1960; Frank 1961, 1973, 1991; Hamilton 1961, 1974; Rinkel 1963; Kissel and Barrucand 1964; Rickels 1968; May and Wittenborn 1969; Clark and Guidice 1970; Levine et al. 1971; the papers include Lasagna et al. 1954; DeMaar and Pelikan 1955; Koteen 1957; Sainz et al. 1957; Freyhen 1958; Koelle 1958; Sleisenger 1958). It is also reflected in the proliferation of papers on the placebo effect: eight prior to 1949, forty-six between 1950 and 1957 (Shapiro 1960a), and almost one thousand by 1980 (Turner et al. 1980). These developments parallel the slow but increasing acceptance of the double-blind procedure (*Lancet* 1954). However, other physicians and investigators opposed the use of the double-blind method, feeling that it was less reliable than a clinical appraisal, added little information, could be dangerous, generally was unnecessary for the evaluation of drugs, was indicated only in specific situations, and so on (Batterman, 1955; Pfeiffer 1957; Tomenius 1958; Anonymous 1964c; Reinharez 1978).

From this review of the literature, it appears that major changes in attitude were taking place in medicine. Not obvious from the published record, however, is the fact that interest in the placebo effect, controlled clinical trials, and use of the double blind was confined to a small group of data-oriented researchers who lived under the usual academic pressure to publish or perish. The majority of other physicians, clinical internists, surgeons, and psychiatrists were more concerned with private practice than with publishing and were unaware of these developments. In fact, they thought them to be unimportant or unnecessary, or believed that these innovations would interfere with treatment and objective evaluation. These attitudes are less apparent in the published literature than in opinions expressed informally and at meetings by many physicians. An indication of this undercurrent is the perplexity expressed by Gold: "I am not sure why it is that the use of a placebo is considered by many physicians objectionable as a method of clinical evaluation and why there seems to be so much resistance to the idea that the experimenting doctor and the patient should remain in the dark about the identity of the agent until the comparison is finished" (1954, 724). The persistent resistance to controlled studies is also revealed by Jerome Levine's reaction to comments solicited about the comprehensive and important work *Principles and Problems in Establishing the Efficacy of Psychotropic Agents* (Levine et al. 1971). Some "were hostile and paranoid" (Levine et al. 1971).

These different theoretical orientations continued over the next fifteen to twenty years, only to dissolve slowly as the use of double-blind methodology increased in published studies, was deemed necessary for publication in peer-reviewed journals, was endorsed by important journals, and became the required methodology for grants and approval of new drugs by the FDA.

A review of the literature beginning in the late 1950s and continuing to the present reveals that psychiatrists, and later, psychologists, were the major contributors to further refinements in methods for conducting clinical trials. Some of the obvious factors related to their ascendancy include problems regarding how to evaluate new drugs and the psychological therapies, psychiatrists' interest in psychological factors of experimentation, and governmental agencies' and pharmaceutical companies' extensive financial support of research.

The Influence of Psychology

Psychologists should have been the first contributors to the methodology of controlled clinical trials and the double-blind method because of their greater awareness of the influence of subject and examiner variables on responses and the need to control these effects. Ironically, they were among the last. The first uses of control groups in psychological studies were by Edward L. Thorndike and R. S. Woodworth (1901) and by W.H.R. Rivers (1908). However, these were isolated studies, and as Edwin G. Boring's (1954) review of psychological research shows, it was many years before most studies used controls. In 1916, none of the articles published in the *Journal of Experimental Psychology* used controls; in 1933, 11 percent used them; and as late as 1951, only 52 percent did so.

Psychologists were also latecomers to the double-blind method. Although the double-blind procedure was first developed in psychophysiological studies by Rivers (1908) and Hollingsworth (1912), these studies are not referred to by Solomon (1949) and Boring (1954) and are not cited thereafter in the medical or psychological literature. Pharmacologists clearly were the first to recommend and use blinding. Sollmann strongly recommended its use in papers written from 1913 to 1930, although only one double-blind study (Hewlett 1913) was published under the aegis of the AMA Committee on Research. Three double-blind studies appear to be separate developments: the study by Adolf Bingel (1918) in Germany, those by Diehl (1933, 1935; Cowen et al. 1942) in the United States, and the study by E. Elovainio and Gustaf Ostling (1948) in Finland. Credit for the major contribution to the development of controlled clinical trials and the double-blind procedure clearly goes to Gold, who, as we have shown, described the procedure extensively, added refinements to the method, and published many double-blind studies between 1934 and 1957. Psychiatrists followed soon thereafter, and psychologists were the last group to become aware of and use the double-blind method. It should have been the other way around. Although the second double-blind study in psychiatry (Hampson et al. 1954) was designed by a psychologist (Rosenthal), most psychologists, except for those involved in clinical studies—primarily of psychotropic drugs—had little knowledge of the double-blind procedure and used the method infrequently until well after its use was accepted in medicine and psychiatry. Once involved, however, psychologists brought their special training and competence to the conduct of studies and creatively contributed to further refinement of the controlled clinical trial and the double-blind method. They published numerous studies and papers on the methodology of clinical trials, the placebo effect, and the double blind. Psychologists, whose training is much more thoroughly grounded in the details of psychological experimentation and the statistical analysis of data, contributed substantial refinements such as careful description of independent and dependent variables, methods of data reduction, the use of factor analysis, evaluation of the reliability and validity of variables, power analysis, multiple regression, and most recently, meta-analysis.[5]

Psychologists also contributed indirectly, but by no means unimportantly, to the development of clinical trials by calling attention to specific psychological variables that often influence psychological studies.[6] And especially as statistical methods became more powerful and complicated and computer use became widespread, statisticians became essential collaborators (Beecher 1957).

5. Some of the many psychologists who contributed over many years to the methodology of clinical trials, the placebo effect, and the double-blind include R. Lipman, S. Fisher, D. McNair, E. Nash, S. Imber, R. Downing, F. Evans, M. Rosenthal, M. Orne, X. Barber, G. Honigfeld, and M. Jospe.

6. These include ascertainment bias (Berkson 1946; Cohen and Cohen 1984); demand characteristics (Orne 1962); experimenter effects (Rosenthal 1966); expectations (Goldstein 1962; Evans 1985); the volunteer subject (Rosenthal and Rosnow 1975); therapeutic suggestibility and psychotherapy (Calestro 1972); the placebo effect (Jospe 1978; Ross and Buckalew 1985; White et al. 1985); and also the possible mechanisms to explain placebo response: endogenous opioids and placebo analgesia (Levine et al. 1978).

The methodology of clinical trials was further enriched by the interaction among pharmacologists, internists, psychiatrists, statisticians, psychologists, and members of governmental agencies and industry in meetings and symposia, through publication of their proceedings, and through collaborative studies. This allowed an exchange of concepts, ideas, and techniques among the specialties which otherwise might have been unavailable if each had worked in isolation. The introduction of cooperative clinical trials or multi-institutional therapeutic studies in Great Britain and the United States provided further stimulus. The history of clinical trials, described by Harry M. Marks (1988), began with the study of syphilis treatment from 1928 to 1935, followed by studies of penicillin initiated during World War II, and studies of streptomycin treatment of tuberculosis in the United States and Great Britain after World War II. The convening of panels of experts in various specialties, and the problems encountered in conducting useful and reliable trials, helped stimulate the development and use of procedures such as randomization, standardized outcome measures, controls, statistics, and other methodological safeguards. The airing of the deliberations and results in publications, the ability to obtain fast and reliable results, and the feasibility of such studies increased clinicians' and researchers' awareness of the need for carefully controlled clinical studies. Although the use of cooperative, multi-institutional studies evolved slowly, the last twenty years have witnessed an increase in their use and in their success.

Critique of the Double-Blind Procedure

The number of drugs and treatments in all branches of medicine, and the number of papers on the placebo effect and the methodology of clinical trials, have escalated since the 1950s. Researchers were the first to use the double-blind procedure in the mid-1950s. Use of the procedure increased over time as governmental agencies required that it be used in clinical studies. However, as more and more published papers extolled the virtues of the double blind, others appeared critical of and rejected its use methodologically and ethically.

Clinicians attacked the new methods of conducting clinical trials as inhumane, contending that they sought to replace humanism with mathematical formulas. They feared that this could lead to the physician's shirking the responsibility to return the patient to health. Among those responding to the criticism was Hill, who noted that sound statistical methods are necessary to determine whether a particular treatment is helpful to patients. He quoted an editorial in the *British Medical Journal* with which he concurred: "In treating patients with unproved remedies we are, whether we like it or not, experimenting on human beings, and a good experiment well reported may be more ethical and entail less shirking of duty than a poor one" (Hill 1952, 118).

The initial criticism tended to reject the use of the double blind outright. Interestingly, some former proponents of the double blind later challenged its use. For example, Batterman (1955, 1547) commented "that data from placebo trials may be misleading" and that enthusiastically endorsed artificial experimental procedures are "rarely confirmed when tested by the general practitioner. . . . Since the bulk of therapy depends on him, testing of drugs should follow conditions he will encounter in treating the average patient." Batterman, who claimed to have used the double-blind technique for eighteen years (although to our knowledge no studies of his have been published), stated that if the double-blind method was used to evaluate an effective accepted drug, an unknown drug, or a placebo, it was impossible to distinguish in terms of effectiveness or action the three types of medication under investigation. Oddly, Batterman did not consider the possibility that the results of the double-blind procedure were valid (i.e., that the two active drugs were not significantly better than placebo).

Hoffer, one of the first psychiatrists to participate in a double-blind study, advanced several arguments against the use of the double-blind method (Hoffer 1967). He noted, for example, that this method makes no allowance for the heterogeneity of the psychiatric population, and that an essential element of the physician–patient relationship (the physician and patient's faith and trust in each other) is violated by the double blind and negates the placebo effect. A. Auerbach, refuting Hoffer's arguments, stressed the importance of the double blind: "Without the double-blind or preferably the triple-blind control in tests of the efficacy of medical and especially psychiatric treatment, results may be attributed to the effects of experimenter bias and subject expectation" (1967, 1482). Nevertheless, Auerbach raised two ethical problems related to double-blind methodology: namely, the question of whether inert material should be administered to seriously ill medical patients, and the need for obtaining informed consent from patients.

Other physicians objected to the double-blind method, believing that it deprived them of information required to make informed judgments, that it was an intrusion on medical practice, and that it was unethical because it deprived patients of treatment with active medication (Nash 1962). Still others cited the possible influence of patient participation on the outcome of a study. For example, a change in the behavior of the control group (such as altering their diet or life style) can affect outcome, especially if the randomization of patients is to a no-intervention group. In the Multiple Risk Factor Intervention Trial, investigators failed to find significant differences in cardiovascular death rates favoring the intervention group. They suspected that patients in the no-intervention group had altered their behavior to lower their risk for cardiovascular mortality (Kramer and Shapiro 1984). John Tomenius (1958, quoted by Sleisenger [1958, 416]) objected to the double-blind study because "the patient's faith in the drug or the prescribing doctor was strong enough to render even a completely inactive placebo abnormally effective." In contrast, Marvin H. Sleisenger came to the opposite conclusion, that the example "eloquently justifies the need for the double-blind procedure for evaluation of the test agents" (Sleisenger 1958, 416). An editorial in *Medical Science* (Anonymous 1964a) described double-blind studies as yielding only minimal information, since the expense of such studies precludes adequate selection of homogeneous subjects, sufficiently detailed observation, and sufficient duration of observation. W. J. Guy and colleagues (1967) recommended that improvement be evaluated by a blinded, independent trained assessment team instead of the treating clinician. Albert Kligman (1973) characterized double-blind studies as "the blind leading the blind," impairing clinical evaluation by locking the investigator into a fixed dosage regimen (although the double blind can be used with a titrated flexible dosage); he asserted that side effects of the active drug always break the double-blind code and stated further that "in the end, efficiency studies stand or fall on the perspicacity of clinicians." Morris Weinberger (1973) expressed reservations about a proposal made by Robert Elashoff, a statistician, that pathology slides be evaluated blindly. Fears and Schneiderman (1974) disagreed with Weinberger. They believed (and we agree) that blind technique helps reduce bias and that all evaluation, whether of judgments or even of laboratory studies, including the statistical analysis by the statistician, should be done blind, to ensure that all potential variables except for the specific effect being tested are identical in all groups.

With increased acceptance of the double blind and the principles of the controlled clinical trial, papers veered away from rejection to discussions of ways to improve the double-blind procedure. Modell and Houde (1958) cautioned that the double-blind method was in fact no guarantee of the reliability of the data and that other factors in the clinical evaluation of drugs could influence the data, and pointed out that the use of the double-blind technique will not validate otherwise poorly designed experiments but in fact may lead to a false-negative interpretation.

Other investigators have recommended the use of the "triple-blind" procedure (a title more euphemistic than descriptive). This method has been used in two ways. Some investigators have attempted to exclude or minimize placebo effects by conducting a preliminary study with placebos. Placebo reactors are then excluded from the definitive study that follows. But placebo effects may occur in as high a percentage of cases in the definitive study as in the preliminary study. A second use of the term *triple-blind* refers to blindness about the design of the study: only investigators who do not treat patients or evaluate outcome are aware of the design, or investigators are not informed of the name of the active drug or of its probable effects. Another suggestion is that the medication or placebo be given in food or fluids, so that all participants in the drug study are unaware that a medication has been administered (Wilkins 1985). Paul Hoch (1956), somewhat earlier, described the ideal experimental setting in similar terms. L. Tetreault and J. M. Bordeleau (1971) extolled the usefulness of the placebo and double-blind techniques for obtaining objective conclusions in clinical psychopharmacology but felt that a policy of using a placebo at all costs is an exaggerated policy. The researcher should determine when a placebo is called for and whether it is ethically acceptable to use one. Many articles have addressed some of the potential bias that may be inherent in controlled trials. Steven M. Zifferblatt and Curtis S. Wilbur (1978) discussed some of the psychological factors operating on both patients and physicians participating in controlled studies. G. Rose (1982) discussed the bias that is possible unless certain basic rules and procedures are observed. Michael S. Kramer and Stanley H. Shapiro (1984) critically reappraised some of the scientific issues involved in the controlled clinical trial.

Another criticism of the double-blind procedure has been that it is possible for both the physician and the patient to break the blind. In particular, many investigators question whether the double-blind procedure is truly blind. Many early papers on the double blind noted that active drug and placebos could be differentiated because of different physical characteristics, taste, dissolubility, and so forth, and because of the telltale side effects of active drugs (Rivers 1908; Gold et al. 1937; Lasagna 1955; Palmer 1955; Fischer and Dlin 1956; Mason-Browne and Borthwick 1957). The extent of this concern is illustrated by the publication of twenty-seven papers on this issue. These studies, including three of our own, are discussed extensively in chapter 9, and recommendations are proposed for improving double-blind studies. Also discussed is the failure of most studies to match active and placebo agents adequately.

A personal experience illustrates the change in attitude about the use of methodology, statistics, the double-blind procedure, and the controlled clinical trial, and their eventual acceptance. As part of my academic responsibilities, beginning in 1960 I (AKS) gave yearly lectures to residents, medical students, and medical staff, as well as many invited lectures at other institutions, about the placebo effect, double-blind methodology, and the evaluation of psychotropic drugs and other psychiatric and medical therapies. These included two hour-long lectures about the placebo effect and the advantages and necessity of using the double-blind procedure in studies. During my lecture to residents on the double blind in 1975, I detected perplexity and restlessness among some of them. I asked what was wrong and was surprised, as well as pleased, to hear that they had never thought there was any other way of doing a study and wondered why so much time had been spent trying to convince them about what they already knew.

By 1975, the vehement and acrimonious debate about these issues had begun to abate. One could discern a beneficial effect on research from the use of controlled methodology. With the use of placebo controls, the primary function of research became the detection of change in efficacy. To facilitate this, more accurate diagnostic and research criteria for disorders were developed, as were sophisticated statistical methods for analysis of data, and multiple rating scales and checklists to ensure the reliability of variables reflecting improvement.

The Food and Drug Administration and the Double Blind

The FDA's recommendations about using stringent methodology and the double blind lagged behind the use of these procedures in medicine. Once established, however, the FDA policies strongly influenced how studies of drugs were done, with ripple effects influencing studies of psychotherapy, surgery, instruments, and all other therapies.

The emphasis of the 1906 Food and Drug Act was on measures to ensure the purity of foods, and although drugs were placed under federal control, the act had little effect on drugs. In 1938, drug manufacturers were required to conduct tests to ensure the safety of drugs before marketing. The Kefauver-Harris Amendment in 1962 required the sponsor of a new drug to submit "adequate and well controlled experiments by experts qualified by scientific training and experience to evaluate the effectiveness of the drug involved." However, the principles and procedures for an adequate study were not defined or implemented, although by this time researchers routinely evaluated drug efficacy using developing methodology and the double blind. The shift to more specific criteria and guidelines is indicated by "Guidelines for Psychotropic Drugs," a 1974 publication by the FDA in conjunction with the American College of Neuropsychopharmacology. In 1978 another set of guidelines was published by the FDA: "Guidelines for the Clinical Evaluation of Psychotropic Drugs: Antidepressants and Antianxiety Drugs," which called for controlled studies and mandated the use of placebo controls.

The FDA's criteria for an adequate study became more rigorous about 1978, requiring that studies be done so as to minimize bias; the double blind could be used but was not required. The term *minimize bias* was used to accommodate studies that could be done only using historic controls such as the numbers of deaths and permanent disability endpoints. However, double-blind studies were increasingly recommended by the FDA beginning in about 1975, and by about 1980, use of the double blind in studies was essentially required to satisfy the criterion of minimizing bias. Applications for FDA approval of new drugs, with rare exceptions, now require studies using the double-blind method as well as randomization and other methodological safeguards.

Papers criticizing the use of the double blind gradually decreased in number, and virtually disappeared after about 1980. Since that time, unless there was some good reason for doing otherwise, the use of the double-blind procedure has been required for those seeking grants to support studies evaluating treatment; FDA approval of new drugs; and acceptance of papers for publication by academic journals.

Thus, although the FDA lagged behind methodological developments that were apparent perhaps twenty years earlier, its imprimatur, once it had been granted, essentially resolved all controversy about the necessity of using carefully controlled methodology, which includes the use of the double-blind procedure for evaluating the effectiveness of medical and psychological treatment. This is illustrated by the work of a large group of distinguished investigators and the publication of an important book, *Principles and Problems in Establishing the Efficacy of Psychotropic Drugs* (Levine et al. 1971). Its importance was underscored by the fact that it was a joint publication of the Psychopharmacology Research Branch of the National Institutes of Health, the Public Health Service, the U.S. Department of Health, Education, and Welfare, the Health Services and Mental Health Administration, the American College of Neuropsychopharmacology, and the Government-Industry Liaison Committee. This multiauthored volume, written by experts who were at the cutting edge of clinical psychopharmacological research, comprehensively discussed state-of-the-art methodological principles, many of which are still current, and strongly recommended the use of the double-blind procedure. Grants for the study of psychotropic drugs now increasingly required the use of the double-blind procedure, and this requirement then spread to most grants for the study of any type of treatment.

Conclusion

Improved methodology served as a buffer against the placebo effect and improved the sensitivity of research in general. However, it also began to stimulate concern about the ethics of using control groups and placebos.

Despite its potential limitations, however, the double-blind procedure is an indispensable tool to control for bias. A biased experiment cannot establish the effectiveness of a new treatment. Whatever the faults and limitations of the controlled experiment, it should not be abandoned; rather, the design and methodology should be improved.

chapter eight

Ethical Controversies about the Use of Placebos, the Double Blind, and Controlled Clinical Trials

Early Ethical Attitudes

Ethical concerns about the use of placebos are implicit in the early and frequently repeated definition of placebo: "I will please, an epithet given to any medication adopted more to please than benefit the patient" (Fox 1803). Robert Cabot was one of the first to refer to placebos as the use of "methylene blue . . . bread pills, subcutaneous injections of a few drops of water (supposed by the patient to be morphine), and other devices for acting upon a patient's symptoms through his mind" (1915, 158). Although Cabot had used placebos "pretty often" in the past, he realized, after a patient caught him substituting water for a morphine injection, that placebos worked only if deception was used and the physician misled the patient. Cabot emphasized the harm to the patient-physician relationship if the physician was discovered using placebos; he advocated avoiding falsehoods, lies, and deception, and recommended telling patients the truth about their diagnosis, prognosis, and treatment, even if it took more time. His injunction about the use of placebos is not absolute, however. Although he stated that "no patient whose language we can speak, whose mind we can approach, needs a placebo," he still gave "placebos now and then (I used to give them by the bushel) to Armenians, Greeks, and others with whom I cannot communicate, because to refuse to give them would then create more misunderstanding, a falser impression, than to give them. If I give nothing at all the patient will think I am refusing to treat him at all" (168).

Very little was published about the ethics of using placebos during the ensuing fifty years, except, you will recall, that clinicians considered *placebo* an objectionable term and rejected the use of placebos. As interest in the placebo effect and recognition of the usefulness of placebos in treatment, the double-blind procedure, and clinical trials greatly increased during the 1950s and 1960s, discussion ensued in the literature about the ethics of using placebos. However, the papers were not systematic or scholarly and were largely confined to brief, anecdotal, clinical impressions and comments in papers usually devoted to other aspects of placebos. An unsystematic review of the literature during this period revealed attitudes varying from enthusiastic endorsement to rejection of placebos; many authors expressed reservations about their use.

We analyzed attitudes about the use of placebos in the published literature up to 1958 by twenty-three nonpsychiatrists and sixteen psychiatrists (Shapiro 1960a). There were many divergent, strongly held views, and the attitudes of psychiatrists differed from those of nonpsychiatrists. The attitudes of nonpsychiatrists were randomly distributed between the extremes (wholehearted endorsement or rejection of placebo use), with the majority having neutral attitudes. Psychiatrists, in contrast, were markedly against the use of placebos, regarding their use as poor medicine, inexcusable, and unethical.

Several explanations for these differences of opinion are possible. Nonpsychiatrists had greater skepticism about psychiatric treatment, tended to substitute nonspecific placebo treatment (inactive or active placebos) for psychotherapy, were experienced in the successful use of placebos, and were not defensive about acknowledging the nonspecificity of their treatment. Psychiatrists, however, believed that psychotherapy was a specific and nonplacebo therapy. Supportive, hypnotic, drug, placebo, and other therapies were derogated as inadequate substitutes for psychotherapy. Psychiatrists believed that psychotherapy was specific and that it was not a placebo treatment, excluded it from the definition of placebo, and claimed, therefore, that they did not use placebos.

Similar attitudes and ideas were expressed again and again in discussions with colleagues and during many of my (AKS's) lectures on the history of the placebo effect. For example, Milton Rosenbaum, chair of the Department of Psychiatry at Albert Einstein College of Medicine in 1958, commented during one of my talks, "No one in this department can use placebos; if you have to give something, give nicotinic acid because it causes a physiologic flushed feeling." In 1969, Oskar Diethelm said that placebos were never used at the Payne Whitney Psychiatric Clinic during his chairmanship from the early 1930s to early 1960s, despite the fact that since the majority of the treatments used during this period were ineffective, they were, in fact, placebo treatments.

It was predictable that in the discussions after my (AKS) lectures, psychotherapeutically oriented psychiatrists would disdainfully refer to many of the treatments used by biologically oriented psychiatrists (such as minor and major tranquilizers, ECT and ICT) as placebos. When challenged about the possibility that psychotherapy was a placebo, they disagreed, commenting that psychotherapy is specific and is effective, by getting to the underlying causes, using the scientific principles underlying blind use of the placebo. Psychotherapy, they asserted, cannot be a placebo because a placebo is defined as a drug; and so on. Such reactions were not limited to psychotherapists but were also made by biologically oriented psychiatrists. The principle underlying the reactions of both groups was identical, although the content changed. At first the biological group humorously derogated psychotherapy as a placebo. But when asked about the possibility that insulin coma therapy (ICT), electroconvulsive therapy (ECT), Sedac (a form of ECT), and minor tranquilizers (such as meprobamate [Miltown], chlordiazepoxide [Librium], and nonbarbiturate hypnotics) were placebos, their response was similar to that of the psychotherapeutic group, namely, that these treatments do something physiologically and are not inert like psychotherapy; and since the placebo is defined as inert, biological treatments cannot be placebos. Incredibly, these ostrich-like (head-in-the-sand) responses occurred at every lecture. Even after I related to each group how they were characterized by the other group, their opinions did not change.

We were impressed with these differences in opinion and curious about what factors related to the way in which physicians in various specialties define the placebo. We designed several studies to review physicians' attitudes and ethics about the use of placebos and the way in which they define the placebo (Shapiro and Streuning 1973a, 1973b, 1974). Questionnaires—containing twenty-two statements about the definition of the placebo, the ethics and attitudes of using placebos, feelings and biases about placebos, and attitudes toward controlled studies and the double-blind procedure—were sent to 240 physicians in seven clinical specialties who were clinicians or researchers. The response rate was 82.9 percent (i.e., 199 physicians returned usable questionnaires). The sample, collected in 1962–63, was composed of 240 physicians (81% of the physicians known to us at the Massachusetts Mental Health Center, the Albert Einstein College of Medicine, the Montefiore Medical Center, and the New York University Medical School).

As hypothesized, the results suggest that critical ethical attitudes characterize physicians who are older (older physicians are linked to older ideas, while younger physicians are more apt to absorb new ideas about placebos), who do more private practice and less research activity (i.e., who have a vested interest in maintaining the stability of private practice and rejecting concepts or procedures that may interfere with it, and who are less aware of and interested in new, evolving methods of conducting clinical trials), who have a more restricted definition of placebo (the older definition supports the stability of private practice, which may be threatened by an extended definition), and who estimate that they themselves make less use of placebos than do other physicians (i.e., who have an exaggerated belief in the effectiveness of therapy by private practitioners). By contrast younger physicians have more tolerant ethical attitudes because they have been exposed to new ideas by their education, are not financially dependent on private practice, spend less time in private practice, and possibly have a vested interest in research, which is necessary for academic advancement. A still more parsimonious interpretation of these results is that demographic, professional, economic, social, and other variables may strongly determine or influence ethical ideas, attitudes, and principles.

The Growth of Ethical Principles Governing Clinical Research

With growing acceptance of randomization, placebo controls, the double-blind procedure, and controlled clinical trials, the importance of principles governing the avoidance of deception, the obtaining of full and adequate informed consent, and the protection of patient autonomy increased. The need to formulate ethical guidelines for clinical research was initially raised in the 1960s by Sir Austin Bradford Hill and Henry Beecher, two individuals who contributed most to the development and adoption of controlled clinical trials. Their stellar reputations lent credibility to the significance of this issue.

Hill's contribution to the introduction of controlled clinical trials is universally acknowledged (Silverman and Chalmers 1992). Hill, an epidemiologist and statistician, was firmly committed to using placebos, the double-blind method, and controlled clinical trials when necessary. He stated, "It may well be unethical . . . not to institute a proper trial" (1951, 11). Witts, a participant in the conference of the Council for International Organization of Medical Scientists, commented, "Placebos rarely cause any ethical misgivings. . . . As we start with the premise that the value of the remedy or its superiority over its counterpart is in dispute, it is difficult to see that there is any ethical or legal dilemma" (1960, 11). At the same time, Hill (1970) expressed concern about the welfare of patients who participated in trials. His personal experience of being a patient (described in chapter 7) may have increased his sensitivity to ethical issues in clinical trials. Certainly it contributed to his decision to compromise the design of the 1948 streptomycin tuberculosis study (Medical Research Council 1948, 1950) by not subjecting severely ill control patients to multiple daily placebo injections. He felt that "it must be possible ethically to give every patient admitted to a trial any of the treatments involved," and "that if the doctor does not believe that, if he thinks even in the absence of any evidence that for the patient's benefit he ought to give one treatment rather than another, then that patient should not be admitted to the trial. Only if, in his state of ignorance, he believes the treatment given to be a matter of indifference can he accept a random distribution of the patients to the different groups. . . . The ethical obligation always and entirely outweighs the experimental" (Hill 1963, 1047).

Beecher documented examples of unethical behavior by investigators involved in clinical trials and called for ethical guidelines. This paper was considered so important that it was adopted by the Committee on Research of the Council on Drugs and published in *JAMA* (Beecher 1959a). After briefly reviewing the history of experimentation, he concluded that "it becomes apparent that added controls are mandatory. Chief among these is the use of the double-unknowns approach to eliminate bias" (462). He then discussed the scope of human experimentation; the goals of investigators; the protection of subjects; the responsibility and safeguards of subjects, volunteers, and investigators; the justification for human trials (permissible and nonpermissible); the types of human experimentation; ethical, moral, and legal aspects of experimentation; the necessity of adequate informed consent; justification for the use of placebo controls in studies; and review of previous codes regulating experimentation; and he concluded with guidelines approved by the AMA.

In a 1963 editorial he again addressed the issue of ethics and experimental therapy. The fact that he was one of the pioneers in the modern development of controlled clinical trials, was professor of research in anesthesia at Harvard Medical School, and had impeccable research credentials added credibility to his charges.

In his important 1966 paper, Beecher highlighted the neglected area of unethical experimenter behavior in clinical research. He challenged the long-held assumption that patient and physician had similar roles in experimentation and argued that the experimental situation was characterized more by an inherent conflict of interest. He pointed out that "experimentation on a patient" is "not for his benefit but for that . . . of patients in general [and] that [experimenters'] patients would not have been available if they had been truly aware of the uses that would be made of them" (Beecher 1966, 1354). He urged serious attention to the problem because of the increase in ethical errors, and anticipated that the number of such errors would continue to increase because of the rise in experimentation.[1]

---

1. More experimentation would be necessary because of the greater need for studies before the approval of new drugs. Moreover, the 624-fold increase in the availability of funds from the National Institutes of Health between 1945 and 1965 would attract many

Beecher documented his concern by referring to a sample of one hundred consecutive studies, twelve of which seemed to be unethical, published in a journal in 1964; a sample of fifty studies, only two of which mentioned informed consent; and a report by Pappworth in England of more than five hundred unethical studies. From the sample of fifty cases, he described twenty-two in his paper. Some withheld known effective treatment: in a study of military personnel treated with penicillin or placebo for streptococcal respiratory infections, two cases of acute rheumatic fever and one case of acute nephritis developed in the placebo control group but not in the group treated with penicillin. In another study, although it was known that penicillin effectively prevented rheumatic fever and glomerulonephritis in patients with streptococcal pharyngitis, 500 patients with streptococcal pharyngitis were treated, without informed consent, with sulfadiazine or were no-treatment controls; rheumatic fever developed in 5.4 percent of those treated with sulfadiazine and in 4.2 percent of controls. In a study of the relapse rate of typhoid fever, 251 charity patients were treated with chloramphenicol, and 8 percent of them died; in the group of 157 given symptomatic treatment, 23 percent died.

Other cited studies included one in which a drug with a known adverse effect on the liver was given to 50 mentally defective and juvenile delinquents to treat acne. Most developed significant hepatic dysfunction, and 3 of 4 patients later given challenge doses again developed liver dysfunction. In a double-blind study of the toxicity of two dosages of chloramphenicol (known to cause aplastic anemia) versus placebo, toxic bone-marrow depression occurred in 2 of 20 patients on low dosage and in 18 or 21 on high dosage. A study of cardiac arrhythmias induced by cyclopropane anesthesia and elevated carbon dioxide levels resulted in ventricular extrasystoles. In a study of immunity to cancer, live cancer cells were injected into 22 patients who were told they would be receiving some cells.

Beecher concluded that an ethical approach to experimentation in humans requires "informed consent," with evidence that all hazards have been made clear and are understood by the patient or guardian, and "the more reliable safeguard provided by the presence of an intelligent, informed, conscientious, compassionate, and responsible investigator" (Beecher 1966, 1360). His papers influenced the National Institutes of Health (NIH) and the FDA to require that the ethical standards and appropriate methods of securing informed consent be reviewed by institutional review boards rather than by governmental granting

---

new investigators and increase the number of studies. In medical schools, researchers had prestige; research faculty increasingly dominated medical schools; and published studies were necessary for academic advancement.

agencies for all federally funded studies (Rothman 1991; see also the 1966 memorandum by the surgeon general cited by Silverman 1989).

Beecher's 1966 paper infuriated colleagues and was severely criticized or ignored by much of the medical community (Rothman 1991). It was rejected by *JAMA* but subsequently was published in the *New England Journal of Medicine*. The paper brought to the attention of the public and the government the failure of physicians and researchers to adequately protect subjects participating in research. It was probably the most important factor leading to the U.S. Public Health Service's proposing the establishment of institutional review boards (U.S. Public Health Service 1966), the NIH's mandating institutional review boards, and the FDA's publishing its rules for "adequate and well-controlled clinical evaluations" (FDA 1970). Human experimentation, according to David J. Rothman, changed during World War II from a cottage industry to an extensive, well-funded national program. Beecher's paper marked the next important critical period of change in medicine, which occurred from 1966 to 1976, according to Rothman (1991), with the doctor now having a very circumscribed role owing to the number of parties and procedures participating in medical decisions.[2]

Two strikingly unethical studies were published in the early 1970s. They were reported extensively in the lay press, and they increased public awareness of the potential dangers of unmonitored controlled clinical trials. In the first study, seventy-six women who came to a clinic to obtain birth control pills received contraceptive hormones or placebos instead. The women were not informed, nor did the attending physician know what they had received. The purpose of the study was to evaluate side effects caused by the hormone and placebo. There were seven unwanted pregnancies in the placebo group. To make matters worse, the

---

2. Rothman eloquently and persuasively described the profound transformation of every aspect of the relationship between physician and patient and between medicine and society—for instance, the sacred trust between physician and patient, and the patient's reliance on the discretion of the physician about medical and ethical decisions. "The image of a physician alone with a patient was being supplanted by one of an examining room so crowded that the physician had difficulty squeezing in and of a patient surrounded by strangers" (Rothman 1991, 2). The strangers are lawyers, judges, journalists, philosophers, bioethicists, clerics, community people, federal and state legislators, hospital administrators, insurance clerks, institutional review boards, and committees to ensure adequate informed consent.

Medicine and demoralized physicians are increasingly enmeshed in bureaucracy, committees, forms, regulations, contracts, and procedures. Rothman viewed these as permanently changing the fabric of medicine. Events since the publication of Rothman's book (1991) confirm his prediction. It seems as though we might be witnessing the death of a noble profession.

responsible physician could only express regret that the law prevented him from giving the women abortions (Goldzieher 1971).

Equally sensational was the "Tuskegee Study," begun in the 1930s as a treatment program for black patients with syphilis. The patients were never told that they had syphilis, nor were they given the option of nonplacebo treatment. The program was discontinued due to a loss of funds during the Depression, but four hundred patients who had enrolled in the study between 1930 and 1972 continued to be treated, to document the course of the illness. The patients were told that they had "bad blood" and were treated with placebos. At the time the study began, and for many years afterward, there was no effective treatment for patients in the later (tertiary) stages of syphilis. However, the Tuskegee Study was not discontinued until 1972, long after penicillin had become available as an effective treatment (Jones 1981; White 1985).

Benevolent paternalism had been the prevalent ethical principle guiding the doctor-patient relationship throughout medical history as far back as the time of Hippocrates, who wrote: "Naught should be betrayed to the patient of what may happen or of what may eventually threaten him, because many patients have been driven in this way to extreme measures," and advised the physician to "calmly and adroitly, [conceal] most things from the patient while . . . attending him. Give encouragement to the patient to allow himself to be treated, turning his attention away from what is being done to him; sometimes reprove sharply and emphatically, and sometimes comfort with solicitude and attention, revealing nothing of the patient's future or present condition" (Castiglioni 1947, 4). Essentially similar views have been expressed until recently (Rawlinson 1985). Beecher's 1966 paper represented a shift from benevolent paternalism to the principle of informed consent and patient autonomy. The paper helped bring about the development of methods to obtain informed consent and make research grants contingent on the use of informed consent, and it stimulated discussion about informed consent among academicians. The ethics of medicine was largely the province of physicians until the 1970s, when there was an assault—largely by ethicists—on benevolent paternalism (Rothman 1991). Ethicists began a more systematic dissection of the issues, at a higher level of scholarship than previously.

The Upsurge of Interest in Medical Ethics

Always in the background after World War II was the barbarous abrogation of human rights by Germany, which led to international concern about denial of human rights. Publications of ethical principles protecting human subjects participating in clinical trials included the Nuremberg Code (U.S. Office of the Adjutant General 1947), the Declaration of Helsinki (World Medical Association 1964), the Declaration of Tokyo (World Health Assembly 1976), and the Declaration of Hawaii (World Psychiatric Association 1977).

Other, more relevant factors also contributed to changing the face of medicine. These factors included the sense of alienation associated with the Vietnam War, the drawing together of patients on Medicare, Medicaid, and prepaid and managed care, the increased costs of medical care, and mistrust of authority (Rothman 1991). Other factors included the growing counterculture, the civil rights movement, the women's movement, and concern about the rights of minorities, women, and children, as well as concern about civil liberties. Also of concern were investigators' vested interests (which may conflict with the best interest of patients and subjects in studies) and a marked increase in the need for and the availability of research funding that could support prestigious research careers and academic advancement. Concern about the protection of subject rights became increasingly important with the proliferation of studies of experimental drugs using placebo controls. The definition of ethical standards shifted from physicians to practitioners of other disciplines, such as clerics, legal scholars, philosophers, and ethicists, and to lay people. In turn, increased dialogue between ethicists and physicians clarified the responsibility of physicians to patients and the obligation to respect patient autonomy (Rawlinson 1985).

The public, ethicists, patients, and even physicians—especially younger physicians—began to replace time-honored principles of benevolent paternalism with what came to be known as patient autonomy. Any and all deception of clinical and research patients was rejected, as was any compromise of the requirement to obtain full and adequate informed consent about research participation and to fully inform patients about their clinical diagnosis, prognosis, and treatment if the patients so requested. Likewise, concern about the ethics of using placebos, the double-blind procedure, and the randomized controlled clinical trial began in the 1970s and has not abated.

Ethical issues were examined primarily with regard to the need to avoid deception about using placebos clinically and in research; the need for adequate informed consent during randomized, placebo-controlled, double-blind clinical studies; and complete disclosure about medical evaluation and treatment, and other aspects of the physician-patient interaction. The use of the double-blind procedure in itself was not seen as violating ethical precepts among most ethicists into the early 1970s as long as the informed consent included a full disclosure of the procedure and its purpose. In fact, it was often thought, although more frequently by researchers and physicians than by ethicists, that not doing a placebo-controlled double-blind study was unethical (Fried 1974; Chalmers 1975). Charles Fried at the time thought that it was often preferable and not unethical for patients to be kept in the dark about some aspects of a study, including the fact that some patients might receive a placebo. Considered unethical, however, was the use of homeopathic doses of a drug as a placebo, or the practice of disguising the placebo treatment as a standard and time-honored remedy that is safe and has been proven to help many people.

By the middle of the 1970s, discussion of medical ethics was becoming more popular, more frequent, and more sophisticated. Differences of opinion revolved around benevolent paternalism or beneficence versus respect for the autonomy of patients; around patient ethics (full disclosure to the patient to protect his or her right of self-determination and human dignity) versus experimental ethics (with general agreement that the former has priority over the latter); and most frequently around the ethics of controlled clinical studies, clinical treatment, and methods of obtaining adequate informed consent. Some criticized the therapeutic use of placebos and the use of placebos in studies. However, as would be expected, solutions to various issues became more complicated. Ethicists, who began with different assumptions, who emphasized different aspects of the problem, and who had more knowledge about particular areas, came to different conclusions than did physicians, experimenters, and others.

The first salvo was fired by Sissela Bok (1974), who published her paper "The Ethics of Giving Placebos," in *Scientific American.* The paper called attention to the unethical use of placebos at a time when there was a greater readiness to react to the disclosure of unethical behavior than there had been in 1966, when Beecher published his paper. Bok discussed the deceptive use of placebos in clinical treatment—that is, physicians who knowingly or intentionally use placebos (inert substances) without informing patients during clinical treatment, double-blind studies, or clinical trials.

An important omission by Bok and many other ethicists is the exclusion of placebo treatments with active medication used in placebo dosages, which are much more frequent and far more important than the knowing use of inert placebos. In the clinical treatment of patients the knowing prescription of placebos, such as an inert substance like lactose, was not extensive in past or in recent medical history. The most frequent use of placebos (the use of drugs that do not have a specific effect on the condition being treated) has been the prescribing of a drug that, unknown to the physician, is in fact a placebo, or the prescribing of a drug at a low dosage that does not have a specific effect.

In a subsequent book, *Lying* (1978), Bok raised the issue of deceit or trickery in giving a patient a placebo. She argued that the physician must take into account the physical risks to the patient (whether a clinical patient or an experimental subject) as well as to the medical profession. It is true that in the past patients were not usually informed that they had been given a placebo. Today, however, all patients must be informed if placebos are to be used and must acknowledge in writing that they understand the experimental design, the advantages and disadvantages of the proposed therapy, their right to refuse treatment, and the physical risks involved, if any. Informed consent ensures that physicians can no longer deceive their patients when placebos are knowingly administered.

Beth Simmons (1978) described roughly similar conclusions. Both Simmons and Bok provide examples of grossly unethical behavior as background for their views. They reject deception associated with benevolent paternalism as unethical and emphasize that physicians must respect patients' autonomy by fully informing them about all facts associated with their treatment in lay language so that the patients can make decisions about informed consent. Knowingly giving a placebo may be justifiable only "where the patient agrees to therapy *understanding* that the physiological benefit may be triggered by a psychological response" (Simmons 1978, 179). In such a case, there is no deception.

Confusion about the Ethics of the Placebo

The literature discussing the ethics of using randomized controlled clinical trials, placebos, and the double-blind procedure has grown explosively during the 1980s and 1990s. On the whole, it is not possible to conclude that there is a consensus about these issues. Differences of opinion among ethicists and between ethicists and physicians about almost every ethical issue are much more common than agreement. However, it appears that most ethicists strongly reject benevolent paternalism and staunchly endorse patient autonomy. They often appear almost reluctant to acknowledge circumstances in which the use of placebos, the double-blind procedure, and other randomized control procedures are justified. Most ethicists condemn the use of any type of deception and urge that patients be fully informed about the treatment they receive in studies, research, and private clinical situations. They also question whether subjects understand the statements in the informed consent documents declaring that placebos are to be used and describing other aspects of the research design. For example, Lee C. Park and Linio Covi (1965) reported that although a group of patients with neurotic anxiety were told they were to be treated with placebos, many of them refused to believe it. P. S. Appelbaum and colleagues (1987) reported that over 40 percent of patients in studies did not understand that some of them who wanted treatment would not receive it. One way to bypass this problem is to assure participating patients in placebo-controlled trials that if they receive placebos during the clinical trial, at the completion of the study they will be treated in an open trial with the standard medication. We used this method successfully in our study comparing haloperidol, pimozide, and placebo in Tourette syndrome (Shapiro et al. 1989). The issue of whether patients understand the informed consent documents is still problematic, however, if the patients are of limited intelligence or have significant psychiatric problems that interfere with reality testing.

Many ethicists believe that it is the patient's right to know that treatment will be chosen according to a randomizing formula, and that the patient should be so informed. Failure to do so, they believe, usurps the patient's autonomy. In addition, they believe, all risks must be stated in the informed consent documents to help subjects make a rational decision about whether or not to participate in the trial (Schafer 1982). Most clinical researchers, and many but not all ethicists, believe that it is ethical to randomize patients in clinical trials involving placebos, especially when data on which to base rational decisions are unavailable and when there is insufficient knowledge to determine whether the new therapy or the standard therapy is more harmful than beneficial.

Clinical researchers, statisticians, and methodologists, however, are more likely to endorse patient autonomy publicly but to support it less strongly privately. They generally approve of stringent control procedures embodied in randomized, double-blind, placebo-controlled clinical trials. In fact, many would label as unethical studies not including these controls (Klerman 1986; Leber 1986; Rickels 1986; Klein 1995).

Paul Leber of the FDA did not find the ethical arguments against the use of placebo controls persuasive. He not only endorsed the use of placebo controls but also stated that they are virtually indispensable to the intelligent assessment of the efficacy of most psychopharmacological drug products. Placebo-controlled trials are able to provide unambiguous evidence of efficacy, and thus, from a regulatory point of view, they are an indispensable tool for the assessment of the efficacy of psychopharmacological drug products. Leber (1986, 32) argued that "placebo controls are our surest protection against fads and fashions that come and go in pharmacology, against the reckless claims of therapeutic enthusiasts, and most important against our own mistaken beliefs and prejudices."

Thomas Chalmers, unlike most clinicians, researchers, and ethicists, strongly recommended the use of multiple studies using randomized controlled methods when drugs are first introduced, even before information about dosage and toxicity is available (Chalmers 1975).

Some argue that the use of placebos is unethical because it withholds effective therapy and may thus endanger the life and welfare of patients. The opponents of placebo use are convinced that placebos are ineffective and that experimental drugs can be clinically evaluated as safe and effective without the use of placebos and double-blind studies. But there is substantial evidence that patients can derive benefits from placebos. Beecher (1959b), for example, reported substantial relief of pain by placebos, in as many as 35 percent of patients. Shapiro and Shapiro (1984a) reported that twenty patients with Tourette syndrome averaged 36 percent improvement in seven dependent variables after six weeks of treatment with placebo. Evans (1985) concluded that placebo is about 55–60 percent as effective as active medication and that the percentage is unrelated to the potency of the active medications. Alan Roberts and co-workers (1993) reported good to excellent results in 70 percent of patients treated with drugs that were previously thought to be effective but were subsequently evaluated as placebos. Prien, discussing the ethical concerns of using placebos, argued that "the difference in improvement rates for drug-treated patients and placebo-treated patients is not so great as to make placebo an unethical control for evaluating the therapeutic efficacy of antidepressant drugs" (1988, 4). In addition, those patients receiving placebos may be subject to less risk than those receiving the active drug being investigated, since an investigational agent may be not only ineffective but also dangerous because of great toxicity or serious side effects.

In situations where a known effective treatment exists and a new drug is proposed, the American College of Gastroenterology recommends that the researcher consider the severity of the illness when making a decision about whether to use a placebo. Three factors are emphasized: (1) it may be more difficult to justify using a placebo if the illness is life threatening; (2) it may also be less important to use placebo controls in conditions that have a predictable and stable course than in those that are plagued by remissions and exacerbations; and (3) the efficacy of the standard treatment must be taken into account (the use of placebo controls would have greater justification if the treatment were of low efficacy) (Stanley 1988).

Some of the ethical constraints about using placebos can be bypassed by variations in experimental design. For example, if the patient's clinical status worsens or the patient fails to improve or develops adverse effects during the clinical trial, the clinician could remove the patient from the clinical trial, but "the criteria for removal should be operationally specified in advance, preferably in quantitative terms" (Klerman 1986, 27).

Karl Rickels (1986) recommended the use of an escape clause that would allow a subject to resume active drug therapy after signs of relapse occurred. He also proposed that trials comparing a standard drug with an experimental agent should be done without a placebo control. However, he noted that forgoing the use of a placebo control is not without problems. For example, it is the use of a placebo control that makes possible the interpretation of the study results if an experiment fails to demonstrate a difference between the experimental and standard medication. If the experimental agent turns out to be inferior to the standard medication in a study without a placebo control, it is impossible to say whether the test medication has any activity at all. Such information would be important, especially if the experimental agent had many fewer side effects than the standard medication.

As drug regulatory bodies in most advanced countries increasingly required randomized, double-blind, controlled studies employing placebos, the Federal Republic of Germany passed a new drug law in 1978 no longer demanding controlled studies as qualification for the acceptance and registration of new drugs. Responsibility for approving the effectiveness and safety of a new drug would be based on more or less clear evidence for the efficacy of the drug. Controlled clinical trials, however, were not to be considered proof of efficacy. Following the passage of the new law, the ethical problems of controlled clinical trials were discussed: some writers rejected the need for controlled studies as unethical; others held that reliable and valid controlled studies could not be done and that such studies could result in investigators being charged with murder if patients died; and still others asserted that physicians have an ethical obligation to conduct controlled trials (Burkhardt and Kienle 1978, 1980; Silverman 1979).

Mary Ann Rawlinson (1985) did not agree with the absolute prohibition on the therapeutic use of placebos in medical practice, an outgrowth of the idea that their use implies deception of the patient. She argued that there are some controls and considerations that ought to regulate the physician's judgment when the "duties of beneficence and veracity conflict" (416), and she enumerated five tests to determine whether placebos should be used clinically.

Conclusion

These examples illustrate the differences of opinion about ethical attitudes to the use of placebos, the double-blind procedure, and randomized clinical trials which can be found in the literature. We concur with William A. Silverman (1989, 10) that "a way must be found. . . . to experiment with various discretionary approaches that would strike a realistic balance among the competing interests. We need an approach that would conserve the spirit of informed consent without snuffing out the flame of responsible clinical study." The current consensus, however, is that it is impossible to control nondrug factors without the use of the double-blind, placebo controls, and other appropriate methodological procedures. These procedures are likely to be controversial until new and better techniques can be developed.

chapter nine

How Blind Is Blind?

The double-blind procedure was the most important methodological innovation leading to the end of the hegemony of the placebo effect of medical treatment. Although acceptance of the double blind method evolved slowly, by the end of the 1970s the method was used routinely. There is now general recognition that in controlled studies the use of this method is necessary to minimize treatment bias and placebo effects. Despite this, questions have been raised about whether double-blind studies fully accomplish their purpose. In particular, many investigators question whether the double-blind procedure is truly blind. The extent of this concern is reflected in published studies that conclude that physicians, patients, or staff members can correctly guess drug assignment in double-blind studies. This is an important issue. If drug assignment inadvertently is revealed in a double-blind study, the study is worse in some sense than one not using a double-blind design, because the study's design may encourage an unjustified faith in the results.

This issue of correct guesses of drug allocation in double-blind studies was first addressed in a brief study of thirty volunteers given phenobarbital or placebo on alternate nights (Goodnow et al. 1951). The number of such studies as of 1991 totaled twenty-seven, and the studies cover a broad spectrum of drugs (table 9.1). The data shown in table 9.1 encompass double-blind studies comparing placebo with one or more drugs, and analysis of guesses by physicians, staff members, patients, or relatives about whether a patient is on active drug or placebo. (In the discussion that follows, guessing that a patient is on an active drug is referred to as "guessing drug"; guessing that a patient is on a placebo is referred to as "guessing placebo.") All patients (except for the incarcerated adolescents in study 10) were treated as outpatients. The studies are loosely grouped by diagnosis, type of drug, number of comparison drugs, and year of publication. Because of the large number of comparisons, only percentages and overall chi squares are cited for descriptive purposes. All studies of guesses by physicians, nurses, and staff members (except for study 12) include more than one physician. Analyses of differences among staff members are described in studies 4, 6, and 8–10. All of the studies are retrospective, and none of them corrected significance levels for multiple tests, except for studies 4, 6, and 8, and study 27, which cited percentages but not significance levels. Study 25 addressed the question of whether placebos and active drugs had identical detectable properties such as vehicle, size, color, etching, texture, taste, and dissolvability.

For each study, table 9.1 reports the overall significant correct guessing of drug allocation, the percentage of subjects who guessed drug more than 50 percent of the time, the percentages of correct guesses in three categories (drug guesses, placebo guesses, and total guesses—either of drug or placebo allocation), and any significant association of drug guessing with clinical improvement and/or adverse effects. The results of all the studies are summarized in table 9.2.

The Determinants of Guesses about Medication Assignment

We studied the guessing of medication allocation in three double-blind studies, part of a larger study carried out at the Special Studies Laboratory (SSL) at the Payne Whitney Psychiatric Clinic (Shapiro et al., 1980, 1983; see also chapter 10). These studies of drug guessing were designed in 1969 and completed in 1974 but not analyzed until 1991. The a priori hypotheses were that physicians would correctly identify drug and placebo more frequently than would be expected by chance; that correct guesses of drug and placebo allocation would be associated with patient improvement (because patients on drugs are more likely to improve than those on placebos), with the occurrence of adverse effects (because drugs are more likely to cause adverse effects than are placebos, and cause a different pattern of adverse effects), and with lower drug dosages and higher placebo dosages (because placebo dosages are more likely to be increased to higher levels because of the absence of clinical response and of severe side effects). We predicted that an enhanced ability to identify drug allocation would be associated with the number of clinical visits (a longer time on drug would enhance drug effects compared to placebo effects among patients). To evaluate whether physicians' ability to guess was a relevant variable, we hypothesized that physicians would not differ significantly in their ability to guess correctly. Finally, we compared these results to those reported in the literature to evaluate to what extent our results replicated previously published results.

The three samples included 222 anxious neurotic patients treated weekly with brief psychotherapy and with diazepam or placebo for six weeks, 88 depressed patients treated weekly with brief psychotherapy and with doxepin or placebo for six weeks, and 119 patients with both depression and anxiety treat-

Table 9.1 Studies Examining Guessing of Drug and Placebo Allocation in Double-Blind Studies

Study	Sample Size/Diagnosis/Length of Treatment/Type of Evaluation (Endpoint or Completers)[a]	Active Drug(s) Used in Study[b]	Individual Guessing	χ^2 $P <$ [c]	% Guessing Drug	% Correct Guesses — Drug Guesses	Placebo Guesses	Total Guesses	Significance of Association of Drug Guess with — Improvement	Adverse Effects
1. Goodnow et al. 1951	30 / normal volunteers / 2 days / crossover / completers	phenobarbital	patient	.01	—	—	—	~75	—	—
2. Denhoff and Holden 1955	18 / cerebral palsy / 2 weeks / crossover / completers	chlorpromazine	occupational therapists	.01	—	—	—	83	—	—
3. Rickels et al. 1970b	138 / anxiety neurosis / 6 weeks / completers	meprobamate	physician	.01	64	76	50	64	.001	.01
4. SSL anxiety study	222 / anxiety neurosis / 6 weeks / endpoint	diazepam	physician	.000	61	74	52	64	.02	.01
5. Rickels et al. 1965	376 / anxiety and depression / 4 weeks / completers (for 7 drugs from 9 studies)	meprobamate, chlordiazepoxide, tybamate, etc.	physician	.001	61	68	49	61	.000	NS
6. SSL depression study	88 / depression / 6 weeks / endpoint	doxepin	physician	.06	83	90	26	61	.003	NS
7. Rabkin et al. 1986	100–137 / mixed depression / 6 weeks / completers	imipramine, phenelzine	physician / patient	.000 / .000	63 / 63	90 / 76	82 / 79	87 / 78	.01 / .000	NS / NS

Study	Sample	Drug	Rater							
8. SSL depression study	119 / mixed depression / 4 weeks / endpoint	amitriptyline, bromazepam	physician	.000	66	82	65	73	NS	.0001
9. Stallone et al. 1974	57 / affective disorder / median 15 months / endpoint	lithium	1 nurse	Sig	—	Sig	NS	—	—	NS
			2 nurses	NS	—	NS	NS	NS	—	NS
			patient	NS	96	NS	NS	NS	Yes	NS
			relatives	.001	—	.001	.001	.001	—	NS
10. Marini et al. 1976	67 / incarcerated aggressive adolescents / 4–12 weeks / endpoint	lithium	physician	NS	34	41	72	56	—	—
			physician	NS	47	54	60	57	—	—
			patient	.02	62	80	59	70	—	Sig
11. Engelhardt et al. 1969	311 / chronic schizophrenia / 3 months / endpoint	chlorpromazine, promazine	physician	.000	71	85	60	77	.001	.001
12. Shapiro and Shapiro 1984a	20 / Tourette disorder / 6 weeks crossover / endpoint	pimozide	physician	.0000	—	95	95	95	—	Yes
13. Munjack et al. 1989	43 / panic disorder and agoraphobia with panic attacks / 5 weeks / completers	alprazolam, propranolol	physician	.05	70	79	50	70	—	—
14. Margraf et al. 1991	59 / panic disorder / 8 weeks / endpoint	alprazolam, imipramine	physician	.000	73	95	72	88	.001	.001
			patient	.000	80	95	56	83	.001	.001
15. Dalby et al. 1978	127 / hyperactive children / 1 day / crossover / completers	methylphenidate	patient	NS	—	—	—	56	—	—
			observers	.01	—	—	—	—	—	—
16. Brownell et al. 1982	57 / obese women / 4 months / completers	fenfluramine	physician	.002	48	73	75	74	Yes	Yes
			patient	.002	54	86	84	85	Yes	Yes

continued

Table 9.1—continued

Study	Sample Size/ Diagnosis/Length of Treatment/Type of Evaluation (Endpoint or Completers)[a]	Active Drug(s) Used in Study[b]	Individual Guessing	χ^2 $P <$ [c]	% Guessing Drug	% Correct Guesses			Significance of Association of Drug Guess with	
						Drug Guesses	Placebo Guesses	Total Guesses	Improvement	Adverse Effects
17. Moscucci et al. 1987	78 / mild obesity / 12 weeks / completers	phenyl-propanolamine	patient	NS	35	43	74	58	.05	.05
18. Hughes and Krahn 1985	99 / smokers / 4 days abstinence / completers	nicotine gum	patient	.000	66	85	56	72	NS	NS
19. Anderson et al. 1972	818 / common cold / 51 days / endpoint	vitamin C	patient	NS	~50	~50	~50	~50	NS	NS
20. Anderson et al. 1974	2,349 / common cold / 90 days / endpoint	6 vitamin C 2 placebos	patient	NS	~67	~66	~33	—	—	—
21. Karlowski et al. 1975	190 / common cold / 9 months / endpoint	vitamin C	patient	.000	50	78	77	77	—	—
22. Anderson et al. 1975	424 / common cold / 15 weeks / endpoint	vitamin C capsule and tablet	patient	—	—	—	—	52	—	—
23. Lewis et al. 1975	190 / common cold/ 9 months / endpoint	vitamin C	patient	.000	50	77	78	77	.05	.01

Study	Sample / condition / duration / endpoint	Drug	Rater	P					
24. Longstreth et al. 1981	60 / irritable bowel / 12–33 months / endpoint	psyllium	patient	NS	—	31	32	32	—
25. Howard et al. 1982	380 / post–heart attack / 3–4 years / endpoint	aspirin	patient	.000	48	63	67	65	.05
26. Lipid Research Clinics Program 1984	3,806 / hyper-cholesterolemia / 7.4 years / endpoint	cholestyramine	patient	.000	—	56	55	55	—
			staff	.000	—	55	53	54	—
27. Byington et al. 1985	3,230–3,551 post–heart attack / 12–40 months / endpoint	propranolol	patient	.000	62	68	44	56	Sig
			physician	.000	73	74	72	73	Sig
			coordinator	.000	49	72	74	73	Sig

Note: Percentages and significance tests are recorded as cited in the studies or were derived from the raw data. Significance tests are cited as: $P \le .05 = \star$, $P \le .01 = \star\star$, $P \le .001 = \star\star\star$, $P \le .0001 = \star\star\star\star$, or as P levels; NS = not significant; Sig = significance cited by the authors or apparent but probability not specified or derivable from data; — = data not available. Percentages, without significance tests, are recorded for correct guess of drug, placebo, and both drug and placebo because of the large number of comparisons. The design, presentation, and analysis of selected studies are discussed in the Appendix at the end of this chapter.

[a]Completers = participants who remained in the study till its completion; endpoint = all patients were evaluated at the last week of treatment.

[b]The proportion is approximately 50% chance of guessing drug and placebo in most studies of one drug and one placebo; approximately 66% chance of guessing drug and 33% chance of guessing placebo in studies of two drugs and one placebo; and so on.

[c]Probability of χ^2 comparing drug and placebo guess with actual drug or placebo received, omitting "don't know," "uncertain," or guessing of irrelevant drugs.

Table 9.2 Compilation of Results from Published Studies Examining Guessing of Drug and Placebo Allocation in Double-Blind Studies

| | Significant Overall Guessing[a] | | More Drug Guesses than Placebo Guesses[b] | | Proportion of Studies Reporting Correct Identification of[c] | | | | | |
| | | | | | Drug | | Placebo | | Drug and Placebo | |
Subject	Fraction[d]	%	Fraction	%	Fraction	%	Fraction	%	Fraction	%
Physician	11/14	83	10/13	77	13/14	93	10/14	71	13/13	100
Patient	12/17	63	8/11	73	11/15	73	10/15	67	13/14	93
Other[e]	5/7	72	0/1	0	4/6	67	3/5	60	3/4	75

Source: This table is based on the published studies listed in table 9.1.
[a] Chi-square analysis of the probability of correct and incorrect drug-placebo guesses. Some of the studies included more than one active drug, and included guesses of "don't know" or "uncertain," and guesses of irrelevant drugs.
[b] Percentage of studies in which subjects guessed drug more often than would be expected by chance.
[c] The columns summarize the percentage of studies exceeding the expected proportion of correct identification of drug, placebo, and both drug and placebo. The expected proportion is about 50% for studies of one drug and placebo, 67% for studies of two drugs and placebo, and so on.
[d] Numerator is the number of studies reporting statistically significant occurrence; denominator is total number of studies.
[e] "Other" includes occupational therapists, nurses, relatives, observers, staff, and coordinators.

ed weekly with brief psychotherapy and with amitriptyline, bromazepam, or placebo for four weeks. Patients were assigned randomly, and the drug allocation was double blind. Each of the three treating psychiatrists had an eclectic, psychodynamic, and psychopharmacological orientation and fifteen years of clinical experience. At each visit, the psychiatrists guessed whether patients were receiving active drug(s) or placebo (referred to as Drug Guess), from which the Correct Guess of Drug versus Placebo Scale was derived. The physicians also completed a Confidence about Drug and Placebo Scale (definitely active drug = 7; probably active drug = 6; possibly active drug = 5; don't know = 4; possibly inactive drug = 3; probably inactive drug = 2; and definitely inactive drug = 1). Nine of the 429 guesses were rated "don't know" on this scale: five of the nine patients that these guesses applied to were on placebo, four were on active drug, and three had missing data. The Correct Guess of Drug versus Placebo Scale and the Confidence about Drug and Placebo Scale were highly correlated, indicating that the degree of certainty about guessing indicated the correctness of the guess. Improvement was rated on the Physician Global Evaluation of Improvement Scale at endpoint (patient's final score in the last week of participation). Adverse effects were rated on a Clinical Global Adverse Effects Scale (no adverse effects = 0; slight adverse effects not interfering with functioning and not requiring remediation = 1; moderate adverse effects requiring remediation but not interfering with treatment = 2; adverse effects nullifying treatment = 3).

Two of our SSL studies confirmed that physicians correctly guessed whether patients were on drug or placebo. Although this was not confirmed in the third study, the trend in the third study was in a similar direction.

How accurate were the guesses? Did the physicians correctly identify which patients were on a drug and which were on a placebo? Physicians correctly guessed that patients were receiving a drug more often than they guessed correctly that patients were receiving a placebo (80% of drug guesses, but only 50% of placebo guesses, were correct); overall, 69 percent of the guesses were correct.

How similar are physicians in their guesses and in their ability to identify drug and placebo correctly? (Physicians 1 and 2 participated in all three studies; physician 3 participated in only the first and third studies.) Physician 3 differed from the two other physicians by guessing 54 percent of the time that active drug was allocated and 46 percent of the time that placebo was allocated; physicians 1 and 2 guessed drug 80 percent of the time and guessed placebo 20 percent of the time. Although all three correctly guessed drug allocation more accurately than placebo allocation, perhaps related to a bias to guess drug in general, physician 3 correctly guessed placebo 31 percent of the time, compared to 12 percent for physician 1 and 14 percent for physician 2. Moreover, physician 3 identified both drug and placebo correctly 73 percent of the time, compared to 64 percent for physician 1 and 55 percent for physician 2.

Similar differences in guessing have been reported in studies of judges (Agnew 1963), physicians (Marini et al. 1976), nurses (Stallone et al. 1974, 1975), and participants in a large-scale study of aspirin from different clinics (Howard et al. 1982). Therefore, some of the variance in guessing is apparently due to rater differences. This suggests that rater differences should be included as a variable in studies of drug guessing.

Four variables—clinical improvement, adverse effects, dosage, and number of visits—were hypothesized a priori to be associated both with physicians' likelihood of guessing drug, and with correct guessing of drug allocation. The results of two SSL studies indicate that adverse effects and lower dosages were the strongest predictors of guesses of active drug allocation and of correct guesses of drug compared to placebo; the results of the third were in a similar direction. Guesses of active drug allocation were associated with patient improvement in only one sample. The number of visits was not significant in any of the samples.

Although the results varied for the three SSL samples, combinations of the predicted variables, which are present in most studies and are difficult to control, are associated with correct drug guessing. In double-blind studies, these variables are likely to unmask the blind and affect the validity of the results.

Comparison of Our Results with Published Studies

The results for our three SSL studies are strikingly similar to those seen in other studies reported in the literature. Physicians correctly guessed drug allocation in 83 percent of fourteen published studies, patients did so in 63 percent of seventeen published studies, and others did so in 72 percent of seven published studies. Both physicians and patients guessed drug more often (73–77% of the time) than they guessed placebo. This tendency to guess drug more often than placebo may contribute to more correct guessing of drug administration by 93 percent of physicians, 73 percent of patients, and 67 percent of other raters. Correct guessing of placebo administration is slightly lower but significantly high: 71 percent for physicians, 67 percent for patients, and 60 percent for other raters. When patients in the study were administered both active drugs and placebos alternately for a fixed number of weeks (e.g., in crossover studies), physicians guessed drug and placebo correctly 100 percent of the time; patients, 93 percent of the time; and other raters, 75 percent of the time.

The factors influencing a physician's ability to correctly identify drug administration more often than placebo administration include the type of drug (i.e., whether the drug is weak or potent), the severity and pattern of adverse effects (i.e., whether there are few, many, or specific adverse effects), a more specific pattern of improvement, drug dosage, and differences between the responses of patients on drugs and those of patients on placebos. For example, patients may report improvement and adverse effects on placebo, but the adverse effects may be less specific than those associated with specific drugs (e.g., the orthostatic hypotension associated with antidepressants and the bradycardia associated with propranolol).

The Relationship of Hypothesized Variables to Drug Guessing

Physicians and patients guessed drug more frequently and correctly guessed drug (above 50%) on the basis of patient improvement (89% of physicians and 75% of patients in the twenty-seven reviewed studies; see table 9.3). This is in contrast to our own SSL finding: improvement was related to guesses that patients were receiving a drug in only one of our studies (the study of doxepin in depressed patients) but not in the other two. We found that adverse effects (side effects) of the drug but not improvement are associated with correct drug guessing in the two other studies. Thus, patient improvement is associated with correct drug guessing in some but not all studies.

Table 9.3 Compilation of Results from Published Studies Reporting Significant Relationships of Drug Guesses with Clinical Improvement and Adverse Effects

| | Proportion of Studies Reporting Significant Relationships of Drug Guesses with | | | |
| | Clinical Improvement | | Adverse Effects | |
Subject	Fraction[a]	%	Fraction	%
Physician	8/9	89	8/11	73
Patient	6/8	75	7/11	64
Other[b]	—	—	1/3	33

Source: This table is based on the published studies listed in table 9.1.

[a]The numerator is the number of studies reporting statistically significant relationship; the denominator is the total number of studies.

[b]Includes occupational therapists, nurses, relatives, observers, staff, and coordinators.

One study (Engelhardt et al. 1969) reported drug guessing to be related to a global but not to a more specific or structured measure of improvement. This finding was not confirmed in another study (Rickels et al. 1970a), which reported that global and structured measures of improvement were correlated, or in our studies, which compared drug guessing to measures of improvement derived from global clinical scales, the Hopkins Symptom Check List, the Psychiatric Outpatient Mood Scale, and the Hamilton Anxiety and Depression Scales. Medication guess has been suggested as a sensitive measure to differentiate clinically active drugs from placebo or as an indirect criterion of clinical improvement, especially in the absence of major adverse effects (Rickels et al. 1965). This idea requires modification, however, because the dosage of the drug and of the placebo, rater differences, and physical characteristics of the drug and the placebo, as well as even minor adverse effects could reveal drug allocation. In fact, our studies indicate that drug guessing, although related to improvement, may not reflect the superiority of an active drug. Although there were no significant differences on improvement measures between active drugs and placebo in our three studies, drug guessing was related to the occurrence of improvement.

The most clinically sensitive method to determine an effective drug dosage that will ensure minimal adverse effects is to initiate treatment at a very low dosage and slowly titrate the drug to an effective dosage. In clinical trials that compare an active drug to an inactive placebo, the active drug frequently has more adverse effects than the placebo. Thus, the SSL study of amitriptyline and bromazepam in depressed patients and the study of diazepam in anxious patients confirmed our hypotheses that the occurrence of more adverse effects would be associated with drug guesses rather than placebo guesses, would be significantly associated with confidence about guessing drug and placebo allocation, and would be significantly associated with correct guessing of drug and placebo allocation. Similar results were obtained for physicians in 73 percent of the twenty-seven reviewed studies and for patients in 64 percent of the studies. In one study, both physicians' and patients' correct guesses of drug administration were associated with significantly lowered heart rate due to treatment with propranolol (Byington et al. 1985). The relationship of side effects of drugs to drug guessing has been extensively discussed in the literature (Nash 1962; Stallone et al. 1975; Thomson 1982).[1]

1. An interesting paper about adverse effects and drug guessing (White et al. 1992) came to our attention subsequent to our literature review. A double-blind study compared thirty-four patients treated with either the putative antidepressant etoperidone or placebo. A blind evaluator who was not associated with the study was provided with adverse effect and dosage information about each patient but no information on therapeutic effects.

It is likely that the drug dosage, expressed in units or number of tablets, would be lower for active drug than for placebo. The dosage of the active drug would not be increased if the patient improved or if adverse effects began to occur. Conversely, if the patient is on placebo, the dosage is more likely to be increased in the absence of improvement and adverse effects. Dosage levels, therefore, might contribute to correct guessing of whether a patient is being treated with active drug or placebo. This expectation was confirmed in the SSL studies of amitriptyline bromazepam in anxious patients and diazepam in anxious patients. The relationship between the dosage levels of drugs and placebos and correct guessing has been reported by others (Engelhardt et al. 1969; Rickels et al. 1970b; Nassif et al. 1981).

Contrary to expectations, our study did not confirm that the length of the study and the length of time patients remained in the study would be correlated with correctness of guessing. A possible explanation for this negative result was that in these studies, average improvement over all visits and improvement at endpoint were not significantly different for active drugs and placebo (Shapiro et al. 1983). Several studies in the literature also support this finding (Rickels et al. 1965, 1970a; Howard et al. 1982).

Physicians in our study responded "don't know" for nine patients (five receiving a drug and four receiving a placebo), which is less often than this response is reported in most other studies. Physicians' confidence about guessing (67%) was greater when they were guessing drug, but "definite" confidence was more frequent with placebo. An association between physician's confidence about guessing, overall drug guesses, and correct drug guesses was reported in a study of treatment with psychotropic drugs (Rickels et al. 1965) but not in a study of nicotine gum (Hughes and Krahn 1985).

Correct guessing by physicians is greater in crossover than in parallel studies (Agnew 1963; studies 1, 2, and 12 in table 9.1), probably because raters have the opportunity of observing the effect of both drugs rather than one or another, as in parallel studies. A report that past use of psychotropic medication was associated with accuracy of physician guess about assignment to active medication or placebo (Rabkin et al. 1986) was not confirmed in our three SSL studies. A retrospective report that accuracy in identifying active drug and placebo was greater among subgroups who were younger, male, employed, married, and had at least

---

The evaluator correctly guessed active drug assignment 73 percent of the time and correctly guessed placebo assignment 67 percent of the time. The dosage levels and certainty about guesses were not significant. This technique provides a useful method of excluding selected variables, such as clinical improvement, from the assessment of study blindability.

a high school education than among other subgroups has not been replicated (Byington et al. 1985).

Only one study attempted to evaluate the blindness of a study of psychotherapy (Carroll et al. 1994). Successful guessing was evaluated for four interacting treatment conditions: active psychotherapy, control or placebo psychotherapy, active drug therapy, and placebo drug therapy. Seventy-six percent of the guesses correctly identified active and placebo psychotherapy, and 75 percent of the guesses correctly identified drug and placebo treatment—which is comparable to the results reported in the literature. Successful guessing was associated with subjective but not with objective measures of improvement. In the study by K. M. Carroll et al. (1994) as in our SSL studies, the accuracy of clinical raters guessing treatment assignment varied from 40 percent to 100 percent. Successful guessing was unrelated to completion of treatment or to improvement. Although most of the analyses were *post hoc* and the sample size should have been larger, the study illustrates the usefulness of sophisticated statistical analysis and the consistency of the findings with those generally reported in other studies.

The Validity of "Identical Matching Placebos"

An essential requirement of the double-blind design is that the active and inactive medications be identical in all respects except for the specific therapeutic component of the active drug to be evaluated. They should be identical in size, color, etching, texture, taste, dissolvability, and pattern of adverse effects, to ensure that the patient and physician cannot discriminate between active and inactive medication. We observed while conducting six double-blind studies through 1972 that, despite the assumption that "an identical matching placebo" had been used as a control in most studies, the active drug was in fact distinguishable from the placebo because of different physical properties. To test this observation, we designed a study to determine whether placebos have significantly different physical characteristics from active medication and can be differentiated by participants in a double-blind study (Blumenthal et al. 1974).

The drugs and placebos that were compared included tablets in the study of diazepam use in anxiety, capsules in the study of amitriptyline and bromazepam use in depression, liquid in the study of doxepin use in depression, and tablets in three previous studies (a meprobamate-versus-placebo study, an amitriptyline-versus-placebo study, and an antipsychotic-versus-placebo study). In the study of identical matching placebos (Blumenthal et al. 1974), thirty-two subjects were designated the patient-simulating group and were given instructions to evaluate whether the medications they were to be given (drugs and placebos) were different or the same. Twenty subjects, comprising the experimenter-simulating group, were given similar instructions but in addition were informed that there were definitely two or three drug types in each of the drug categories (two minor tranquilizers, one major tranquilizer, and three antidepressants; some of these were in tablet form, some in capsule form, and some in liquid form).

The subjects differentiated active and placebo drugs for five of the drug groups, but none differentiated the two active and placebo capsules used in the study of amitriptyline-bromazepam in depression. The basis for successful differentiation, when it occurred, included a more granular texture for placebo, sharper etching and edges for placebo, lighter color for active drug, thicker size for the active drug than placebo, and the fact that the placebo, but not the two active capsules, floated in water.

The importance of using identical matching placebos or control substances was discussed in the first experimental double-blind study by Rivers (1908), in studies of alcohol between 1912 and 1959 (Hollingsworth 1912; Nash 1962; Gadow et al. 1986a, 1986b), in several more recent studies (Anderson et al. 1972; Howard et al. 1982; Hughes and Krahn 1985), and in many other studies.

Breaking of the blind due to differences in taste between active drug and placebo is frequently cited in the literature (Baker and Thorpe 1957; Karlowski et al. 1975; Lewis et al. 1975; Miller et al. 1977; Dalby et al. 1978; Howard et al. 1982; Rose 1982). Aware of this problem, investigators required taste tests to ensure that the active drug and the placebo were similar in taste (Anderson et al. 1972, 1974, 1975). Several comprehensive reviews of the double-blind design highlight the need to control for differences in taste (Nash 1962; Gadow et al. 1986a, 1986b; Fisher and Greenberg 1989).

Important physical and pharmacological differences between active drug and the placebo tablets, capsules, and liquid preparations include differences in size, etching, texture, consistency, dissolvability, smell, and general appearance, and the differences revealed by simple chemical tests such as acid tests, and sometimes by complicated laboratory tests (Blumenthal et al. 1974; Hill et al. 1976; Howard et al. 1982).

A review of twenty-two double-blind studies reported similar results (Hill et al. 1976). Only two of sixteen active capsules or tablets had acceptable matching with placebos; two aerosols, two ointments, and a nasal spray had acceptable matches. One liquid preparation was poorly matched. Eight crossover studies used capsules or tablets that were poorly matched. The cues for differentiation included taste, color, appearance, shape, consistency, and smell. In our study of identical matching placebos, observers differed in their ability to detect differences. The authors discussed the difficulties of formulating identical active and inactive preparations and provided useful recommendations about how to minimize differences.

Similar findings have been reported in clinical trials. At the conclusion of a clinical trial of prophylactic use of aspirin for heart attacks (Howard et al. 1982), investigators asked 271 patients about the basis for their guesses. The findings revealed a startling and surprising array of techniques and procedures used to uncover drug allocation. Tasting was associated more with aspirin guesses than with placebo guesses. Other attempts to identify the capsules included inspecting and smelling the contents, testing the physiological effects, doing acid tests or having the capsules analyzed professionally, evaluating the bleeding time and the blood aspirin level, and seeking professional help to identify substances. Sixty-five percent of the 95 patients who tested the capsules correctly identified aspirin, compared to 47 percent of 285 nontesters. In another study, differences in taste were associated with correct guessing of vitamin C and placebo in 42 percent of 190 subjects (Lewis et al. 1975), and taste was noted by participants in other studies (Karlowski et al. 1975; Miller et al. 1977; Dalby et al. 1978). The importance of formulating identical and indistinguishable drugs and placebos for use in double-blind trials is underscored by two large studies of the prophylactic use of vitamin C for the common cold. The investigators took special precautions to formulate drug and control substances that were indistinguishable in appearance and taste, and tested to ensure that they were indistinguishable. Patients were not able to guess drug allocation correctly (Anderson et al. 1972, 1974, 1975).

Attempts by patients to break the blind are frequent in studies that include a placebo control. Attempts to break the blind even occurred (surprising the investigators) among 311 "well-educated, well-motivated, medically sophisticated . . . volunteers employed at the National Institutes of Health" who participated in a study of vitamin C versus placebo for the common cold (Lewis et al. 1975). Because of haste to begin the study and the nature of the sample, little thought had been given to the formulation of the vitamin and placebo capsules, which were easily distinguishable by taste. The investigators reported that tasting was quite frequent, that dropouts were more frequent in the placebo group, and that tasting was a reliable basis for guessing.

It is likely that most double-blind studies can be unblinded to some extent. Correct guessing of drug and placebo allocation by physicians and patients exceeds chance expectations in most double-blind studies. Physicians and patients tend to guess active drug more frequently than they guess placebo, and their drug guesses are more often correct than their placebo guesses. If drug allocation is guessed more frequently than placebo allocation, there may be a greater likelihood that drug allocation will be guessed correctly. Erroneously attributing improvement and placebo-induced adverse effects to a drug also contribute to the greater frequency of guessing drug. Guesses that a drug is being administered, as well as correct drug guessing, are less likely with drugs that have weak effects (such as the subtle benefits of vitamin C in prevention of colds), and with drugs that have few adverse effects.

The variables that appear to affect guessing include patient improvement, adverse effects, dosage units of active drug and placebo, differences among raters, differences between the control substance and the active medication used in studies, and occasionally the length of the study. Any of one of these factors, or their combination, can contribute to unblinding the double blind, making a study prone to placebo effects. In the absence of other clues, however, the effect of improvement alone on medication guess is not an adequate indication that a study has been unblinded.

Studies indicate that patients frequently attempt to identify whether they have been given a placebo or active drug, that patients who realize they are receiving a placebo tend to drop out, and that patients, physicians, and staff are able to identify active drug and placebo. The failure to completely match drug and placebo often compromises or unblinds the double-blind design.

Discussion of Methods to Improve Blind Studies

Our studies and others have identified variables that often compromise or unmask the double blind. The discussion that follows focuses on these variables and suggests methods to improve and control the variables that can result in the unblinding of a study.

Identical Matching Placebos

Inherent in the double-blind procedure is the recognition that the active treatment or drug being evaluated should be identical to the comparison treatment. When we became aware that discernible differences between the active drug and placebo could break the blind (Blumenthal et al. 1974), we discussed this problem with drug company officials. They told us that it was difficult to physically match drug and placebo tablets because different constituents and presses were used in their manufacture, and that it was difficult as well to formulate placebo tablets (or liquid) with the same taste as the active drug. However, it was our impression that drug companies thought the problem unimportant and were unwilling to do anything about it.

There are various solutions to this problem. One method is the use of capsules containing a powdered drug and an obfuscating flavored filler (Gadow et al. 1986a, 1986b). Liquid medications are even more easily disguised. A preliminary test should be done to ensure that the trial substance is identical to the placebo in appearance and taste (Rivers 1908; Nash 1962; Dalby et al. 1978).

Active Placebos

The adverse effects of active drugs and the contrasting inactivity of placebos also contribute to the unblinding of studies (Gadow et al. 1986a, 1986b; Fisher and Greenberg 1989; Margraf et al. 1991; White et al. 1992). Studies demonstrate that it is easier to break the double blind when potent drugs such as neuroleptics and beta blockers are used than when less-potent drugs such as aspirin or vitamin C are used (table 9.1).

A critical review of the evidence for the efficacy of biological therapies for mental disorders emphasizes the importance of this factor. Seymour Fisher and Roger Greenberg (1989) and Greenberg et al. (1992) highlighted the problems caused by the fact that inactive placebos are used in most of the reviewed studies and the fact that the difference in effectiveness between active drug and placebo is markedly less when an active drug is compared to an active placebo. They concluded that because of these factors the effectiveness of psychoactive drugs cannot be established until more studies are done using active placebos as controls.[2] They cited a study stating that forty (59%) of 68 of the antidepressant studies published between 1958 and 1972 using an inert placebo control reported the antidepressant as effective, compared to only one (14%) of seven studies using an active placebo (atropine) (Thomson 1982). Similar results are described by Fisher and Greenberg in four additional studies (Fahy et al. 1963; Weintraub and Aronson 1963; Friedman 1975; McLean et al. 1979) comparing an antidepressant with an active placebo. Also cited by Fisher and Greenberg were other studies indicating that adverse effects may enhance the therapeutic efficacy of active drugs (Penick and Fisher 1965; Dinnerstein and Halm 1970) and of the placebo effect (Baker and Thorpe 1957; Kast 1961; Shapiro et al. 1975; Moertel et al. 1976).

It may be difficult to formulate active placebos, and using them may involve ethical problems. Finding active placebos to resemble some categories of drugs

---

2. Noted without comment is the failure of Greenberg and Fisher to level similar criticism about the use of inadequate waiting-list, attention, and other nonequivalent placebo controls in studies of psychotherapy.

appears to be simple. The use of a barbiturate, meprobamate, hydroxyzine, glutethimide, ethchlorvynol, chloral hydrate, or paraldehyde would effectively mimic the sedative effects of antianxiety drugs such as the benzodiazepines. In studies of tricyclic antidepressants, adverse effects could be mimicked with atropine, which causes the anticholinergic adverse effects of xerostomia and constipation; sedatives, to mimic sedation from monoamine oxidase (MAOI) antidepressants; and clonidine in studies of tricyclic antidepressants, for lowered blood pressure and sedation. Methylphenidate could be used for drugs such as fluoxetine that can induce akathisia. Tylenol could be used in studies of vitamin C for the common cold. However, mimicking the adverse effects of some drugs would be difficult. Ethically, it would be hard to justify using a placebo with pulse-lowering effects in studies of beta blockers for coronary and other problems, or using a placebo that mimics the effects of drugs that reduce prothrombin time or induce orthostatic hypotension, and so on. An alternative would be to use ineffective or only marginally effective drugs such as meprobamate for anxiety, promazine for psychosis, nialamide for depression, and caffeine for the study of stimulants.

Ethical attitudes about how to conduct studies change. Thirty years ago it was not considered unethical to evaluate new drugs in open studies. For example, the FDA approved haloperidol for the treatment of adult Tourette syndrome patients as late as 1968, and for children with Tourette syndrome in 1978, on the basis of the clinical experience of a few physicians (Shapiro et al. 1988).

If there were agreement within the scientific and lay communities that active placebos are necessary if one is to derive valid conclusions about the efficacy of a drug or any other treatment, governmental agencies, drug manufacturers, hospital research advisory committees, patients, physicians, and ethicists would accept and require such studies, as they have accepted the use of double-blind studies.

Identical Units of Active Drug and Placebo

Three of our studies and many others (e.g., Sixty Plus Reinfarction Study 1980; Nassif et al. 1981; Howard 1982; Hughes and Krahn 1985) have demonstrated that when the physician titrates the dosage (both of active drug and of placebo) until the therapeutic response is adequate or until the onset of adverse effects, the dosage of the active drug is invariably lower than the placebo dosage. In fact, the dosage increase for placebo often is continued to the maximum. The difference in the number of pills dispensed makes it more likely that physicians or staff members will be able to guess drug allocation. There are two ways to avoid this problem. For studies that use standard dosages, standard dosages should be used for both active drug and placebo, and increases in dosage should be the same for all patients throughout the study. For studies that do not use standard dosages, different dosages can be formulated for use in one capsule or in several (Howard 1982; Gadow et al. 1986a, 1986b). However, most clinical studies require the titration of dosage because the effective dosage and the dosage that induces adverse effects vary considerably among patients, on the basis of age, sex, and weight, and genetic, metabolic, and pharmacodynamic factors. In titration studies, to avoid revealing drug allocation, the record can be reviewed by a physician who is not associated with the study to determine the appropriate dosage, which then would be formulated by a pharmacist within one or more standard units or standard quantities of tablets, capsules, or suspension (Sixty Plus Reinfarction Study 1980). These methods, however, especially the last, might interfere with the full participation and clinical effectiveness of the treating physician.

Length of Treatment

We expected that correct guessing would be related to the length of treatment. The more experience physicians have with patients and with patients' response to treatment, the more likely they would be to guess correctly. Our expectation was not confirmed in our three SSL studies, which extended over four to six weeks of treatment. A possible explanation is that the difference between active drugs and placebos decreased over time in these studies. In fact, there was a trend for improvement to increase with placebo more than with active drugs with more visits and at endpoint (at four or six weeks). Thus, improvement on placebo and placebo-induced adverse effects would make it difficult to differentiate between active drug and placebo. However, similar results are reported in most of the studies that did report significant improvement in patients receiving the active drug. There is no apparent explanation for the lack of association between the length of studies and correct guessing.

Compliance

Noncompliance can also interfere with correct guessing. In one of our double-blind studies comparing diazepam with placebo, which included drug counts at each visit and intensive weekly psychotherapy, a patient revealed to the psychiatrist at the end of treatment that she had entered the study only to be treated with psychotherapy and had never taken the prescribed medication, although drug counts at each visit had been correct. To increase the likelihood of compliance, current studies obtain blood levels. However, this method does not always ensure compliance, since it is reported that some patients do not take their drugs except on the days that blood levels are scheduled. Nevertheless, the use of blood levels is the best method at this time to ensure compliance.

Differences between Physicians

We and others have demonstrated that physicians differ in their ability to correctly guess drug allocation. This may suggest that, to ensure the integrity of the blind procedure, patients should be treated only by physicians who fail to correctly identify drug allocation.

Patients Who Guess Incorrectly

What about patients who do not guess drug allocation correctly? Are they a special group who may be useful in determining whether the response to treatment is independent of compromise of the double-blind design? On the basis of the hypothesis that bias should be suspected among patients who guess correctly and improve, and that patients who do not guess correctly are unbiased, several authors suggested an interesting method of analysis using patients who could not guess drug allocation (Howard et al. 1982; Kramer and Shapiro 1984; Hughes and Krahn 1985; Gadow et al. 1986a, 1986b).

Not Informing Patients about the Design of Studies

Several authors have suggested that bias can be minimized if physicians, staff, and patients are not informed about the design of a study or the treatments being evaluated (Nowlis and Nowlis 1956; Nash 1962). The disadvantage of this procedure is that it deprives most participants of motivation to participate in the study. Moreover, such a design would be seen as unethical because today it is mandatory that patients be fully informed about the design of studies.

The Use of the Double-Blind Design in Nontreatment Studies

Similar problems compromise nontreatment studies (Fears and Schneiderman 1974). The essential feature of all controlled studies is that the design, execution, and statistical analysis should result in conclusions that are associated only with the variable or hypothesis being evaluated. In fact, the principle of the double-blind procedure should be extended to all studies to ensure that the results are not biased. This would include blinding the investigator about experimental and control variables during all stages of the study, including the statistical analysis of the data, which is also subject to bias (Rosenthal 1985). The code for random and blind allocation to the experimental and control groups should not be revealed until all the data are collected and the statistical analysis is completed. Only after the results are analyzed should the code be revealed. This procedure should be used in biological studies such as chemistry and neurohormone determinations, computerized axial tomography and magnetic resonance imaging studies of schizophrenia, psychological studies of diagnosis using projective tests and other scales, genetic studies of comorbidity, and so on.

Other Methodological Safeguards

The use of the double-blind procedure is obviously not the only methodological requirement for an adequate study. Double-blind methodology is highlighted because it has been a neglected problem in research and is associated with the general area of placebo effects. The underlying principles and concepts of the randomized clinical trial—the gold standard for studies—include the use of the double-blind procedure, sometimes referred to as masking (Standards Reporting Trials Group 1994). The other methodological principles included in the use of the term *randomized clinical trial* vary with different authors. Well-controlled studies usually include random assignment of appropriate subjects to experimental and control groups to avoid ascertainment bias and satisfy probability requirements for appropriate statistical analysis; a priori specification of hypotheses; independent and dependent variables; specification of statistical procedures to be used; adequate sample size; the use of measures with demonstrated reliability and validity, to control for errors in measurement; assessment of statistical power; clear differentiation between a priori hypotheses and *post hoc* hypotheses; the use of adjusted probability values based on the number of variables tested, to avoid errors; and subsequent replication of results. There have been advances in statistical analysis, and controlled clinical trials now usually require sophisticated statistical collaboration.[3]

The reader is referred to other papers listed in table 9.1. For interesting observations and data, creative suggestions about how to minimize compromise of

3. The increased complexity of statistical analyses and methodological problems is illustrated in the many papers about the use of statistics published in *JAMA* and *Science* in recent years. These papers include Cohen and Cohen 1984; Mann 1990; Yusuf et al. 1991; Ottenbacher 1992; Guyatt et al. 1993; Guyatt and Rennie 1993; Jaeschke et al. 1993; Nowak 1994; Cohen 1994; and Schulz et al. 1995.

the blind design, and recommendations about methods to control potential unblinding variables and improve methods of analysis of studies, see particularly
Levine et al. 1971; Fears and Schneiderman 1974; Nash 1962; Zifferblatt and
Wilbur 1978; Howard et al. 1982; Kramer and Shapiro 1984; Gadow et al. 1986a,
1986b; Fisher and Greenberg 1989; and White et al. 1992.

Conclusion

There is little doubt that unblinding a double-blind study compromises the
method. The extent of the unblinding determines the validity of the results. The
basic principles of the double-blind procedure are that the active treatment or
drug being evaluated should be identical to the comparison treatment, placebo,
or substance in all respects except for the specific effects or pharmacological
properties of the active treatment or drug; that patients should be randomly allocated to treatment with the active treatment or the control; and that the patient, the clinician, and other staff members be blind to the allocation. These features are accepted as important and necessary for evaluating the efficacy of a
treatment or drug. Studies, however, indicate that subtle and multiple features of
controlled trials may allow clinicians, patients, and staff members to discern drug
allocation, thus unmasking the double blind. Because small significant differences between an active drug and placebo are frequent, compromising the design could influence the results and lead to the finding of spurious significant
differences between active drug and placebo. To prevent this, adequate methods
to ensure the double blind are important. The extent to which blindness is necessary or achievable varies with the drug, the subjects, and other characteristics
of the study. The principles of an adequate double-blind design apply not only
to drug studies but also to studies of psychotherapy, psychopathology, biology,
and so on. Tests to measure the degree of blinding are necessary in all studies,
and conclusions about the results should be modified if unblinding has occurred.

Ensuring the integrity of the double blind, however, is complicated, time
consuming, and expensive. Some of the procedures the method entails seem to
be more important to some drug categories or types of studies than to others;
empirical studies are required to determine the extent to which each or even all
of the procedures are important, and whether added scientific rigor results in
meaningful differences. Such studies, which have not yet been done, would include comparisons of studies differing with regard to the degree of blinding and
other methodological features. They would include comparisons of the results
for data from a family of studies identical except for the method used: a nonblind or open study, a single-blind study, a double-blind study using an inert

placebo, and a double-blind study using an active placebo that mimics all adverse effects of the experimental drug. Such studies might also include comparison of a placebo and an experimental drug that have an identical physical appearance and physiological characteristics with other placebo-drug sets that differ from each other to varying degrees. Until such studies are done, potential factors that threaten the anonymity of the blind allocation and facilitate successful guessing of drug allocation should be evaluated during the design stage before a study is begun and should be examined again after the study is completed.

Current legal, ethical, and economic factors are likely to prevent the study and development of optimal methods of designing inviolable double-blind studies. Physicians and investigators are legally and ethically required to fully inform patients about the design of studies. This requirement has already decreased the number of patients available for some types of studies, such as studies of the efficacy of bone transplants for breast cancer. Conducting such studies is further complicated by ethical concerns. Critical articles have been published about the use of placebos and the double-blind method. These concerns were exaggerated, distorted, and extensively publicized in lay periodicals. A final deterrent to development of a foolproof double-blind procedure is the marked decrease in funds for medical research. We may be stuck, therefore, with an imperfect instrument, which in the foreseeable future is likely to remain imperfectly known.

A remote hope of solving the problem has been provided by the initiation of a serious scientific program that resembles science fiction. The Human Brain Project has been established to create a federation of computer databases that will tie together disparate strands of brain research, ranging from molecular biology to computer science. The database is increased as new data and information become available, ultimately creating a retrievable multimedia atlas of the brain, which may be extended to other physiological systems in the body.

If this project is successful, one may speculate that in the future it may become unnecessary to conduct expensive, inefficient, inadequate, and possibly unethical clinical trials to evaluate whether potentially useful drugs and treatments are effective. We may be able to merely submit the formula for a new psychopharmacological treatment to the database atlas of the brain and receive a dynamic multimedia picture and printout of the treatment's effectiveness, side effects, interactions, advantages, and disadvantages, and the way in which the treatment compares to placebo and other available treatments.

This may be the future, but for the time being we must carry on with the randomized clinical trial, and double-blind methodology. It is the best method we have, and the procedure should be improved rather than abandoned. An obvious way to improve studies is suggested by a survey of placebo-controlled double-blind studies over four years, in which less than 5 percent of the studies involved blindness checks (Ney et al. 1986). Given the extensiveness of the problem illustrated in this review, we cannot assume that blindness regarding patients' allocation to treatment or control groups is always maintained. It is highly desirable, therefore, to develop procedures to evaluate the success of blinding in studies, ascertain the sources of unblinding, and determine the extent to which unblinding influences the results of studies.

Appendix: Comments about Selected Studies Examining Guessing of Drug and Placebo Allocation in Double-Blind Studies

This appendix discusses the design, presentation, and/or analysis of certain of the studies listed in table 9.1.

STUDY 1. Thirty volunteers received either placebo or phenobarbital on the first night and were crossed over to the alternative drug on the second night. Both nights were guessed by subjects.

STUDY 3. Adverse effects increased with the duration of the study.

STUDY 4. Correct guesses were associated with lower dosage units for diazepam and higher dosage units for placebo. There were no significant changes in correct guessing over visits, and the correctness of guesses did not differ significantly between subjects at endpoint and completers.

STUDY 5. The STUDY included data derived from nine studies of seven drugs. The drugs were classified as effective (meprobamate, chlordiazepoxide, and tybamate) or ineffective (amphenidone, hydroxyzine, nialamide, and phenobarbital). Correct guessing of ineffective drugs was similar to the pattern for placebo. Because information was not provided about how many studies included two or more active drugs, in some of the studies the proportion for random drug and placebo may not be 50 percent. Guessing drugs was associated more with the certainty of the guess. Having very few adverse effects is not associated with correct guessing. The authors suggested that correct drug guessing may be a sensitive measure of drug efficacy.

STUDY 7. The study design included two antidepressants—imipramine and phenalzine—and placebo. The participants were instructed to expect a one-in-three chance of receiving each drug, leading to a 66 percent chance of receiving an active drug and a 33 percent chance of receiving a placebo. One hundred patients made a guess about treatment condition. Responders to treatment were more accurate than nonresponders, and the accuracy of guesses by physicians was associated with a past history of psychotropic drug use ($P < .07$).

STUDY 9. Correct guess rates for nurses were significant for patients whose treatment exceeded the median of fifteen months.

STUDY 10. It is difficult to compare the data reported in this study to the data from the other studies in the table. The other studies compared guesses of one physician for all subjects. In this study, three physicians made 141 guesses for 67 patients; thus, an unknown number of patients were rated by more than one physician. The physicians made 61, 51, and 9 guesses, respectively, and the patients made 37 guesses. The derived data in table 9.1 are presented only for physician and patient guesses, omitting a large number of uncertain and unscorable responses, and only for the first two physicians, since only 9 patients were rated by the third physician. With these limitations, overall, with a Bonferonni correction, the results are essentially negative for physicians and positive for patients. The placebo and lithium preparations were not identical and the taste was different. Six of thirteen interviewed patients opened the capsules, and one did a chemical test. The authors recommended the use of an active placebo control.

STUDY 11. The authors recommended a structured rating scale instead of global ratings of improvement, a triple-blind procedure (which was defined as not informing physicians about the nature of the medications), and the use of more than one drug.

STUDY 12. The study is a six-week crossover study of pimozide and placebo; guesses were by one physician who treated all patients.

STUDY 16. Patients reported that the informed consent procedures alerted them to the possibility that they might receive placebos and to possible specific side effects, which challenged them to guess and contributed to their guessing. The study recommended active placebos.

STUDY 17. Placebo was more easily identified than active drug. The authors concluded that blindness depends on pharmacodynamics, the toxicity of the active drug, and the outcome measured (e.g., appetite versus future heart attack, or cholesterol values), and discussed the ethics and difficulty of formulating an active placebo.

STUDY 18. The authors noted that active drug was more frequently guessed than placebo. Uncertainty about guess occurred for nine patients on nicotine gum and sixteen on placebo gum (total 25.3%). Although 84 percent used perceived benefit as the basis for their guess, compared with 22 percent who based their guess on adverse effects, it was concluded, on the basis of a proposed method demonstrating that drug effects differ between correct and incorrect identifiers, that blindness was maintained. A level-of-confidence measure was not different for the active and placebo gum, and most patients who stated a belief were confident about their belief.

STUDY 19. Placebo and active tablets were indistinguishable in appearance and taste. This factor and the weakness of the active drug led to correct and incorrect guesses about having received placebo or active drug being about 50 percent, and contributed to the intactness of the double-blind procedure.

STUDY 20. About one-half the sample of 2,349 subjects did not guess. Chances of guessing active vitamin C were 75 percent (there were six vitamin and two placebo preparations). The vitamin tablets were described as being similar in size and shape and were judged in a taste test by colleagues as reasonably well matched in flavor, texture, and appearance.

STUDY 21. Of the total sample of 190 subjects, 88 (46%) did not guess. The taste of the placebos was different than that of the vitamin C capsules. Some of the subjects tasted the contents and professed to know what they were being given. Dropouts were higher in the placebo group. The placebo capsules were not identical to the vitamin C capsules.

STUDY 22. Sixty-eight percent of the sample did not guess whether they had received active or placebo vitamin C. Of the remaining 137 subjects, 52 percent guessed vitamin C or placebo correctly: that is, 17 percent of the total sample guessed correctly.

STUDY 23. The taste of the different-tasting placebo and vitamin C preparations was associated with correct guessing, $P < .001$. Forty-two percent of the volunteers entering the study tasted their medication. Of the sample of 190 subjects, 88 (46%) did not guess.

STUDY 25. Of the sample of 380 subjects, 49 (13%) did not guess, and 27 (7%) guessed extraneous substances. The range for correct guessing of aspirin and placebo varied considerably, from 25 percent to 67 percent, averaging 52 percent, among the sixteen participating clinics. Each clinic, however, had a larger number of correct than mistaken guesses, the magnitude of the differences varying from 4 percent to 48 percent. Correct guessing was associated with certainty of guessing. No trend was apparent in correct guesses over time. Up to 27 percent of subjects tasted the capsules, the proportion varying from 13 percent to 43 percent among the sixteen clinics. Subsequent inquiry about the basis for guessing by 271 subjects revealed a surprising array of techniques and procedures. Tasting was associated more with guessing aspirin than with guessing placebo ($P < .05$). Other attempts to identify the capsules were made by 9 who smelled the contents, 8 who inspected the contents, 13 who tested the physiologic effects, 5 who did acid tests or had the capsules professionally analyzed, 1 who evaluated the bleeding time, and 1 who evaluated the aspirin level in his blood. Twenty of 101 testers sought professional help to identify substances. Of 95 testers, 67 percent correctly guessed aspirin, compared to 47 percent of 285 nontesters ($P < .001$).

STUDY 27. This study is one of the few that acknowledge that statistical testing would be inappropriate because of the large number of retrospective multiple comparisons. Only percentages are cited; statistical tests were done by us for descriptive purposes only. Higher percentages are reported for correct identification of propanolol for men who were employed and married, and who had at least a high school diploma. Correct identification of placebo was more frequent among patients who were younger than 60 years, employed, and had a high school diploma, and who had not had a heart attack before the study.

chapter ten

Predicting Placebo Response

The history of the placebo effect reveals several major themes. For a long period, the persistent theme was the quaint, interesting, often dramatic, and frequently unbelievable examples of the placebo effect that dominated medical treatment. From the 1930s to the 1950s, the theme shifted to the exploration of different methods of controlling the placebo effect, primarily by the use of the double-blind procedure, in studies of treatment effectiveness. After 1950, improved documentation of the extent and power of the placebo effect was stressed. Over time, an increasing number of studies, usually retrospective analyses using small samples and primitive statistics, focused primarily on the evaluation of drugs. Many variables were identified as being associated with the placebo effect, but there was little or no agreement about which variables contributed to the understanding of the placebo reaction.

With the advent of more sophisticated methodology after the 1950s, the quality of all studies, including those of the placebo effect, improved, but the studies continued to be retrospective analyses. Placebo controls were used to evaluate treatments; initially these were drug treatments, but soon they included nondrug treatments, such as insulin coma treatment, electroconvulsive therapy, lobotomy, and psychotherapy. Very few studies were hypothesis oriented, and it is difficult to determine whether those studies that claimed to be hypothesis oriented were actually formulated to test hypotheses. The result was that dramatic reports of variables associated with the placebo effect could not be replicated, and they simply disappeared into the wastebasket of history, never to be heard of again.

Interest in the placebo effect increased, as did the number of papers published on all aspects of the placebo reaction. This accumulation of literature made it possible to review and evaluate areas of agreement about variables associated with the placebo effect. The number of variables thought to be associated with the placebo effect increased with each study that was reviewed. We published our results over the years (Shapiro 1959, 1960a, 1960b, 1963, 1964a, 1964b, 1971; Shapiro et al. 1968, 1975, 1980, 1983; Shapiro and Morris 1978). Many others also reviewed this literature, both briefly and extensively, but most reviews were primarily reworked versions of previously published papers and contributed little new knowledge about the placebo effect.

Our original plan for our studies was exceedingly ambitious. We were going to collect all papers in the placebo literature that described variables associated with placebo reactions. The data from studies fulfilling the criteria for an adequate study would be considered. The sample of studies would be divided into demographic, socioeconomic, diagnostic, and other relevant groupings. The goal of the review was to determine whether we could identify variables that would be consistently associated with positive placebo reaction, absence of placebo reaction, negative placebo reaction, or placebo-induced side effects.

Although this goal was laudable, it was destined to fail: the studies in the literature were done in so many different ways, and included so many different samples, so many types of variables, and so much *post hoc* manipulation in the analysis of the data that it was impossible to draw conclusions and make generalizations. Moreover, evaluation of these studies clearly indicated to us and others that agreement about what variables were consistently and meaningfully associated with placebo reaction could not be achieved. These conclusions confirmed our impressions that previous reviews attempting to achieve this goal had also failed.

Recognizing that the studies were not done adequately, we entertained the possibility that we could do them better. To achieve this end, we designed better studies—we thought—than those done previously, expecting the answers to come tumbling out of our methodologically sophisticated efforts. We planned to describe the results of our studies very carefully and completely in detailed chapters: one chapter for the design of the study, and other chapters describing the relationships between the placebo effect and demographic, socioeconomic, diagnostic, psychiatric, personality-related, and psychological variables, and selected situational and interactional variables.

We were young, rash, and overly optimistic. Careful, sophisticated analysis of the data failed to provide definite answers to our questions. We considered numerous hypotheses, looking for the answers that we felt sure were there but that continued to elude us. Some of the results were published in 1980 and 1983.[1] Here we will describe the overall method and the results, using common parlance and avoiding descriptions of complex data analyses for different samples

---

1. The evidence, support, and rationale for the selection of variables thought to be associated with positive placebo effects have been described elsewhere (Shapiro et al. 1980, 1983).

and different placebo variables. By so doing, we will more adequately reflect our conclusion about what is known and unknown.

Studies at the Special Studies Laboratory

At the Payne Whitney Psychiatric Clinic, New York Hospital–Cornell University Medical Center, we established a Placebo Studies Laboratory (renamed the Special Studies Laboratory in 1966). Our primary purpose was to study the placebo effect of treatment and to improve the methods of evaluating the efficacy and adverse effect of new drugs. The studies were conducted between 1972 and 1976.

We studied 753 subjects (of a total of 1,070 evaluated who fulfilled criteria for initial testing): 352 anxious outpatients, 272 depressed outpatients, and 129 outpatients from the mixed depression and anxiety sample. At the first visit, the patients completed the Preference about Therapy Scale. Patients rated items indicating their desire or preference for several types of therapy (medicines or drug therapy, psychotherapy or talking treatment, group therapy, and six other items) on a seven-point scale varying from "prefer strongly" to "do not prefer strongly." They then rated thirty-six items about their attitudes toward treatment (such as "I would like to be treated with drugs for my troubles," and "To become dependent on a drug is no solution") on a seven-point scale varying from "disagree strongly" to "agree strongly." Following this, they rated the sixty-four items of the Hopkins Symptom Check List, a self-report scale of symptomatic discomfort, on a five-point scale varying from "not at all" to "extremely," and the seventy items of the Psychiatric Outpatient Mood Scale, using the same five-point scale. They also filled out a demographic scale, completed a questionnaire about previous drug usage, and rated whether or not the medications they had taken had been beneficial. They completed the thirteen standard and nine experimental scales of the Minnesota Multiphasic Personality Inventory. Finally, they were scheduled for another appointment, usually in about one week.

At the second visit, before taking the drug placebo test, the patients again completed the Hopkins Symptom Check List and the Psychiatric Outpatient Mood Scale, rating the symptoms that had been present during the previous week, and a 140-item scale about how they felt at the time of testing. They rated the general intensity of their current symptoms on a four-point scale ("none," "a little," "quite a bit," and "extremely").

The drug placebo test (DPT) was administered during the next hour. The clinician placed a cup of water and a green capsule on the desk and asked the patient to read the instructions. Patients were asked to ingest the capsule, to concentrate on the effects of the medication on their previously described symptoms, and to rate the degree of change in these symptoms. Within five minutes after ingesting the green capsule, they were asked to guess what type of medication they had received (the premedication guess). Ratings of symptom change were made at thirty and sixty minutes, and the overall effect of the medication was rated at the end of the hour. The overall effect was rated on a seven-point scale that varied from "feeling markedly worse" to "feeling markedly better." After one hour, patients were again asked to guess what type of medication they had received (the postmedication guess).

Following the DPT, patients rated 52 statements comparing how they felt now to how they had felt before they took the medication, using a seven-point scale varying from "strongly disagree" to "strongly agree." (The statements included items such as "The medicine made me feel calmer" and "The medicine was probably a sugar pill.") They completed the Attitude to Psychiatrist Scale, on which they evaluated the psychiatrist's likability, physical attractiveness, and competence. Psychiatrists completed a forty-five-minute screening interview for additional diagnostic and clinical information, rated patients on the Hamilton Anxiety and Hamilton Depression Scales (HAS-HDS), and evaluated the patients' likability, physical attractiveness, and suitability for treatment.

Selected Variables for Use in Predicting Positive Placebo Effects

Patients in the samples fulfilled the following criteria: they were between sixteen and seventy years of age; they had completed the sixth grade and were capable of completing forms and testing procedures; they were not diagnosed as organic, senile, or alcoholic and were not addicted to narcotics or barbiturates; they were not on anticonvulsive drugs and not on high or moderate doses of psychotropic drugs; they had had fewer than six treatment sessions during the past six months and had not been hospitalized during the same time period.

In analyses of the data from a number of samples, we found theoretically meaningful and significant relationships between the placebo effect, measured by the DPT, and seven variables: patient's preference for treatment with drugs and psychotherapy; patient's desire to leave the choice of treatment to the physician; drug expectations; patients' attitudes; physicians' attitudes; anxiety; and depression.

Patients' Preference about Therapy

From a large and comprehensive scale indicating the patient's preference for different types of therapy, two variables were selected. The first was a preference for both drugs and psychotherapy. Since the placebo stimulus was a drug, one would expect that patients preferring drug therapy would likely have a more positive placebo reaction when presented with a drug placebo stimulus than they would when presented with a group therapy stimulus; likewise, patients preferring drug therapy would have a more positive placebo effect when given a drug placebo than would patients who preferred psychotherapy exclusively. Therefore, patients preferring both drugs and psychotherapy were expected to have a positive placebo reaction to the DPT because they preferred drug treatment, indicating a desire to be treated with drugs.

The second variable was a preference for leaving the choice of treatment to the physician. A sizable number of patients preferred to leave the choice of therapy to the treating physician. This may represent passivity, dependence on the physician, or faith in the physician's judgment; but in fact, one may wonder why patients would select a type of therapy before they knew anything about what the clinic or physician would select or recommend. If a patient preferred a drug or left the decision to the physician, we hypothesized that either option would be associated with a positive placebo reaction. Our interpretation is that patients had an a priori assumption that drugs would be helpful to them and therefore they preferred to be treated with them. When they were presented with a drug placebo stimulus, it may have confirmed to them that the clinic and physicians were in some way "on track" and were recommending an appropriate treatment. Those expressing a preference for leaving the decision about treatment to the physician might have a tendency to trust physicians or might have faith in the reputation of the clinic, in comprehensive clinical testing and evaluation, in the professional demeanor of the staff, or in the competence of the physician.

For these reasons, we hypothesized that both of these variables would be associated with a positive placebo reaction.

Drug Expectations

Studies of the expectation of types of treatment and subsequent outcome have been extensively reported in the literature, although it is not clear from the reports what constitutes the best measure of expectation, or what are the various meanings of expectation. Patients and subjects may enter therapy or an experiment with preconceived notions derived from past experience. Experimenters may communicate expectations about treatment in both intended and unintended ways. Patients' attitudes toward treatment may also be important. At this point in the evaluation (visit 2), the only thing the patients knew was that they had completed various symptom scales, had been given minimal information about the placebo test, and had been asked to ingest a green capsule. The patients were then immediately asked to guess what kind of drug they had been given. It was expected that their guesses about the category of the drug would be related to the kind of drug they probably required for treatment, and that they would expect to be treated appropriately—they would expect an antianxiety or tranquilizer drug if they were anxious, or a stimulant or antidepressant if depressed, and in neither case would they expect a placebo. Treatment consistent with their expectations would indicate to the patients that the clinic was treating them seriously by evaluating what they needed in the way of treatment. When patients guessed correct drug assignment (antianxiety or antidepressant drug), it confirmed their own expectations that they would be given the appropriate drug, even though they did not know what drug they had been given, or whether or not treatment would be with an active drug specific for their symptoms.

We expected (though we did not formally hypothesize this before the study) that the guesses that patients made post-ingestion, even though they now had the experience of ingesting the inert placebo, with no telltale effects indicating what it was, would resemble the premedication guess.

The evolving pattern of responses by the patients to our various questions suggested a building up of positive responses. Patients had a positive perception of the clinic, the personnel, and the treatment program and had decided what was most appropriate for their treatment. What derives from this indication is a desire and readiness for treatment and a belief or expectation that the physician or clinic would treat them appropriately.

Patients' Attitudes and Physicians' Attitudes

Using numerous studies, especially studies employing the Rogerian nondirective psychotherapeutic approach, we examined the relationship between positive placebo effects and patients' positive attitudes to the therapist and to psychotherapy. Rogerian therapists have demonstrated in many studies that the following therapist variables are positively associated with a positive response to psychotherapy: genuineness, empathy, and unconditional positive regard for the patient. We measured attitudes in a very simple form by asking the patients after the placebo test was completed to rate the psychiatrist who had administered the drug. The questions were the following: Was the psychiatrist who administered the drug test likable? Was the psychiatrist who administered the drug test physically attractive? Was the psychiatrist who gave the drug test competent? Ratings varied from "strongly agree" to "strongly disagree" that the psychiatrist was likable, physically attractive, and competent. A statement was added to the form assuring patients that their responses would be confidential and would not be revealed to the physician. We expected that patients' favorable attitudes toward the psychiatrists would be associated with positive placebo responses.

The same questions were asked of the psychiatrists about the patients. The responses were unrelated to the placebo response, so we discontinued asking the psychiatrists these questions.

Thus, although patients' ratings indicated that they viewed the psychiatrists as likable, physically attractive, and competent, it was not clear whether psychiatrists were displaying these favorable attributes or whether patients were erroneously interpreting the psychiatrists' behavior on the basis of other factors, such as improvement. In a study by Chassan et al. (1980), positive correlations were found between the patients' evaluation of their own progress and their view of the therapist as likable and interested in them. In contrast, the correlation coefficients were low between the therapists' rating of how likable the patients found them and the patients' rating of how likable they found the therapist.

Symptoms: Anxiety and Depression

The presence of symptoms is important for the study of the placebo effect. They provide an index of severity and of discomfort. Some types of symptoms are more closely related to the placebo effect than others. Several symptoms have come to the attention of researchers over the years as factors predisposing the patient toward a positive placebo response.

Anxiety is the symptom most frequently reported in the literature as being related to placebo effects. Therefore, the SSL study first examined the relation between positive placebo effects and the presence or absence, and the severity, of anxiety. Although identified less frequently than anxiety, depression is also reported in the literature as being associated with a positive placebo response. We included this symptom, but with the expectation that the results would not be as strong as those with anxiety. We hypothesized that patients with symptoms of anxiety or depression would have a positive placebo response.

Results of the Study at the Special Studies Laboratory

Before the SSL study, we had hypothesized that the previously described seven independent variables selected for evaluation would best predict positive placebo response to the DPT. The results for the correlation of the seven predictor variables with the overall measure of placebo effect are presented in table 10.1.

Table 10.1 Test of Hypotheses: Correlation of Independent Variables with Positive
Placebo Response for the Total Sample ($N = 753$) at the Special Studies Laboratory

Independent Variable	r^a	P
Therapy preference		
Patient prefers to be treated with both drugs and psychotherapy	0.26	0.0001
Patient prefers to leave the decision about therapy to the psychiatrist	0.19	0.0001
Drug expectation		
Patient expects the placebo test drug to be a sedative-tranquilizer, not a placebo	0.28	0.0001
Patient-physician attitude		
Positive attitude of patient to physician	0.16	0.0001
Positive attitude of physician to patient	−0.06	NS
Symptoms		
Anxiety	0.13	0.0002
Depression	0.09	0.0076

Note: Total sample is composed of an anxious sample (352 subjects), a depressed sample
(272 subjects), and a mixed depressive-anxious sample (129 subjects).
[a] Abbreviations: N = total number of subjects; r = correlation coefficient; P = probability; NS = not significant.

It is clear that all of the predictor variables (with the exception of positive attitude of the physician to the patient) were significantly correlated with a positive placebo reaction. The magnitude and direction of the relationships of the predictor variables with the overall rating of placebo reaction were consistent with the hypotheses about the three samples (anxious outpatients, depressed outpatients, and mixed depression-anxiety sample).

After the placebo test, 429 patients were assigned to treatment with four to six weeks of weekly drug treatment and brief psychotherapy, or with placebo drug treatment and brief psychotherapy. The drugs used in the studies were diazepam (Valium) versus placebo, amitryptyline (Elavil) versus placebo, and doxepin (Sinequan) versus placebo. Patients were evaluated by psychiatrists for both active drug and placebo, and for whether they responded better to active drug or placebo. Surprisingly, there were no differences among the evaluations. Separate analyses were done for the relationship between outcome and placebo effect in both the drug treatment group and the placebo group. The a priori prediction that positive placebo response would be associated with positive treatment outcome was confirmed in both treatment and placebo groups.

Thus, improvement after treatment was significantly linked with positive responses to a drug placebo stimulus in all three studies. Although the correlations were low, they were replicated across the three samples. The current studies suggest that the likelihood that a test of placebo reactivity will be related to clinical course is increased if placebo testing is done in a clinical context, and that positive placebo reactivity is more likely to be found if the form of the placebo test is consistent with the patient's preference for therapy. Other factors linked to placebo reactivity include the strength of the instructions about an expected effect, expectations about the effect of the placebo, positive attitudes of the patient to the physician, and clinical discomfort (particularly anxiety).

We expected that the correlation of negative placebo response, nonresponse to placebo, and placebo-induced side effects with the variables we examined would in general be opposite to the correlation of positive placebo reaction with those variables. Thus, patients with a neutral placebo response would not prefer treatment with drugs and psychotherapy or would not prefer to leave the decision about therapy to the physician, would not have a positive attitude to the physician, would not have high levels of anxiety or depression, and would have expected to receive a placebo rather than a drug during the placebo test. These hypotheses were confirmed.

One of the striking results of this study was the simple nature of the independent variables. The variables that were not significant to placebo reaction in the composite study of the total sample include scores on the Rod and Frame Test, the Neuroticism-Extroversion Scale, and the Social Desirability and Acquiescence Scales from the Minnesota Multiphasic Personality Inventory.

Interpretation

The correlation between the independent variables and a patient's having a positive placebo response can be interpreted narratively as follows: The presence or absence of symptoms influences the response to the placebo test. Patients with distress, particularly anxiety, are more likely to have positive placebo responses if the form of the placebo is a relevant treatment stimulus for a patient (e.g., a drug stimulus if the patient believes that he or she needs drug treatment and that drugs are effective). Patients who express a preference for treatment with drugs and psychotherapy might interpret receiving a drug placebo stimulus as acknowledgment and confirmation of their need, desire, and preference for treatment. Those expressing a preference for leaving the decision about treatment to the physician might have a tendency to trust physicians or might have faith in the reputation of the clinic, comprehensive clinical testing and evaluation, the professional demeanor of the staff, and the competence of the physician.

Positive placebo responses are likely if patients have positive expectations about treatment, as reflected by their guessing that the placebo stimulus is a relevant, active drug for their symptoms, and not a placebo. A positive placebo response may mean that the patient has a positive expectation, and believes that his or her symptoms have been evaluated as serious and warrant real clinical treatment with a drug. Additionally, patients with a positive reaction to a drug placebo may have believed that they would be treated with an appropriate and effective drug related to their symptoms. Positive placebo response is also related to a general positive attitude to the physician, who is seen as likable, attractive, and competent, reflecting positive expectations that he or she would be helpful.

Preference for a particular therapy is an important variable for the study of the placebo effect. If no therapy is given—if patients are simply asked to sit in a room—many feel worse than before. We had previously used a control group of patients but discontinued using this type of control procedure. Patients in the Control Placebo Test group (CPT) had applied for treatment of their symptoms and were expecting treatment. It is likely that when they were told that they were being tested to observe spontaneous variation, such information stimulated fantasies about the procedure. Therefore, they may have had a less favorable therapeutic response and more frequent new symptoms because they saw the CPT as a noxious stimulus. In addition, the form of the placebo must be consistent with the patient's assumptions, beliefs, religion, culture, and preferences about therapy, and often with current societal preferences and enthusiasms for therapeutic modalities. An appropriate placebo stimulus for an organic food and vitamin enthusiast might be a tablet with only neutral and natural substances, such as vitamins or a concentrated extract of fruits and vegetables. Those with a penchant for psychoanalysis are not likely to have positive placebo reactions to a drug, nor are Christian Scientists. A long-distance runner might have positive placebo effects if asked to run around the hospital for an hour, and so on. The form of the placebo stimulus has not been explicitly included in previous studies of the placebo effect or in studies of treatment.

Conclusion

We have considered nonpositive types of placebo reaction (negative and neutral) and have also discussed several important factors related to positive placebo test results. They include the pivotal relationship of high levels of symptom distress (especially anxiety) to positive placebo effects, the need for the therapeutic stimulus to be a relevant one that meets patients' expectations, the importance of a favorable attitude to the physician, and the relation between positive placebo test results and improvement. These findings have been replicated in studies (Shapiro et al. 1980). In addition, we believe that our results may be attributed to our having maximized, in the therapeutic setting of our studies, nonspecific factors tending to favor positive expectations in the patient. These factors include giving patients an appointment within one week, conducting a comprehensive evaluation, using efficient procedure, seeing patients punctually at the appointed time, offering a pleasant atmosphere at a prestigious psychiatric clinic, using experienced research assistants and psychiatrists who were both drug oriented and psychodynamically oriented, and using staff members who were interested in the specific drugs being tested, as well as in nonspecific or placebo effects of treatment. To enhance positive therapeutic outcome, therefore, treatment should include, at a minimum, these nonspecific therapeutic factors.

chapter eleven

Summary and Conclusions

Psychological factors have always been important in medicine. Until the middle of the twentieth century, treatment was primitive, unscientific, for the most part ineffective, and often shocking (to the modern mind) and dangerous. Useful drugs or procedures appeared infrequently in medical history, and for thousands of years physicians prescribed what we now know were useless and often dangerous medications. We know today that the effectiveness of these procedures and medications was due to nonspecific factors: the placebo effect. In fact, the history of medical treatment, until recently, has been essentially the history of the placebo effect. Despite the use of ineffective methods, physicians have been respected and honored because they have been the therapeutic agents for the placebo effect. The placebo effect flourished as the norm of medical treatment at least until the beginning of modern scientific medicine.

As late as the twentieth century, patients continued to submit to purging, puking, poisoning, cutting, cupping, blistering, bleeding, freezing, heating, sweating, leeching, and shocking. Cure-alls and other nonspecific remedies were used for centuries, and some of these noxious methods and bizarre substances continue to be used by healers today. Healers have used methods such as dehydration—whether by leeching, scarification, bloodletting, clysterization, stomachics, vomitives, purgation, or sweating—to effect a cure (although every modern hospital and physician now recognizes that it is necessary to do the exact opposite by hydrating patients as a life-saving procedure). A common underlying theme for such treatments was the removal of the bad, evil, or diseased, both psychological and physiological; this rationale reassured patients, mobilizing their hope and helping them to feel better. Since the language for expressing emotional problems was limited, it is likely that psychological problems were expressed in somatic complaints. For example, depressive symptoms could be experienced as symptoms of exhaustion, insomnia, or decreased libido. If treated medically, these depressive symptoms would have been treated with cathartics such as purging, bleeding, and enemas. Religious expiation, by contrast, would serve the function of psychological catharsis by expelling bad, unacceptable impulses and evil thoughts. This could also result in clinical improvement, which could be seen as a placebo effect.

What useful drugs did exist were often used inappropriately, in inappropriate dosages, for scores of conditions, and physicians lacked the capacity to evaluate their specific usefulness, thus contributing to the loss of the benefit of these drugs for future generations. Despite this, historians continue to exaggerate the effectiveness of primitive medicine, without regard to its proven usefulness. The only possible resolution to the question of the efficacy of ancient drugs is to accurately determine the putative name of each ancient drug, its chemistry and methods of preparation, how it was used, and for what illnesses; to translate this information into current pharmacological knowledge; and to conduct in vitro and in vivo clinically controlled studies—a task not likely to be done anytime soon. Without such proof, the claims about the efficacy of ancient remedies have yet to be proved.

There were some useful drugs prior to the nineteenth century, although their discovery was erratic and sporadic: quinine was discovered in 1632, and digitalis, smallpox immunization, and Lind's lemons for scurvy in the eighteenth century. Only with the onset of scientific medicine in the middle of the nineteenth century did treatment improve somewhat (as shown by the discovery of vitamins, hormones, anesthesia, aseptic surgery, and smallpox immunization). Nevertheless, placebos continued to dominate treatment for the next one hundred years. Therapeutic nihilism characterized medicine as late as the beginning of the twentieth century. Even as late as 1950, a placebo medication was given to 40 percent of general practice patients, and the majority of published studies used uncontrolled or inadequately controlled research designs.

Very slowly, progress was made in improving clinical trial methodology: initially the use of the single-blind method and placebo controls, and finally, in the 1950s, the increasing acceptance and use of the double-blind method. The development of the double-blind procedure and other advances in clinical trial methodology were major steps toward weakening the hegemony of the placebo effect. The contributions of H. L. Hollingsworth, Torald Sollmann, and Harry A. Gold in this major revolution in scientific methodology were highlighted because of their incredible prescience. Gold developed the double-blind method virtually alone beginning in 1937, using it relentlessly and uncompromisingly in his many studies and proselytizing about the necessity of controlling for the placebo effect. Although strongly resisted for many years, the double-blind method has since the 1960s been a requirement for NIH funding of studies and for FDA approval of new drugs or instrumentation; since the 1980s it has been required for the publication of scientific papers.

Our studies and those of others have demonstrated that the double-blind method is not infallible. Frequently, the double blind can be unblinded. The method can be compromised if the active drug and the placebo are not identical in etching, embossing, color, taste, and dissolubility. In addition, physicians can often guess what type of drug the patient received (active drug or placebo) on the basis of the type of drug being studied, the side effect patterns of the active drug, higher dosage units for patients receiving placebo, and patient improvement; but physicians vary in their ability to guess correctly. We and others have suggested methods to ensure that blinding is not violated. Blinding can be protected by using capsules that have been carefully formulated and matched so that research assistants and patients will be unable to detect physical differences between drug and placebo. Another possible answer is the use of liquid solutions. Personnel should have no contact with the medicine except for its dispensation in closed containers. Personnel independent of the study should be employed in counts of returned medication.

The placebo effect is ubiquitous, and despite significant advances in clinical trial methodology, nonspecific or placebo effects have not disappeared from clinical trials. Estimates of the prevalence of placebo response rates are mainly derived from studies that include a placebo control group, and range from 21 to 58 percent. In psychopharmacology, placebo response rates vary from 30 to 50 percent in depression, and placebos have been found to be 59 percent as effective as tricyclic antidepressant, 65 percent as effective as lithium, 58 percent as effective as nonpharmacological treatment of insomnia, and 55 percent as effective as injected morphine and common analgesics. But placebo effects do not occur only in drug therapy. Surgery is not subject to controlled studies, primarily because controlled trials in surgery (e.g., the use of invasive procedures such as sham surgery as a control for transplants) are technically more difficult to devise and ethically more difficult to justify. The result is that surgery, because it is difficult to subject to clinical trial, is more prone to placebo effects than medicine. Serious questions about the overuse, effectiveness, safety, and benefit of cesarean sections, hysterectomies, spinal fusions, transplants, and surgery for cardiac problems are documented in the literature.

The greatest prevalence of the placebo effect occurs in uncontrolled clinical reports because in uncontrolled studies placebo mechanisms are maximized. Reviews of studies of enthusiastically endorsed but later abandoned treatments reported an average improvement in 82 percent of patients treated for angina pectoris and in 70 percent of patients in a series of recent studies of medical treatments (Roberts et al. 1993). Reports of higher percentages are particularly common in studies of illnesses whose symptoms wax, wane, fluctuate, and spontaneously remit. The percentages are smaller, of course, in studies of serious illnesses (e.g., malignancies) with infrequent spontaneous remission, but even here placebo effects are reported anecdotally.

Psychiatry and psychotherapy are rife with placebo effects. As it became increasingly possible to control the physical environment, somatic displacement became a less adequate and less necessary outlet for psychological problems. Today, with increased emphasis on rationality, understanding, and open discussion, it is possible to approach psychological problems more directly. When traditional religious and other explanations failed, the human capacity for fantasy and projection focused increasingly on self-understanding, and psychoanalysis and psychotherapy became the institutional outlet for psychological problems. Placebo effects, which were formerly associated with physical illness and treatment, are now also commonly associated with psychological treatment. A controlled study of the efficacy of psychoanalysis has never been done. Without such evidence, the effectiveness of that form of therapy cannot be convincingly evaluated.

Although psychotherapy has been reported to be more effective than placebo, its efficacy has yet to be proven. Most of the studies of psychotherapy that attempt to use controls are flawed. When the evidence is examined, it is clear that the placebo controls are usually inadequate. One method that has been proposed for evaluation of the efficacy of psychotherapy has been to contrast one therapy with another, but few studies support the superiority of one therapy over the other. Moreover, most studies report that differences in the training and experience of therapists, the nature of the patients' problems, the length of sessions, the number of sessions, and the duration of therapy do not result in different therapeutic effects. Meta-analysis has been used to discriminate between the effectiveness of various schools of therapy and has clearly demonstrated the superiority of various types of therapies over a host of placebo treatments. Although it is a powerful technique, it is not free of defects, including the use of questionable data.

There are now more than 250 different schools of psychotherapy, and data supporting the theories and efficacy of any particular school are absent. Psychotherapy appears to mix ill-defined nonspecific elements indiscriminately in the hope that some will be effective. There appears to be general consensus that psychotherapy is useful, beneficial, and effective for many patients, but this is true of many notable placebo treatments. Additional studies are needed before we can say with certainty that psychotherapy is more than a placebo.

Placebo treatment is easy to transmute into new forms. We have seen this in the repeated repackaging of types of psychotherapy and in the fraud, faith, fallacies, and fads that still flourish. The ubiquity of fraudulent treatments and other ineffective treatments is reflected in the amounts spent annually: $30 billion for fraud and religious and psychic healing; $13.9 billion for vitamins, organic diets, and holistic and alternative treatment; and untold amounts for fads such as New Age, lifestyle-related, or self-help modalities (such as ecotherapy, or communing with nature; and meditative immunotherapy, which is believed to encourage the growth and strength of good white blood cells and destroy malignant cells).

Successful therapies, too, inevitably become associated with placebo effects. And it is reasonable to assume that the placebo effect has become associated with the placebo itself. Whereas *placebo* was formerly a pejorative word and treatment with placebos was seen as unethical, the placebo has now become respectable. Today there is growing appreciation of its power to heal; its therapeutic power has become exaggerated and its effect increased. Thus, individuals often submit to or seek treatments that have only anecdotal support and have not been scientifically validated. In fact, even when told that the treatment may be a placebo, they continue to tout its effectiveness if they improve.

Megavitamins, nutrition and organic foods, stress reduction, holistic medicine, and even the concept of behavioral health may be examples of recent popular placebos. There is no definitive evidence demonstrating that these techniques are clinically useful or effective. Psychotherapy and other psychological procedures, even biological psychiatry, are not exempt from the placebo effect. Many psychotherapists believe that the placebo effect does not apply to psychotherapy because both are psychological procedures, and psychotherapy is characterized by others as the ultimate placebo.

Belief in the positive effect of placebos even extends to biological psychiatry. When patients applied to a prominent university study center for the treatment of depression, they were told that if they were to get better on placebo it would mean that the placebo had a beneficial effect on their neurotransmitters—certainly a preposterously premature conclusion that exploits the credulity of patients volunteering for treatment in a study. This explanation to patients may be based on provocative studies by Levine et al. (1978, 1981, 1984), Fields (1997), and others supporting the hypothesis that placebos decrease pain by increasing endogenous opioids. However, these studies are difficult to interpret, often are inadequately replicated, may explain some but not all types of analgesia, have not evaluated the effect of other psychological variables such as fear and anxiety, did not clearly identify the mechanism of the decrease in pain, and provided no evidence supporting a relationship of the opioid system to placebo effects other than analgesia (Grevert and Goldstein 1985; Fields 1997).

Another reflection of the placebo's popularity is the current interest in mind-body relationships, which includes speculation about the effects of stress, depression, social isolation, personality, and other psychological and psychosocial factors on the body. An extension of these speculations is the belief that placebos, nonspecific behavioral therapies, and improved immunological functioning can reduce the risk, morbidity, and mortality of infections, heart attacks, autoimmune disorders, and cancer (Temoshok et al. 1985; Eli et al. 1992; Lee et al. 1992; Mulder et al. 1992; Waxler-Morrison et al. 1992; Fawzy et al. 1993; Gellert et al. 1993; Spiegel 1993; Stein et al. 1993). The literature examining these speculations demonstrates that nonspecific therapeutic procedures improve mood, coping, and other psychosocial factors, as well as compliance with medical management. In some studies, but not in others, these factors are reported to prolong survival in cancer patients. Treatments that are nonspecific may reduce the reaction to distress; decrease depression, demoralization, and hopelessness; and promote health-enhancing behavior; and thus secondarily may have a favorable effect on illness (Beecher 1959b, 1959c; Shapiro and Shapiro 1984b; Frank and Frank 1991). Increase in survival rates, therefore, may be related primarily to psychosocial intervening variables such as compliance with medical management; improved diet, exercise, and sleep; abstinence from alcohol, smoking, and addictive, nonaddictive, and neuroleptic drugs; increased assertiveness with physicians about treatment; and the ability to cope with illness better (House et al. 1988; Cohen et al. 1991; Williams et al. 1991; Perry et al. 1992; Frasure-Smith et al. 1993; Horwitz and Horwitz 1993; Perry and Fishman 1993; Spiegel 1993; Stein et al. 1993).

We cannot yet answer the question of whether placebos and other nonspecific treatments have specific, meaningful effects on physical illness. To date, such effects have not been substantiated by well-controlled and replicated studies in humans, free of *post hoc* analyses of nonhypothesized variables, subgroup analyses, and other methodological shortcomings—all of which contribute to the reporting of chance, nonreplicated relationships. Our critical, data-oriented review of the literature does not substantiate the belief that placebos and psychological factors have specific physiological effects on physical illness.

We are also still beset by the problem that the mechanism by which psychological factors, placebos, and psychological therapies may affect physical illness and disease is unknown. It has been proposed that psychological factors such as depression or stress can impair immune function, cause or cure illness, and delay or hasten death. These interrelationships fall within the province of psychoimmunology. But this discipline appears to be characterized more by creative speculation about the interaction of psychological, immunological, and brain relationships than by critical studies in human beings. The extensive findings reported are more like neuropsychophysiological perturbations that do not have significant, prolonged, and important clinical effects. At present, the data provide no support for the hypothesis that changes in immune parameters have any clinical use or relevance (Evans et al. 1989; Darko et al. 1991; Stein et al. 1991; Perry et al. 1992; Stein 1992; Perry 1994).

What is known about the placebo effect? The published studies of the placebo effect reveal an absence of a systematic approach. Characteristically they are anecdotal reports, clinical impressions, theoretical formulations, or *post hoc* extrapolations of chance significant findings from many variables in which a placebo was used as a control for the study of specific treatment. There is in the literature little consistency about placebo stimuli, methods of administration, and duration of treatment with placebo. In addition, many of the studies use measures with inadequate reliability and validity, subjects who are volunteers, and/or therapists with varied or inadequate training. As a result, the findings vary from study to study and cannot be replicated, thus making it difficult to compare the results and derive general conclusions.

Positive placebo effects were described in the literature more frequently than other types. Our research studies (Shapiro et al., 1980, 1983) identified four types of placebo reactors: positive placebo reactors, who reported decreased symptoms; negative placebo reactors, who described exacerbation of their symptoms; neutral or nonplacebo reactors, or patients with no change in their symptoms; and a fourth group who reported new symptoms or side effects, referred to as placebo-induced side effects. Those patients reacting negatively or positively to a placebo tended to develop placebo-induced side effects more frequently than did neutral reactors. In one controlled study (Shapiro et al. 1974), patients given placebos in the form of a drug tablet reported significantly more somatic side effects, whereas cognitive and affective side effects were reported by those given a psychotherapeutic-type placebo stimulus or patients in the control condition. Placebo response was positive in 51 percent of patients receiving placebos (symptoms decreased; the patient felt better); negative in 12 percent (symptoms increased; the patient felt worse); and absent in 37 percent (there was no change); and placebo-induced side effects (new unpleasant symptoms) occurred in 57 percent of the total sample (86% of negative placebo reactors, 63% of positive placebo reactors, and 40% of nonplacebo reactors) in our 1980–83 studies.

Demographic variables such as age, sex, intelligence, race, social class, and ethnic or religious background were unrelated to placebo reaction. Clinical placebo effects were not correlated with susceptibility to hypnosis, tests of suggestibility, or the use of volunteer subjects in laboratory studies, and placebo effects were not constant: they varied over time. Several studies reported a relationship between suggestibility and clinical course. However, a stronger relationship was reported when a more clinically relevant placebo test was used to predict clinical course. Placebo stimuli must resemble a credible therapy for the patient. Our studies (Shapiro et al. 1980, 1983) demonstrated a consistent association between positive placebo reaction and the patient's desire for drug treatment, if the placebo was presented as a drug. There was a significant increase in positive placebo effects when the placebo test instructions suggested a favorable response to treatment: "Our evaluation indicated that you should respond favorably to the test drug." There was a weak but significant and consistent relationship between placebo reaction and clinical course in several studies. The amount of improvement in our studies was significant and ranged from 2 percent to 16 percent. This was demonstrated only with regard to short-term treatment.

There was no evidence of a relationship between placebo reaction and personality variables such as field independence or dependence, dominance, compliance, social desirability, introversion, and extroversion. There was some support for a relationship between placebo reaction and some measures of acquiescence.

Positive placebo reactors had high anxiety scores, and this variable was an important determinant of the response to treatment. The pivotal role of anxiety in positive placebo response is supported by numerous citations in the literature and the results of our studies. Although all of the symptom scales (anxiety; depression; somatization; hostility; fatigue; and energy-fatigue, a combination of anxiety and depression) significantly improved during a one-hour placebo test, only moderate to high anxiety correlated with positive placebo response. In a testing milieu, subjects' anxiety may be amplified by uncertainties and fantasies associated with applying for treatment and visiting an impressive hospital or office, by concern about the meaning and seriousness of the symptoms, and by questions about how severe their illness is and what treatment will be recommended. In fact, the greater the degree of anxiety, the stronger the positive placebo response appears to be.

We found it difficult to separate anxiety and depression in our studies. Improvement in the measurement of facets of anxiety and depression may lead to the identification of those specific anxiety-related factors that are associated with placebo responsiveness and may facilitate our understanding of the placebo effect as it is influenced by anxiety and depression.

Other important determinants of the response to treatment are the patient's positive attitude toward the treatment and the patient's response to the physician. As we have shown, there is a significant correlation between the patient's attitude toward the physician (rating the physician as likable, physically attractive, and competent) and improvement. However, when the physicians used the same scale to rate their colleagues, their ratings did not correlate with patients' ratings, suggesting that patients view physicians differently than do other physicians.

Although we did not assess positive expectations about the efficacy of treatment, they were consistently reported as an important nonspecific factor in placebo reaction and treatment outcome. It is posited that the healer's belief in the efficacy of the treatment may have a positive effect on therapeutic outcome. Likewise, patients' positive expectations are seen as important. If a patient believes that he or she needs drug treatment and that drugs are effective and then is treated with drugs, or if a patient trusts, has faith in, or values the decision of the physician about the choice of treatment, that patient is more likely to have a positive placebo response. Positive expectations about choice of treatment may reflect factors such as hope, faith, optimism, and motivation—factors that are difficult to differentiate one from another. Expectations of improvement, however, may either be independent of or may overlap with such factors. Future studies should consider patients' preferences about the type and kind of treatment and the possible role of preferences as important variables in the design of experimental studies of the placebo effect. It is necessary to consider, as a source of placebo response, patients' conception of, preferences regarding, and attitudes toward treatment, and to evaluate the possible interaction of these factors in studies of therapeutic outcome.

There are differences in how patients respond to placebos. Some patients have the capacity to be optimistic or positive placebo reactors; others have little or no capacity to develop optimism and are not placebo reactors; and still others, negative placebo reactors, remain symptomatic and impaired. Positive attitudes may have an evolutionary advantage since they may lead to the maintenance of health, thereby ensuring survival and procreation, whereas negative attitudes may lead to demoralization and increase the probability of chronic illness and even death. Perhaps we should search for ways to enhance the placebo effect, which in turn may stimulate hope, optimism, and the motivation required to deal with a difficult world. Although one study (Fields 1997) cited endogenous, self-induced opiates as a possible candidate for an analgesic hormone providing the pain relief associated with placebos, the findings have not been replicated and require generalization in other areas.

We do know that nonspecific factors involved in the art of medicine, the doctor-patient relationship, and the placebo effect of treatment can be used to improve therapy in largely unknown, nonspecific, and unpredictable ways. As our research demonstrated, certain factors in the doctor-patient relationship augment placebo effects: belief in the effectiveness of the treatment, and the patient's perception of the physician as empathic, physically attractive, likable, and competent. Physicians who are sensitive to these factors, who like their patients, respond positively to them, and use this factor, knowingly or unknowingly, may thereby contribute to a positive therapeutic outcome.

Today more patients are taking a more active role in their treatment. Patients seek greater individual responsibility and an active, independent role. The development of new technologies and a broadening of the scope of medicine to include the concept of prevention may alter how the healer and patient relate to each other. The placebo effect may be the most important determinant in this development, although how it does so is probably multiply determined. Implicit in the placebo effect is the recognition that patients bring to the healing process their own attitudes and belief systems, which can be stronger than the specific action of a drug. Self-help therapies have perhaps unknowingly taken advantage of this factor. In such therapies, the doctor provides a milieu that maximizes the patient's role, changing it from passive to active. Reliance on individual responsibility may also create positive placebo reactions and enhance the possibility of a positive treatment outcome. While the evidence is not yet substantive that these methods can reverse the course of an illness or can otherwise influence health, favorable preliminary reports about self-help methods, holistic medicine, and behavioral health warrant further investigation. The extent to which such methods influence the maintenance and promotion of health are empirical issues that can be tested with appropriately designed controlled studies.

The relationship between the placebo effect and the underlying mechanisms of the body that control and maintain health still eludes us. We hope that our studies, and those of other investigators, will contribute understanding about the laws governing the nonspecific, as yet mystifying, but very powerful therapeutic potential of the placebo effect. If the nonspecificity of the placebo effect can be rendered specific and its strength can be unleashed, the terms *placebo* and *placebo effect* can appropriately disappear into medical history.

References

Ackerknecht, E. H. 1971. *Medicine and Ethnology.* Stuttgart: Verlag Hans Huber Bern.

Ackner, B., Harris, A., and Oldham, A. J. 1957. Insulin treatment of schizophrenia: A controlled study. *Lancet* 2:607–11.

Adams, S. H. 1905. The great American fraud. *Collier's* 36:14, 15, 29.

Agnew, N. M. 1963. The relative value of self-report and objective tests in assessing the effects of amphetamine. *Journal of Psychiatric Research* 2:85–100.

Altman, L. K. 1993. Scientists debate destroying the last strains of smallpox. *New York Times,* August 30, B6.

Amberson, J. B., McMahon, B. T., and Pinner, M. 1931. A clinical trial of sanocrysin in pulmonary tuberculosis. *American Review of Tuberculosis* 24:401–35.

American Psychiatric Association (APA). 1956. *Psychiatric Research Reports of the American Psychiatric Association.* Vol. 4, *An Evaluation of the Newer Psychopharmacologic Agents and Their Role in Current Psychiatric Practice.* Washington, D.C.: APA.

American Psychiatric Association (APA), Commission on Psychotherapies. 1982. *Psychotherapy Research: Methodological and Efficacy Issues.* Washington, D.C.: APA.

American Psychoanalytic Association. 1958. *Central Fact-Gathering Committee: Summary and Final Report.* Mimeographed.

Anderson, T. W., Reid, D.B.W., and Beaton, G. H. 1972. Vitamin C and the common cold: A double-blind trial. *Canadian Medical Association Journal* 107:503–8.

Anderson, T. W., Suranyi, G., and Beaton, G. H. 1974. The effect on winter illness of large doses of vitamin C. *Canadian Medical Association Journal* 111:31–36.

Anderson, T. W., Beaton, G. H., Corey, P. N., et al. 1975. Winter illness and vitamin C: The effect of relatively low doses. *Canadian Medical Association Journal* 112:823–26.

Andrews, G., and Harvey, R. 1981. Does psychotherapy benefit neurotic patients? A reanalysis of the Smith, Glass, and Miller data. *Archives of General Psychiatry* 38:1203–8.

Anonymous. 1931. Clinical trials of new medicines. *Lancet* 2:304.

———. 1954. Controlled trials: Planned deception. *Lancet* 1:534–35.

———. 1955a. The placebo: A neglected agent? pt. 1. *Physician's Bulletin* 20:3.

———. 1955b. The placebo: A neglected agent? pt. 2. *Physician's Bulletin* 20:48.

———. 1955c. Placebos [editorial]. *JAMA* 159:780.

———. 1957a. Mistletoe. *Spectrum* 5:612.

———. 1957b. The placebo. *Spectrum* 5:141.

————. 1960a. Charitable chirurgion. *MD* 4:188–93.

————. 1960b. The placebo. *Spectrum* 8:208.

————. 1962. A plea for the placebo. *Medical Times* 90:161.

————. 1964a. The blind lead the halt [editorial]. *Medical Science,* December.

————. 1964b. The placebo progress. *Hospital Focus,* May 15.

————. 1964c. Placebo reactions and adverse effects of drugs. *Medical Science,* May, p. 24.

————. 1994a. Homeopathy: Much ado about nothing? *Consumer Reports* 59:201–6.

————. 1994b. Psychiatry's match results continue to decline. *Psychiatric News* 29:1, 29.

————. 1995. Mental health: Does therapy help? *Consumer Reports* 60:734–39.

Appelbaum, P. S., Roth, L., Lidz, C. W., et al. 1987. False hopes and best data: Consent to research and the therapeutic misconception. *Hastings Center Report* 17:20–24.

Appleton's Medical Dictionary. 1904. Edited by F. P. Foster. New York: D. Appleton.

————. 1909. Edited by F. P. Foster. New York: D. Appleton.

————. 1915. Edited by E. J. Smith. New York: D. Appleton.

Arieti, S. 1959. *American Handbook of Psychiatry.* Vols. 1 and 2. New York: Basic Books.

Astin, A. W., and Ross, S. 1960. Glutamic acid in human intelligence. *Psychological Bulletin* 57:429–34.

Auerbach, A. 1967. The double-blind design: A theoretical re-examination. *Canadian Medical Association Journal* 97:1480–82.

Austin, S. C., Stolley, P. D., and Lasky, T. 1992. The history of malariotherapy for neurosyphilis. *JAMA* 268:516–19.

Bailey, P. 1965. *Sigmund the Unserene: A Tragedy in Three Acts.* Springfield, Ill.: Charles C Thomas.

Baker, A. A., and Thorpe, J. G. 1957. Placebo response. *Archives of Neurology and Psychiatry* 78:57–60.

Bakst, H., Kissin, M., Leibowitz, S., et al. 1948. The effect of intravenous aminophylline on the capacity for effort without pain in patients with angina of effort. *American Heart Journal* 36:527–34.

Bannerman, R. H., ed. 1983. *Traditional Medicine and Healthcare Coverage.* Geneva: World Health Organization.

Baruk, H. 1957. *Les thérapeutiques psychiatriques.* Paris: Presses Universitaires de France.

Barzansky, B., and Gevitz, N. 1992. *Beyond Flexner: Medical Education in the Twentieth Century.* Westport, Conn.: Greenwood Press.

Batterman, R. C. 1955. Appraisal of new drugs [correspondence]. *JAMA* 158:1547.

Beardsley, R. S., Gardocki, G. J., and Larson, D. B. 1988. Prescribing of psychotropic medication by primary care physicians and psychiatrists. *Archives of General Psychiatry* 45:1117–19.

Beck, A. T., Rush, A. J., Shaw, B. F., et al. 1979. *Cognitive Therapy of Depression.* New York: Guilford Press.

Beecher, H. K. 1952. Experimental pharmacology and measurement of the subjective response. *Science* 116:157–62.

———. 1955. The powerful placebo. *JAMA* 159:1602–6.

———. 1956. The subjective response and reaction to sensation. *American Journal of Medicine* 20:107–13.

———. 1957. The measurement of pain: Prototype for the quantitative study of subjective responses. *Pharmacological Reviews* 9:59–209.

———. 1959a. Experimentation in man. *JAMA* 169:461–78.

———. 1959b. *Measurement of Subjective Responses: Quantitative Effects of Drugs.* New York: Oxford University Press.

———. 1959c. Placebos and the evaluation of the subjective response. In S. O. Waife and A. Shapiro, eds., *The Clinical Evaluation of New Drugs.* New York: Haeber-Harper. Pp. 61–75.

———. 1961. Surgery as placebo. *JAMA* 176:1103.

———. 1963. Ethics and experimental therapy [editorial]. *JAMA* 186:8581.

———. 1966. Ethics and clinical research. *New England Journal of Medicine* 274:1354–60.

Behavioral and Brain Sciences. 1983. Vol. 6.

Bellak, L. 1948. *Dementia Praecox.* New York: Grune and Stratton.

———. 1952. *Manic-Depressive Psychosis and Allied Conditions.* New York: Grune and Stratton.

Bennett, J. H. 1866. *The Restorative Treatment of Pneumonia,* 3d ed. Edinburgh: Adam and Charles Black.

Bergin, A. E., and Lambert, M. J. 1978. The evaluation of therapeutic outcomes. In S. L. Garfield and A. E. Bergin, eds., *Handbook of Psychotherapy and Behavior Change,* 2d ed. New York: McGraw-Hill. Pp. 139–89.

Berkeley, G. 1744. *Siris: A Chain of Philosophical Reflexions and Inquiries Concerning the Virtues of Tar Water.* London: W. Innys.

Berkson, J. 1946. Limitations of the application of four-fold table analysis to hospital data. *Biometrics* 2:47–53.

Bernard, C. 1927. *An Introduction to the Study of Experimental Medicine.* Translated by H. C. Greene. New York: Macmillan.

Bernheim, H. 1889. *Suggestive Therapeutics.* New York: G. A. Putnam's Sons.

Bettmann, O. L. 1956. *A Pictorial History of Medicine.* Springfield, Ill.: Charles C Thomas.

Beutler, L. E. 1991. Have all won and must all have prizes? Revisiting Luborsky et al.'s verdict. *Journal of Consulting and Clinical Psychology* 59:226–32.

Bingel, A. 1918. Treatment of diphtheria with ordinary horse serum. *Deutsches Archiv fuer Klinische Medizin* 125:284–332.

Bloch, M. 1973. *The Royal Touch.* Translated by F. E. Anderson. London: Routledge and Kegan Paul.

Blumenthal, D. S., Burke, R. E., and Shapiro, A. K. 1974. Validity of identical matching placebos. *Archives of General Psychiatry* 31:214–15.

Boardman, R. H., Lomas, J., and Markowe, M. 1956. Insulin and chlorpromazine in schizophrenia: A comparative study in previously untreated cases. *Lancet* 2:487–91.

Bok, S. 1974. The ethics of giving placebos. *Scientific American* 231:17–23.

―――. 1978. *Lying: Moral Choice in Public and Private Life.* New York: Pantheon Books.

Boling, L., Ryan, W., and Greenblatt, M. 1957. Insulin treatment of psychotic patients. *American Journal of Psychiatry* 113:1009.

Bond, E. D., and Morris, J.H.H. 1954. Manic-depressive reactions. *American Journal of Psychiatry* 110:883.

Boring, E. G. 1954. The nature and history of experimental control. *American Journal of Psychology* 67:573–89.

Borkovec, T.C.D., Kaloupek, D. G., and Slama, K. M. 1975. The facilitative effect of muscle tension-release in the relaxation treatment of sleep disturbance. *Behavioral Therapy* 6:301–9.

Boswell, P. C., and Murray, E. J. 1979. Effects of meditation on psychological and physiological measures of anxiety. *Journal of Consulting and Clinical Psychology* 47:606–7.

Bradley, D. 1993. Frog venom cocktail yields a one-handed painkiller. *Science* 261:1117.

Braslow, J. T. 1995. Effect of therapeutic innovation on perception of disease and the doctor-patient relationship: A history of general paralysis of the insane and malaria fever therapy, 1910–1930. *American Journal of Psychiatry* 152:660–65.

Brill, N. G., Crumpton, E., Eiduson, S., et al. 1957. Investigation of the therapeutic components and various factors associated with improvement with electroconvulsive treatment: A preliminary report. *American Journal of Psychiatry* 113:997–1008.

British Medical Association. 1950. Fifty years of medicine. *British Medical Journal* 1:68.

Bromberg, W. 1954. *Man above Humanity: A History of Psychotherapy.* Philadelphia: J. B. Lippincott.

―――. 1975. *From Shaman to Psychotherapist.* Chicago: Henry Regnery.

Brown, S. 1948. Side reactions in pyribenzamine medication. *Proceedings of the Society for Experimental Biology and Medicine* 67:373–74.

Brown, W. A. 1988. Placebo as a treatment for depression. *Neuropsychopharmacology* 10:265–69.

Brownell, K.D., and Stunkard, A.J. 1982. The double-blind in danger: Untoward consequences of informed consent. *American Journal of Psychiatry* 139:1487–89.

Bruce-Chwatt, L. J. 1988. Cinchona and its alkaloids: 350 years. *New York State Journal of Medicine* 88:318–22.

Brush, S. G. 1974. The prayer test. *American Scientist* 62:561–63.

Bull, J. P. 1959. The historical development of clinical therapeutic trials. *Journal of Chronic Diseases* 10:218–48.

―――. 1970. Interview by A. K. Shapiro, London, England, August 20.

Burkhardt, R., and Kienle, G. 1978. Controlled clinical trials and medical ethics. *Lancet* 2:1356–59.

———. 1980. Controlled clinical trials and drug regulations. *Controlled Clinical Trials* 1:153–66.

Byington, R. P., Curb, J. D., and Mattson, M. E. 1985. Assessment of double-blindness at the conclusion of the B-blocker heart attack trial. *JAMA* 253:1733–36.

Cabot, R. C. 1915. *Social Service and the Art of Healing.* New York: Moffat, Yard.

Caldwell, A. E. 1970. History of psychopharmacology. In W. G. Clark and J. del Giudice, eds., *Principles of Psychopharmacology,* 1st ed. New York: Academic Press.

———. 1978. History of psychopharmacology. In W. G. Clark and J. Del Giudice, eds., *Principles of Psychopharmacology,* 2d ed. New York: Academic Press.

Calestro, K. M. 1972. Psychotherapy, faith healing and suggestion. *International Journal of Psychiatry* 10:83–113.

Carpenter, W. T., Buchanan, R. W., Kirkpatrick, B., et al. 1993. Strong inference, theory, testing, and the neuroanatomy of schizophrenia. *Archives of General Psychiatry* 50:825–31.

Carr-Kaffashan, L., and Woolfolk, R. L. 1979. Active and placebo effects in treatment of moderate and severe insomnia. *Journal of Consulting and Clinical Psychology* 47:1072–80.

Carroll, K. M., Rounsaville, B. J., and Nich, C. 1994. Blind man's bluff: Effectiveness and significance of psychotherapy and pharmacotherapy, blinding procedures in clinical trials. *Journal of Consulting and Clinical Psychology* 62:276–80.

Castiglioni, A. 1947. *Adventures of the Mind,* 2d ed. New York: Alfred A. Knopf.

Catholic Encyclopedia. 1911. Vols. 2, 7, and 8. New York: Gilmary Society.

Cattell, M. 1950. Dosage in the therapy of cardio-vascular disease. *JAMA* 144:889–92.

———. 1969. Interview by A. K. Shapiro, New York City, April 2.

Chalmers, T. C. 1975. Ethical aspects of clinical trials. *American Journal of Ophthalmology* 79:753–58.

Charpignon. 1864. *Etudes sur la médecine animique et vitaliste.* Translated in H. Bernheim, Suggestive Therapeutics. New York: G. A. Putnam's Sons, 1889.

Chassan, J., Janulis, P. T., Shapiro, A. K., et al. 1980. Preliminary study of intensive design in psychotherapy research. *Comprehensive Psychiatry* 1:111–25.

Chelimsky, E. 1993. The political debate about health care: Are we losing sight of quality? *Science* 262:525–28.

Chen, K. K., and Schmidt, C. F. 1930. *Ephedrine and Related Substances.* Medicine Monographs, vol. 17. Philadelphia: Williams and Wilkins.

Chlorpromazine and Mental Health. 1955. Proceedings of the Symposium Held under the Auspices of Smith, Kline and French Laboratories, June 6. Philadelphia: Lea and Febiger.

Clancy, J. 1970. Letter to A. K. Shapiro, August 19.

Clancy, J., Hoffer, A., Lucy, J., et al. 1954. Design and planning in psychiatric research as illustrated by the Weyburn chronic nucleotide project. *Menninger Clinic Bulletin* 18:147–53.

Clark, W. G., and del Giudice, J., eds. 1970. *Principles of Psychopharmacology.* New York: Academic Press.

Cobb, L. A., Thomas, G. I., Dillard, D. H., et al. 1959. An evaluation of internal-mammary-artery ligation by a double-blind technic. *New England Journal of Medicine* 260:1115–18.

ℬ   Cohen, J. 1994. Immune response corp.: Take two. *Science* 264:1402.

Cohen, P., and Cohen, J. 1984. The clinician's illusion. *Archives of General Psychiatry* 41:1178–82.

Cohen, S., Tyrrell, D. A., and Smith, P. A. 1991. Psychological stress and susceptibility to the common cold. *New England Journal of Medicine* 325:606–12.

Coleman, W. 1987. Experimental physiology and statistical inferences. In I. Kruger, G. Gigerenzer, and M. S. Morgan, eds., *Ideas in the Sciences.* Cambridge: MIT Press.

Colp, R. J. 1989. History of psychiatry. In H. I. Kaplan and B. S. Sadock, eds., *Comprehensive Textbook of Psychiatry,* 5th ed. Vol. 2. Baltimore: Williams and Wilkins.

The Compact Edition of the Oxford English Dictionary. 1971. New York: Oxford University Press.

Coover, J. E. 1917. *Experiments in Psychical Research at Leland Stanford Junior University,* 1st ed. Psychical Research Monographs. Stanford, Calif.: Leland Stanford Jr. University Publications.

Cope, Z. 1958. The treatment of wounds through the ages. *Medical History* 2:163–74.

Cornell Conferences on Therapy. 1946. The use of placebos in therapy. *New York State Journal of Medicine* 46:1718.

———. 1954. How to evaluate a new drug. *American Journal of Medicine* 17:722–27.

Council on Pharmacy and Chemistry. 1930a. *New and Non-official Remedies.* Chicago: American Medical Association.

———. 1930b. *Useful Drugs.* Chicago: American Medical Association.

Cowan, D. W., Diehl, H. S., and Baker, A. B. 1942. Vitamins for the prevention of colds. *JAMA* 120:1268–71.

Cramp, A. J. 1911. *Nostrums and Quackery,* 2d ed. Chicago: American Medical Association.

———. 1913. *Nostrums and Quackery.* Vol. 2. Chicago: American Medical Association.

———. 1921. *Nostrums and Quackery.* Chicago: American Medical Association.

———. 1936. *Nostrums and Quackery and Pseudo-Medicine.* Vol. 3. Chicago: American Medical Association.

Critelli, J. W. 1985. Placebo effects, common factors, and incremental effectiveness. *American Psychologist* 40:850–51.

Critelli, J. W., and Neumann, K. F. 1984. The placebo: Conceptual analysis of a construct in transition. *American Psychologist* 39:32–39.

Crits-Christoph, P. 1992. The efficacy of brief dynamic psychotherapy: A meta-analysis. *American Journal of Psychiatry* 149:151–58.

Dahl, H. 1983. On the definition and measurement of wishes. In J. Masling, ed., *Empirical Studies of Psychoanalytic Theories.* Hillsdale, N.J.: Erlbaum Associates.

Dalby, J. T., Kapelus, G. J., Swanson, J. M., et al. 1978. An examination of the double-blind design in drug research with hyperactive children. *Progress in Neuro-Psychopharmacology* 2:123–27.

Darko, D. F., Wilson, N. W., Gillin, J. C., et al. 1991. A critical appraisal of nitrogen-induced lymphocyte proliferation in depressed patients. *American Journal of Psychiatry* 148:337–44.

Davanloo, H. 1980. *Short-Term Dynamic Psychotherapy.* New York: Jason Aronson.

Davis, J. M., and Glassman, A. H. 1989. Antidepressant drugs. In H. I. Kaplan and B. J. Sadock, eds., *Comprehensive Textbook of Psychiatry,* 5th ed. Vol. 2. Baltimore: Williams and Wilkins. Pp. 1627–54.

Davis, J. M., Wang, Z., and Janicak, P. G. 1993. A quantitative analysis of clinical drug trials for the treatment of affective disorders. *Psychopharmacology Bulletin* 29:175–81.

DeBakey, M. E. 1993. Medical centers of excellence and health reform. *Science* 262:523–28.

DeMaar, E.W.J., and Pelikan, E. W. 1955. The use of placebos in therapy and clinical pharmacology. *Modern Hospital* 84:108–18.

Denhoff, E., and Holden, R. H. 1955. The effectiveness of chlorpromazine (Thorazine) with cerebral palsied children. *Journal of Pediatrics* 47:328–32.

Deniker, P. 1970. Introduction of neuroleptic chemotherapy into psychiatry. In F.J.J. Ayd and B. Blackwell, eds., *Discoveries in Biological Psychiatry.* Philadelphia: J. B. Lippincott.

Denton, J. E., and Beecher, H. K. 1949. New analgesics. 1. Methods in the clinical evaluation of new analgesics. *JAMA* 141:1051–57.

Deutsch, A. 1949. *The Mentally Ill in America,* 2d ed. New York: Columbia University Press.

Dictionary of Christianity in America. 1990. Edited by D. Reed. Downers Grove, Ill.: Intervarsity Press.

Diehl, H. S. 1933. Medicinal treatment of the common cold. *JAMA* 101:2042–49.

———. 1935. The common cold. *New York State Journal of Medicine* 35:109–16.

Diethelm, O. 1946. Cornell Conferences on Therapy. *New York State Journal of Medicine* 46:1718.

———. 1967. Interview by A. K. Shapiro, New York City, December 23.

Dimond, E. G., Kittle, C. F., and Cockett, J. E. 1960. Comparison of internal mammary artery ligation and sham operation for angina pectoris. *American Journal of Cardiology* 4:483–86.

Dinnerstein, A. J., and Halm, J. 1970. Modification of placebo effects by means of drugs: Effects of aspirin and placebos on self-rated moods. *Journal of Abnormal Psychology* 75:308–14.

Dorland, W.A.N. 1900. *The American Illustrated Medical Dictionary,* 1st ed. Philadelphia: W. B. Saunders.

————. 1901. *The American Illustrated Medical Dictionary*, 2d ed. Philadelphia: W. B. Saunders.

————. 1909. *The American Illustrated Medical Dictionary*, 5th ed. Philadelphia: W. B. Saunders.

————. 1913. *The American Illustrated Medical Dictionary*, 7th ed. Philadelphia: W. B. Saunders.

————. 1915. *The American Illustrated Medical Dictionary*, 8th ed. Philadelphia: W. B. Saunders.

————. 1922. *The American Illustrated Medical Dictionary*, 11th ed. Philadelphia: W. B. Saunders.

————. 1929. *The American Illustrated Medical Dictionary*, 15th ed. Philadelphia: W. B. Saunders.

————. 1932. *The American Illustrated Medical Dictionary*, 16th ed. Philadelphia: W. B. Saunders.

————. 1937. *The American Illustrated Medical Dictionary*, 17th ed. Philadelphia: W. B. Saunders.

————. 1938. *The American Illustrated Medical Dictionary*, 18th ed. Philadelphia: W. B. Saunders.

————. 1941. *The American Illustrated Medical Dictionary*, 19th ed. Philadelphia: W. B. Saunders.

————. 1944. *The American Illustrated Medical Dictionary*, 20th ed. Philadelphia: W. B. Saunders.

————. 1947. *The American Illustrated Medical Dictionary*, 21st ed. Philadelphia: W. B. Saunders.

————. 1951. *The American Illustrated Medical Dictionary*, 22d ed. Philadelphia: W. B. Saunders.

Dubois, E. F. 1946. Cornell conference on therapy. *New York State Journal of Medicine* 46:1718.

DuBois, M. 1837. Report on animal magnetism, made to the Royal Academy of Medicine in Paris. *London Medical Gazette*, September 16 and 23.

Duran-Reynals, M. L. 1946. *The Fever Bark Tree.* New York: Doubleday.

Edelstein, E. J., and Edelstein, L. 1945. *Asclepius: A Collection and Interpretation of the Testimonies.* Vols. 1 and 2. Baltimore: Johns Hopkins Press.

Eisenberg, D. M., Kessler, R. C., Foster, C., et al. 1993. Unconventional medicine in the United States. *New England Journal of Medicine* 328:246–52.

Eli, K., Nishimoto, R., Mediansky, L., et al. 1992. Social relations, social support, and survival among patients with cancer. *Journal of Psychosomatic Research* 36:531–41.

Elkin, I., Tracie Shea, M., Watkins, J. T., et al. 1989. National Institute of Mental Health treatment of depression collaborative research program: General effectiveness of treatments. *Archives of General Psychiatry* 46:971–82.

Ellenberger, H. E. 1970. *The Discovery of the Unconscious.* New York: Basic Books.

Elovainio, E., and Ostling, G. 1948. Observations on preoperative treatment with strophanthin. *Annales Chirurgiae et Gynaecologiae Fenniae* 37:23–35.

Engelhardt, D. M., Margolis, R. A., Rudorfer, L., et al. 1969. Physician bias and the double-blind. *Archives of General Psychiatry* 20:315–20.

Engels, G. I., Garnefski, N., and Diekstra, R.F.W. 1993. Efficacy of rational-emotive therapy: A quantitative analysis. *Journal of Consulting and Clinical Psychology* 61:1083–90.

Estes, J. W. 1989. *The Medical Skills of Ancient Egypt*. Canton, Mass.: Science History Publications.

Evans, D. L., Leserman, J., Pedersen, C. A., et al. 1989. Immune correlates of stress and depression. *Psychopharmacology Bulletin* 25:319–24.

Evans, F. J. 1985. Expectancy, therapeutic instructions, and the placebo response. In L. White, B. Tursky, and G. E. Schwartz, eds., *Placebo: Theory, Research, and Mechanisms*. New York: Guilford Press. Pp. 215–28.

Evans, W., and Hoyle, C. 1933. The comparative value of drugs used in the continuous treatment of angina pectoris. *Quarterly Journal of Medicine* 26:311–38.

Eysenck, H. J. 1952. The effects of psychotherapy: An evaluation. *Journal of Consulting Psychology* 16:319–24.

———. 1961. The effects of psychotherapy. In H. J. Eysenck, ed., *Handbook of Abnormal Psychology*. New York: Basic Books.

———. 1965. The effects of psychotherapy. *International Journal of Psychiatry* 3:150–53.

———. 1966. *The Effects of Psychotherapy*. New York: International Science Press.

———. 1994. Meta-analysis and its problems. *British Medical Journal* 309:789–92.

———. 1995. Meta-analysis squared: Does it make sense? *American Psychologist* 50:110–11.

Fahy, P., Imiah, N., and Harrington, J. 1963. A controlled comparison of electroconvulsive therapy, imipramine, and thiopentone sleep in depression. *Journal of Neuropsychiatry* 4:310–14.

Fawcett, J., Epstein, P., Fiester, S. J., et al. 1987. Clinical management-imipramine/placebo administration manual: NIMH treatment of depression collaborative research program. *Psychopharmacology Bulletin* 23:309–24.

Fawzy, F. I., Fawzy, N. W., Hyun, C. S., et al. 1993. Malignant melanoma: Effects of an early structured psychiatric intervention, coping, and affective state on recurrence and survival six years later. *Archives of General Psychiatry* 50:681–89.

FDA. *See* U.S. Food and Drug Administration.

Fears, T. R., and Schneiderman, M. A. 1974. Pathologic evaluation and the blind technique. *Science* 183:21–22.

Featherstone, R. M., and Simon, A. 1959. *A Pharmacologic Approach to the Study of the Mind*. Springfield, Ill.: Charles C Thomas.

Fenichel, O. 1954. Brief psychotherapy. In *The Collected Papers of Otto Fenichel*. New York: W. Norton.

Ferguson, F. R., Davey, A.F.C., and Topley, W.W.C. 1927. The value of mixed vaccines in the prevention of the common cold. *Journal of Hygiene* 26:98–109.

Fields, H. L. 1997. Toward a neurobiology of placebo analgesia. In A. Harrington, ed., *The Placebo Effect.* Cambridge: Harvard University Press.

Findley, T. 1953. The placebo and the physician. *Medical Clinics of North America* 37:1821–26.

Fink, M., Shaw, R., Gross, G. E., et al. 1958. Comparative study of chlorpromazine and insulin coma in therapy of psychosis. *JAMA* 166:1846.

Fink, P. J. 1994. Are psychiatrists replaceable? *Psychiatric Times,* August, Special Report, p. 22.

Finland, M. 1930. The serum treatment of lobar pneumonia. *New England Journal of Medicine* 202:1244–47.

Fischer, H. K., and Dlin, B. M. 1956. The dynamics of placebo therapy: A clinical study. *American Journal of Medicine Science* 232:504–12.

Fishbein, M. 1925. *The Medical Follies.* New York: Boni and Liveright.

———. 1927. *The New Medical Follies.* New York: Boni and Liveright.

———. 1932. *Fads and Quackery in Healing.* New York: Blue Ribbon Books.

Fisher, J. W. 1970. Letter to A. K. Shapiro, October 22.

Fisher, R. A. 1926. *Statistical Methods for Research Workers.* Edinburgh: Oliver and Boyd.

———. 1935. *The Design of Experiments.* London: Oliver and Boyd.

Fisher, S., and Greenberg, R. P. 1977. *The Scientific Credibility of Freud's Theory and Therapy.* New York: Basic Books.

———. 1989. A second opinion: Rethinking the claims of biological psychiatry. In S. Fisher and R. P. Greenberg, eds., *The Limits of Biological Treatments for Psychological Distress: Comparisons with Psychotherapy and Placebo.* Hillsdale, N.J.: Lawrence Erlbaum Associates.

Flexner, A. 1910. *Medical Education in the United States and Canada.* New York: Carnegie Foundation for the Advancement of Teaching.

Foege, W. H. 1993. A world without polio. *JAMA* 270:1859–60.

Food and Drug Act. 1906. *U.S. Statutes at Large* 34:76.

Food, Drug, and Cosmetics Act. 1938. *U.S. Statutes at Large,* sec. 505, 52:1040; 76:780.

Foster, F. P. 1894. *An Illustrated Encyclopedic Medicinal Dictionary.* New York: D. Appleton.

Foulds, G. A. 1958. Clinical research in psychiatry. *Journal of Mental Science* 104:259–65.

Fox, B. 1961. The investigation of the effects of psychiatric practice. *Journal of Mental Science* 107:1–12.

Fox, J. 1803. *A New Medical Dictionary.* London: Darton and Harvey.

Fox, K. 1993. Light microscopes get a sharper look. *Science* 261:1275.

Frank, J. D. 1958. Some effects of expectancy and influence in psychotherapy. In J. H. Masserman and J. L. Moreno, eds., *Progress in Psychotherapy.* New York: Grune and Stratton.

———. 1961. *Persuasion and Healing.* Baltimore: Johns Hopkins Press.

———. 1970. Letter to A. K. Shapiro, August 31.

———. 1973. *Persuasion and Healing,* 2d ed. Baltimore: Johns Hopkins University Press.

Frank, J. D., and Frank, J. B. 1991. *Persuasion and Healing,* 3d ed. Baltimore: Johns Hopkins University Press.

Frank, J. D., Gliedman, L. H., Imber, S. B., et al. 1957. Why patients leave psychotherapy. *Archives of Neurology and Psychiatry* 77:283.

———. 1959. Patients' expectancies and relearning as factors determining improvement in psychotherapy. *American Journal of Psychiatry* 115:961–68.

Franklin, B. 1757. Letter to John Pringle. In I. B. Cohen, ed., *Benjamin Franklin's Experiments.* 1941. Cambridge: Harvard University Press.

Frasure-Smith, N., Lesperance, F., and Talajic, M. 1993. Depression following myocardial infarction. *JAMA* 270:1819–25.

Freyhen, F. 1958. Symposium: Research in psychiatry with special reference to drug therapy. The neuroleptic action and effectiveness of proclorperozin in psychiatric disorders. In *Psychiatric Research Reports of the American Psychiatric Association.* Vol. 9. Washington, D.C.: APA.

Fried, C. 1974. *Medical Experimentation: Personal Integrity and Social Policy.* New York: Elsevier.

Friedman, A. S. 1975. Interaction of drug therapy with marital therapy in depressive patients. *Archives of General Psychiatry* 32:619–37.

Gaddum, J. H. 1954. Walter Ernest Dixen Memorial Lecture: Clinical pharmacology. *Proceedings of the Royal Society of Medicine* 47:302.

Gadow, K. D., White, L., and Ferguson, D. 1986a. Placebo controls and double-blind conditions: Experimenter bias, conditioned placebo response, and drug-psychotherapy comparisons. In S. E. Breuning, A. D. Poling, and J. L. Matson, eds., *Methodological Issues in Human Psychopharmacology: Advances in Learning and Behavioral Disabilities,* Suppl. 1. New York: JAI Press. Pp. 85–114.

———. 1986b. Placebo controls and double-blind conditions: Placebo theory in experimental design. In S. E. Breuning, A. D. Poling, and J. L. Matson, eds., *Methodological Issues in Human Psychopharmacology: Advances in Learning and Behavioral Disabilities,* Suppl. 1. New York: JAI Press. Pp. 41–83.

Garfield, S. L. 1980. *Psychotherapy: An Eclectic Approach.* New York: John Wiley and Sons.

———. 1983. Does psychotherapy work? Yes, no, maybe. *Behavioral and Brain Sciences* 6:292–93.

———. 1984. Psychotherapy: Efficacy, generality, and specificity. In J.B.W. Williams and R. L. Spitzer, eds., *Psychotherapy Research: Where Are We and Where Should We Go?* New York: Guilford Press. Pp. 295–305.

Garrison, F. H. 1921. *An Introduction to the History of Medicine,* 3d ed. Philadelphia: W. B. Saunders.

———. 1929. *An Introduction to the History of Medicine,* 4th ed. Philadelphia: W. B. Saunders.

Gatchel, R. J., Hatch, J. P., Maynard, A., et al. 1979. Comparison of heart rate biofeedback, false biofeedback, and systematic desensitization in reducing speech anxiety:

Short- and long-term effectiveness. *Journal of Consulting and Clinical Psychology* 47:620–22.

Gellert, G. A., Maxwell, R. M., and Siegel, B. S. 1993. Breast cancer patients receiving adjunctive psychosocial support therapy: A ten-year follow-up study. *Journal of Clinical Oncology* 2:66–69.

Ghalioungui, P. 1963. *Magic and Medical Science in Ancient Egypt.* New York: Barnes and Noble.

Glover, E. 1955. *The Technique of Psychoanalysis.* New York: International Universities Press.

Gold, H. 1930. Recent advances in drug therapy. *International Clinics* 4:88–114.

———. 1946. Cornell Conferences on Therapy: The use of placebos in therapy. *New York State Journal of Medicine* 46:1718–27.

———. 1952. Proper study of mankind is man [editorial]. *American Journal of Medicine* 12:619–20.

———. 1954. How to evaluate a new drug. *American Journal of Medicine* 17:722–27.

———. 1967a. Clinical pharmacology: Historical note. *Journal of Clinical Pharmacology and Journal of New Drugs* 7:309–11.

———. 1967b. Interview by A. K. Shapiro, New York City.

———. 1968. Interview by A. K. Shapiro, New York City, January 23.

———. 1969. Interview by A. K. Shapiro, New York City.

Gold, H., Kwit, N. T., and Otto, H. 1937. The xanthines (theobromine and aminophylline) in the treatment of cardiac pain. *JAMA* 108:2173–79.

Gold, H., Travell, J., and Modell, W. 1937. The effect of theophylline with ethylenediamine (aminophylline) on the course of cardiac infarction following experimental coronary occlusion. *American Heart Journal* 14:284–96.

Goldman, B. L., Domitor, P. J., and Murray, E. J. 1979. Effects of Zen meditation on anxiety reduction and perceptual functioning. *Journal of Consulting and Clinical Psychology* 47:551–56.

Goldstein, A. P. 1962. *Therapist-Patient Expectancies in Psychotherapy.* New York: Pergamon Press.

Goldzieher, D. R. 1971. A placebo controlled double-blind crossover investigation of the side-effects attributed to oral contraceptives. *Fertility and Sterility* 22:609–23.

Goleman, D. 1993. Psychology's new interest in the world beyond self. *New York Times,* August 29, E5.

Goodnow, R. E., Beecher, H. K., Brazier, M.A.B., et al. 1951. Physiological performance following a hypnotic dose of a barbiturate. *Journal of Pharmacology and Experimental Therapeutics* 102:55–61.

Gorman, J. M., and Davis, J. M. 1989. Antianxiety drugs. In H. I. Kaplan and B. J. Sadock, eds., *Comprehensive Textbook of Psychiatry,* 5th ed. Vol. 2. Baltimore: Williams and Wilkins. Pp. 1579–91.

Goshen, C. E. 1967. *Documentary History of Psychiatry.* New York: Philosophic Library.

Greenberg, R. P., and Fisher, S. 1989. Examining antidepressant effectiveness: Findings, ambiguities, and such vexing puzzles. In S. Fisher and R. P. Greenberg, eds., *The Limits of Biological Treatments for Psychological Distress: Comparisons with Psychotherapy and Placebo.* Hillsdale, N.J.: Lawrence Erlbaum Associates.

Greenberg, R. P., Bornstein, R. F., Greenberg, M. D., et al. 1992. A meta-analysis of antidepressant outcome under "blinder" conditions. *Journal of Consulting and Clinical Psychology* 60:664–69.

Greenblatt, D.J., and Shader, R. I. 1971. Meprobamate: A study of irrational drug use. *American Journal of Psychiatry* 127:1217–1303.

Greiner, T. 1959. Problem of methodology in research with drugs. *American Journal of Mental Deficiency* 64:346–52.

———. 1961. Why we rarely know about drugs. *JAMA* 177:42–45.

———. 1962a. The ethics of drug research on human subjects. *Journal of New Drugs* 2:7–22.

———. 1962b. The hypothesis in clinical pharmacology. *Clinical Pharmacology and Therapeutics* 3:147–52.

———. 1962c. Subjective bias of the clinical pharmacologist. *JAMA* 181:120–21.

———. 1969. Interview by A. K. Shapiro, New York City, February 26.

———. 1992. Telephone interview by A. K. Shapiro, Dallas, Tex., August 15.

Greiner, T., Bross, I., and Gold, H. 1957. A method for evaluation of laxative habits in human subjects. *Journal of Chronic Diseases* 6:244–55.

Greiner, T. H., Gold, H., Cattell, M., et al. 1950. A method for the evaluation of effects of drugs on cardiac pain in patients with angina of effort: A study of khellin (visammin). *American Journal of Medicine* 9:143–55.

Greiner, T., Gold, H., Ganz, A., et al. 1959. "Case report" in human pharmacology. *JAMA* 171:290–95.

Grevert, P., and Goldstein, A. 1985. Placebo analgesia, naloxone, and the role of endogenous opioids. In L. White, B. Tursky, and G. E. Schwartz, eds., *Placebo: Theory, Research, and Mechanisms.* New York: Guilford Press. Pp. 332–50.

Grimes, D. A. 1993. Technology follies: The uncritical acceptance of medical innovation. *JAMA* 269:3030–33.

Gross, M. L. 1978. *The Psychological Society.* New York: Random House.

Grünbaum, A. 1984. *The Foundations of Psychoanalysis: A Philosophical Critique.* Berkeley: University of California Press.

———. 1985. Explication and implications of the placebo concept. In L. White, B. Tursky, and G. E. Schwartz, eds., *Placebo: Theory, Research, and Mechanisms.* New York: Guilford Press. Pp. 9–36.

———. 1986. Precis of the foundations of psychoanalysis: A philosophical critique. *Behavioral and Brain Sciences* 9:217–84.

———. 1993. *Validation in the Clinical Theory of Psychoanalysis: A Study in the Philosophy of Psychoanalysis.* Madison, Conn.: International Universities Press.

Guelfi, J. D., Boyer, P., and Dreyfus, J. F. 1983. Placebo use in clinical trials on psychotropic drugs in France. *Neuropsychobiology* 9:20–25.

Guy, W. H., Gross, M., and Dennis, H. 1967. An alternative to the double-blind procedure. *American Journal of Psychiatry* 123:1505–12.

Guyatt, G. H., and Rennie, D. 1993. Users' guides to the medical literature. *JAMA* 270:2096–97.

Guyatt, G. H., Sackett, D. L., and Cook, D. J. 1993. Users' guide to the medical literature. *JAMA* 270:2598–2601.

Haas, H., Fink, H., and Hartfelder, G. 1959. Das Placeboproblem. *Fortschritte der Arzneimittelforschung* 1:279–454.

Hacking, I. 1988. Telepathy: Origins of randomization in experimental design. *Isis* 79:427–51.

Haggard, H. W. 1929. *Devils, Drugs, and Doctors.* New York: Harper and Brothers.

———. 1933. *Mystery, Magic, and Medicine.* New York: Doubleday Doran.

———. 1934. *The Doctor in History.* New Haven: Yale University Press.

Hahn, R. A. 1985. A sociocultural model of illness and healing. In L. White, B. Tursky, and G. E. Schwartz, eds., *Placebo: Theory, Research, and Mechanisms.* New York: Guilford Press. Pp. 167–95.

Hailman, H. F. 1953. The blind placebo in the evaluation of drugs [correspondence]. *JAMA* 151:1430.

Hamilton, M. 1961. *Lectures on the Methodology of Clinical Research.* Edinburgh: E. and S. Livingstone.

———. 1974. *Lectures on the Methodology of Clinical Research,* 2d ed. Edinburgh: Churchill Livingstone.

Hampshire, C. H. 1933. Pharmacy in retrospect and prospect. *Lancet* 2:275–78.

Hampson, J. L. 1970. Letter to A. K. Shapiro, September 22.

Hampson, J. L., Rosenthal, D., and Frank, J. D. 1954. A comparative study of the effect of mephenesin and placebo on the symptomatology of a mixed group of psychiatric outpatients. *Bulletin of the Johns Hopkins Hospital* 95:170–77.

Harriman, P. L. 1947. *The New Dictionary of Psychology.* New York: Philosophical Library.

Hart, P. D. 1946. Chemotherapy of tuberculosis. *British Medical Journal* 2:805–9.

Haygarth, J. 1801. *Of the Imagination as a Cause and as a Cure of Disorders of the Body,* new ed. Bath, England: R. Crutwell.

Hediger, E. M., and Gold, H. 1935. U.S.P. ether from large drums and ether from small cans labeled "for anesthesia." *JAMA* 104:2244–48.

Henn, F. A. 1989. Psychosurgery. In H. I. Kaplan and B. J. Sadock, eds., *Comprehensive Textbook of Psychiatry.* Baltimore: Williams and Wilkins. Pp. 1679–80.

Henney, J. E. 1993. Combatting medical fraud. *New York State Journal of Medicine* 93:86–87.

Herink, R. 1980. *The Psychotherapy Handbook.* New York: New American Library.

Hewlett, A. W. 1913. Clinical effects of "natural" and "synthetic" sodium salicylate. *JAMA* 61:319–21.

Hill, A. B. 1951. The clinical trial. *British Medical Bulletin* 7:278–82.

———. 1952. The clinical trial. *New England Journal of Medicine* 247:113–19.

———. 1963. Medical ethics and controlled trials. *British Medical Journal* 1:1043–49.

———. 1970. Interview by A. K. Shapiro, London, England, August 20.

Hill, L. E., Nunn, A. J., and Fox, W. 1976. Matching quality of agents employed in "double-blind" controlled clinical trials. *Lancet* 1:352–56.

Hilts, P. J. 1995. Health maintenance organizations turn to spiritual healing. *New York Times,* December 27, C10.

Hinsie, L. E., and Campbell, R. J. 1960. *Psychiatric Dictionary,* 3d ed. New York: Oxford University Press.

———. 1970. *Psychiatric Dictionary,* 4th ed. New York: Oxford University Press.

Hippocrates. 1964. *The Theory and Practice of Medicine.* New York: Citadel Press.

Hoagland, R. J., Dietz, E. N., Myers, P. W., et al. 1950. Antihistaminic drugs for colds. *JAMA* 143:157–60.

Hoch, P. 1956. Symposium: An evaluation of the newer psycho-pharmacologic agents and their role in current psychiatric practice. Round-table discussion. In *Psychiatric Research Reports of the American Psychiatric Association.* Vol. 4. Washington, D.C.: APA.

Hoffer, A. 1967. A theoretical examination of double-blind design. *Canadian Medical Association Journal* 97:123–27.

———. 1970a. Letter to A. K. Shapiro, December 21.

———. 1970b. Letter to A. K. Shapiro, May 7.

———. 1970c. Letter to A. K. Shapiro, November 16.

———. 1970d. Interview by A. K. Shapiro, April 29.

Hofling, C. K. 1955. The place of placebos in medical practice. *GP* 11:103.

Hollingsworth, H. L. 1912. The Influence of caffeine on mental and motor efficiency. *Archiv für Psychologie* (Frankfurt am Main) 22:1–166.

Hollon, S. D. 1996. The efficacy and effectiveness of psychotherapy relative to medication. *American Psychologist* 51:1025–39.

Holmes, O. W. 1891. *Medical Essays, 1842–1882.* Cambridge, Mass.: Riverside Press.

Hooper, R. 1811. *Hooper Quincy's Lexicon Medicum.* London: Longman Brown.

———. 1848. *Hooper Quincy's Lexicon Medicum,* 8th ed. London: Longman Brown.

Horowitz, M. J. 1976. *Stress Response Syndromes.* New York: Aronson.

Horwitt, M. K. 1956. Fact and artifact in the biology of schizophrenia. *Science* 124:429.

Horwitz, R. I., and Horwitz, S. M. 1993. Adherence to treatment and health outcomes. *Archives of Internal Medicine* 153:1863–68.

House, J. S., Landis, K. R., and Umberson, D. 1988. Social relationships and health. *Science* 241:540–45.

Houston, W. R. 1938. Doctor himself as therapeutic agent. *Annals of Internal Medicine* 11:1416–25.

Howard, J., Whittemore, A. S., Hoover, J. J., et al. 1982. How blind was the patient blind in AMIS? *Clinical Pharmacology and Therapeutics* 32:543–53.

Huard, P., and Wong, M. 1968. *Chinese Medicine.* Translated by Bernard Fielding. New York: McGraw-Hill.

Hughes, J. R., and Krahn, D. 1985. Blindness and the validity of the double-blind procedure. *Journal of Clinical Psychopharmacology* 6:138–42.

Hume, E. H. 1940. *The Chinese Way in Medicine*. Baltimore: Johns Hopkins Press.

Hunter, R., and Macalpine, I. 1963. *Three Hundred Years of Psychiatry, 1535–1860*. London: Oxford University Press.

Hutt, P. B. 1983. Investigations and reports respecting FDA regulation of new drugs (pt. 1). *Clinical Pharmacology and Therapeutics* 33:537–48.

Imber, S. D., Frank, J. D., Nash, E. H., et al. 1957. Improvement and amount of therapeutic contact: An alternative to the use of no-treatment controls in psychotherapy. *Journal of Consulting Psychology* 21:309–15.

Imber, S. D., Pilkonis, P. A., Sotsky, S. M., et al. 1990. Mode-specific effects among three treatments for depression. *Journal of Consulting and Clinical Psychology* 58:352–59.

Jacobson, N. S., and Baucom, D. H. 1977. Design and assessment of nonspecific control groups in behavior modification research. *Behavioral Therapy* 8:709–19.

Jaeschke, R., Guyatt, G., and Sackett, D. L. 1993. Users' guide to the medical literature. *JAMA* 271:389–91.

Jaffe, J. H. 1970. Narcotic analgesics. In L. S. Goodman and A. Gilman, eds., *The Pharmacological Basis of Therapeutics*, 4th ed. New York: Macmillan.

Janet, P. 1909. *Neuroses*. Translated by E. Flammarin. Paris: F. Alcan.

———. 1924. *Principles of Psychotherapy*. New York: Macmillan.

———. 1925. *Psychological Healing: A Historical and Clinical Study*. Vol. 1. London: George Allen and Unwin.

Jarcho, S. 1993. *Quinine's Predecessor: Francesco Tosti and the Early History of Cinchona*. Baltimore: Johns Hopkins University Press.

Jastrow, M. J. 1913. The medicine of the Babylonians and Assyrians. *Lancet* 2:1137.

Jayne, W. A. 1962. *The Healing Gods of Ancient Civilizations*. New York: New York University Books.

Jevons, W. S. 1874. *The Principles of Science: A Treatise on Logic and Scientific Method*. New York: Macmillan.

Jones, J. 1981. *Bad Blood: The Tuskegee Syphilis Experiment*. New York: Free Press.

Jospe, M. 1978. *The Placebo Effect in Healing*. Lexington, Mass.: Lexington Books, D.C. Heath.

Kahn, R. J., McNair, D. M., Lipman, R. S., et al. 1986. Imipramine and chlordiazepoxide in depressive and anxiety disorders: II. Efficacy in anxious patients. *Archives of General Psychiatry* 43:79–85.

Kalinowsky, L. B. 1970. Biological psychiatric treatments preceding pharmacotherapy. In F.J.J. Ayd and B. Blackwell, eds., *Discoveries in Biological Psychiatry*. Philadelphia: J. B. Lippincott.

Kalinowsky, L. B., and Hoch, P. H. 1952. *Shock Treatments, Psychosurgery, and Other Somatic Treatment in Psychiatry*, 2d ed. New York: Grune and Stratton.

Karlowski, T. R., Chalmers, T. C., Frenkel, L. D., et al. 1975. Ascorbic acid for the common cold: A prophylactic and therapeutic trial. *JAMA* 231:1038–42.

Kast, E. C. 1961. Alpha-ethyltryptamine acetate in the treatment of depression, a study of the methodology of drug evaluation. *Journal of Neuropsychiatry* 1:114–18.

Kay, M. W. 1963. Letter to A. K. Shapiro, February 13 and 25.

Kazdin, A. E. 1988. *Child Psychotherapy: Developing and Identifying Effective Treatments.* Elmsford, N.Y.: Pergamon Press.

———. 1991. Effectiveness of psychotherapy with children and adolescents. *Journal of Consulting and Clinical Psychology* 59:785–98.

Kazdin, A. E., and Wilcoxon, L. A. 1976. Systematic desensitization and nonspecific treatment effects: A methodological evaluation. *Psychological Bulletin* 83:729–59.

Keats, A. S., Beecher, H. K., and Mosteller, F. C. 1950. Measurement of pathological pain in distinction to experimental pain. *Journal of Applied Physiology* 1:35–44.

Kefauver-Harris Amendments of October 10, 1962, to *Food, Drug, and Cosmetics Act. Code of Federal Regulations.* Washington, D.C.: U.S. Government Printing Office.

Kellert, S. R., and Wilson, E. O., eds. 1993. *The Biophilia Hypothesis.* Fort Meyers Beach, Fla.: Island Press.

King, L. S. 1958. *The Medical World of the Eighteenth Century.* Chicago: University of Chicago Press.

———. 1963. *The Growth of Medical Thought.* Chicago: University of Chicago Press.

———. 1966. The road to scientific therapy. *JAMA* 197:92–98.

Kirsch, I. 1985. The logical consequences of the common-factor definition of the term placebo. *American Psychologist* 40:237–38.

Kirsch, I., and Henry, D. 1979. Self-desensitization and meditation in the reduction of public speaking anxiety. *Journal of Consulting and Clinical Psychology* 47:536–41.

Kissel, P., and Barrucand, D. 1964. *Placebo and Placebo Effect in Medicine.* Paris: Masson.

Kitchell, J. R., Glover, R. P., and Kyle, R. H. 1958. Bilateral internal mammary artery ligation for angina pectoris. *American Journal of Cardiology* 1:46–59.

Klein, D. F. 1995. Response to Rothman and Michels on placebo-controlled clinical trials. *American Society of Clinical Psychopharmacology* 6:3–4.

Klein, M. H., Dittman, A. T., Parloff, M. B., et al. 1969. Behavior therapy: Observations and reflections. *Journal of Consulting and Clinical Psychology* 33:259–66.

Klerman, G. L. 1986. Scientific and ethical considerations in the use of placebo controls in clinical trials in psychopharmacology. *Psychopharmacology Bulletin* 22:25–29.

Klerman, G. L., Weissman, M. M., Rounsaville, B. J., et al. 1984. *Interpersonal Psychotherapy of Depression.* New York: Basic Books.

Kligman, A. 1973. The double-blind dilemma [letter]. *JAMA* 225:1658–59.

Kline, N. S. 1956. *Psychopharmacology.* Washington, D.C.: American Association for the Advancement of Science.

———. 1959. *Psychopharmacology Frontiers.* Boston: Little Brown.

———. 1970. Monoamine oxidase inhibitors: An unfinished picaresque tale. In F.J.J. Ayd and B. Blackwell, eds., *Discoveries in Biological Psychiatry.* Philadelphia: J. B. Lippincott.

Knight, R. P. 1941. Evaluation of the results of psychoanalytic therapy. *American Journal of Psychiatry* 98:434–46.

Koelle, G. B. 1958. Symposium: Discussion and critique on methodology of research in psychiatry. Pharmacological approaches to the study of tranquilizing agents. In *Psychiatric Research Reports of the American Psychiatric Association.* Vol. 9. Washington, D.C.: APA.

Koteen, H. 1957. The use of a "double blind" study investigating the clinical merits of a new tranquilizing agent. *Annals of Internal Medicine* 47:978.

Kraemer, H. C., Pruyn, J. P., Gibbons, R. D., et al. 1987. Methodology in psychiatric research: Report on the 1986 MacArthur Foundation Network I Methodology Institute. *Archives of General Psychiatry* 44:1100–1106.

Kramer, H., and Sprenger, J. 1971. *The Malleus Maleficarum.* Translated by M. Summers. New York: Dover Publications.

Kramer, M. S., and Shapiro, S. H. 1984. Scientific challenges in the application of randomized trials. *JAMA* 252:2739–45.

Kremers, E., and Urdang, G. 1940. *The History of Pharmacy.* Philadelphia: J. B. Lippincott.

Kuhn, R. 1958. The treatment of depressive states with G-22355 (imipramine). *American Journal of Psychiatry* 115:459–64.

Kwit, N. 1969. Interview by A. K. Shapiro, October 4.

Landman, J. T., and Dawes, R. M. 1982. Psychotherapy outcome: Smith and Glass' conclusions stand up under scrutiny. *American Psychologist* 37:504–6.

Lasagna, L. 1955. The controlled clinical trial: Theory and practice. *Journal of Chronic Diseases* 4:353–67.

———. 1956. Placebos. *Scientific American* 193:68.

Lasagna, L., and Beecher, H. K. 1954. The optimal dose of morphine. *JAMA* 156:230–34.

Lasagna, L., Mosteller, F., von Felsinger, J. M., et al. 1954. A study of placebo response. *American Journal of Medicine* 16:770.

Laurence, D. R. 1970. Interview by A. K. Shapiro, August 19.

Laurence, D. R., and Bennett, P. N. 1987. *Clinical Pharmacology,* 6th ed. Edinburgh: Churchill Livingstone.

Leake, C. D. 1958. *The Amphetamines: Their Actions and Uses.* Springfield, Ill.: Charles C Thomas.

———. 1970. The long road for a drug from idea to use: The amphetamines. In F.J.J. Ayd and B. Blackwell, eds., *Discoveries in Biological Psychiatry.* Philadelphia: J. P. Lippincott.

Leber, P. 1986. The placebo control in clinical trials (a view from the FDA). *Psychopharmacology Bulletin* 22:30–32.

———. 1992. Telephone interview by A. K. Shapiro.

Lee, L. E., Jr. 1942. Studies of morphine, codeine, and their derivatives: XVI. Clinical studies of morphine, methyldihydromorphinone (Metopon), and dihydrodesoxymorphine D (Desmorphine). *Journal de Pharmacologie* 75:161–72.

Lee, M. S., Love, S. B., Mitchell, J. B., et al. 1992. Mastectomy or conservation for early breast cancer: Psychological morbidity. *European Journal of Cancer* 28A:1340–44.

Leighton, G., and McKinlay, P. L. 1930. *Milk Consumption and the Growth of School Children*. Edinburgh: Department of Health for Scotland, His Majesty's Stationery Office.

Lennox, W. G. 1957. The centenary of bromides. *New England Journal of Medicine* 259:887.

Leslie, A. 1954. Ethics and practice of placebo therapy. *American Journal of Medicine* 16:854.

Lesse, S. 1962. Placebo reactions in psychotherapy. *Diseases of the Nervous System* 23:313–19.

Leuret, F., and Bon, H. 1957. *Modern Miraculous Cures*. New York: Farrar, Straus, and Cudahay.

Levine, J., Schiele, B. C., and Bouthilet, L. 1971. *Principles and Problems in Establishing the Efficacy of Psychotropic Agents*. PHS Publication no. 2138. Washington, D.C.: U.S. Public Health Service.

Levine, J. D., and Gordon, N. C. 1984. Influence of the method of drug administration on analgesic response. *Nature* 312:755–56.

Levine, J. D., Gordon, N. C., and Fields, H. L. 1978. The mechanism of placebo analgesia. *Lancet* 2:654–57.

Levine, J. D., Gordon, N. C., Smith, R., et al. 1981. Analgesic responses to morphine and placebo in individuals with postoperative pain. *Pain* 10:379–89.

Lewis, C. T. 1953. *A Latin Dictionary*. Oxford: Clarendon Press.

Lewis, T. L., Karlowski, T. R., Kapikian, A. Z., et al. 1975. A controlled clinical trial of ascorbic acid for the common cold. *Annals of the New York Academy of Sciences* 258:505–12.

Lidren, D. M., Watkins, P. L., Gould, R. A., et al. 1994. A comparison of bibliotherapy and group therapy in the treatment of panic disorder. *Journal of Consulting and Clinical Psychology* 62:865–69.

Lieberman, M. A., Yalom, I. D., and Miles, M. B. 1973. *Encounter Groups: First Facts*. New York: Basic Books.

Lilienfeld, A. M. 1982. Ceteris paribus: The evolution of the clinical trial. *Bulletin of the History of Medicine* 56:1–18.

Lind, J. 1753. *A Treatise of the Scurvy*. Edinburgh: Sands, Murray, and Cochran.

Lipid Research Clinics Program. 1984. The lipid research clinics coronary primary prevention trial results: 1. Reduction in incidence of coronary heart disease. *JAMA* 251:351–64.

Lipman, R. S. 1989. Pharmacotherapy of the anxiety disorders. In S. Fisher and R. P. Greenberg, eds., *The Limits of Biological Treatments for Psychological Distress: Comparisons with Psychotherapy and Placebo*. Hillsdale, N.J.: Lawrence Erlbaum Associates.

Lipsey, M. W., and Wilson, D. B. 1993. The efficacy of psychological, educational, and behavioral treatment: Confirmation from meta-analysis. *American Psychologist* 48:1181–1209.

Lister, J. 1870. On the effects of the antiseptic system upon the salubrity of a surgical hospital. *Lancet* 1:4.

Loftus, E., and Klinger, M. R. 1992. Is the unconscious smart or dumb? *American Psychologist* 47:761–65.

Longstreth, G. F., Fox, D. D., Youkeles, L., et al. 1981. Psyllium therapy in the irritable bowel syndrome. *Annals of Medicine* 95:53–56.

Louis, P.C.A. 1834. *Essay on Clinical Instruction*. Translated by P. Martin. London: S. Highley.

Luborsky, L. 1984. *Principles of Psychoanalytic Psychotherapy: A Manual for Supportive-Expressive Treatment*. New York: Basic Books.

Luborsky, L., and Spence, D. P. 1978. Quantitative research on psychoanalytic therapy. In S. L. Garfield and A. E. Bergin, eds., *Handbook of Psychotherapy and Behavior Change*, 2d ed. New York: Wiley.

Luborsky, L., Singer, B., and Luborsky, L. 1975. Comparative studies of psychotherapies: Is it true that "everyone has won and all must have prizes"? *Archives of General Psychiatry* 32:995–1007.

Macht, D. I. 1915. The history of opium and some of its preparations and alkaloids. *JAMA* 64:477–81.

Macht, D. I., Herman, N. B., and Levy, C. S. 1916. A quantitative study of the analgesia produced by opium alkaloids, individually and in combination with each other, in normal man. *Journal de Pharmacologie* 8:1–37.

Macht, D. I., Greenberg, J., and Isaacs, S. 1919–20. The effect of some antipyretics on the acuity of hearing. *Proceedings of the Society for Experimental Biology and Medicine* 17:22–23.

Majno, G. 1975. *The Healing Hand*. Cambridge: Harvard University Press.

Major, H.H.A. 1954. *A History of Medicine*. Vol. 1. Springfield, Ill.: Charles C Thomas.

Maloy, B. S. 1942. *A Simplified Medical Dictionary for Lawyers*. Chicago: Callaghan.

Mann, C. 1990. Meta-analysis in the breech. *Science* 249:476–80.

Mann, J. 1973. *Time-Limited Psychotherapy*. Cambridge: Harvard University Press.

Margraf, J., Ehlers, A., Roth, W. T., et al. 1991. How "blind" are double-blind studies? *Journal of Consulting and Clinical Psychology* 59:184–87.

Marini, J. L., Sheard, M. H., Bridges, C. I., et al. 1976. An evaluation of the double-blind design in a study comparing lithium carbonate with placebo. *Acta Psychiatrica Scandinavica* 53:343–54.

Marks, H. M. 1987. Ideas as reforms: Therapeutic experiments and medical practice, 1900–1980. Ph.D. diss. Cambridge: Massachusetts Institute of Technology.

———. 1988. Notes from the underground: The social organization of therapeutic research. In R. C. Maulitz and D. E. Long, eds., *Grand Rounds: One Hundred Years of Internal Medicine*. Philadelphia: University of Pennsylvania Press. Pp. 297–336.

———. 1992a. Letter to A. K. Shapiro, July 10.

————. 1992b. Telephone interview by A. K. Shapiro, June 8.

Marnham, P. 1981. *Lourdes.* New York: Coward, McCann, and Geoghegan.

Mason-Browne, N. L., and Borthwick, J. W. 1957. Effect of perphenazine (Trilafon) on modification of crude consciousness. *Diseases of the Nervous System* 18:2–8.

May, P.R.A., and Wittenborn, J. R. 1969. *Psychotropic Drug Response: Advances in Prediction.* Springfield, Ill.: Charles C Thomas.

McIlmoyl, J. 1953. The staff viewpoint on the nucleotide project. *Saskatchewan Psychiatric Services Journal* 5:13–15.

McLean, P. D., and Hakstian, A. R. 1979. Clinical depression: Comparative efficacy of outpatient treatments. *Journal of Consulting and Clinical Psychology* 47:818–36.

Means, J. O. 1876. *The Prayer-Gauge Debate.* Boston: Congregational Publishing Society.

Medical Research Council. 1948. Streptomycin treatment of pulmonary tuberculosis. *British Medical Journal* 2:769–82.

————. 1950. Streptomycin in Tuberculosis Trials Committee and the British Tuberculosis Association Research Committee. *British Medical Journal* 2:1073.

Medical Research Council, Special Committee. 1950. Clinical trials of antihistaminic drugs in the prevention and treatment of the common cold. *British Medical Journal* 2:425–29.

Medical Research Council, Therapeutic Trials Committee. 1934. The serum treatment of lobar pneumonia. *Lancet* 1:290–95.

Miller, J. Z., Nance, W. E., Norton, J. A., et al. 1977. Therapeutic effect of vitamin C: A co-twin control study. *JAMA* 237:248–51.

Miner, R. W., ed. 1955. Reserpine in the treatment of neuropsychiatric, neurological, and related clinical problems. *Annals of the New York Academy of Sciences* 61:1–280.

Minick, C. R., and Haimowitz, B. 1989. A passion for teaching: A profile of Dr. Walter Riker. *Cornell University Medical College Alumni Quarterly* 50:2–13.

Mitchell, P. 1993. Chlorpromazine turns forty. *Psychopharmacology Bulletin* 29:341–34.

Modell, W. 1955a. *The Relief of Symptoms.* Philadelphia: W. B. Saunders.

————. 1955b. Problems in the evaluation of drugs in man. *Journal of Pharmacy and Pharmacology* 2:577–94.

————. 1962. The protean control of clinical pharmacology. *Clinical Pharmacology and Therapeutics* 3:235–38.

————. 1967. Interview by A. K. Shapiro, New York City, October 31.

————. 1976. Origins and development of pharmacology. In W. Modell, H. O. Schild, and H. O. Wilson, eds., *Applied Pharmacology.* Philadelphia: W. B. Saunders. Pp. 7–28.

Modell, W., and Garrett, M. 1960. Interactions between pharmacodynamic and placebo effects in drug evaluations in man. *Nature* 185:538–39.

Modell, W., and Houde, R. W. 1958. Factors influencing clinical evaluation of drugs. *JAMA* 167:2190–98.

Modell, W., and Lansing, A. 1967. *Drugs.* New York: Time.

Modell, W., Gold, H., and Clarke, D. A. 1945. Quantitative observations on mercuhydrin and mercupurin. *Journal of Clinical Investigation* 24:384–87.

Moertel, C. G., Taylor, W. F., Roth, A., et al. 1976. Who responds to sugar pills? *Mayo Clinic Proceedings* 51:96–100.

Montaigne. 1946. *The Essays of Montaigne.* New York: Modern Library.

Morris, M. G. 1992. Interview by A. K. Shapiro, September 2.

Morse, W. 1934. *"Chinese Medicine" Clio Medica: A Series of Primers on the History of Medicine.* Vol. 7. New York: P. B. Hoeber.

Moscucci, M., Byrne, L., Weintraub, M., et al. 1987. Blinding, unblinding, and the placebo effect: An analysis of patients' guesses of treatment assignment in a double-blind clinical trial. *Clinical Pharmacology and Therapeutics* 41:259–65.

Motherby, G. 1785. *A New Medical Dictionary or General Repository of Physics,* 2d ed. London: J. Johnson.

———. 1795. *A New Medical Dictionary or General Repository of Physics,* 4th ed. London: J. Johnson.

———. 1801. *A New Medical Dictionary or General Repository of Physics,* 5th ed. London: J. Johnson.

Mulder, C. I., Emmelkamp, P.M.G., Mulder, J. W., et al. 1992. Immunological and psychosocial effects of a cognitive behavioral vs. an experiential group therapy program for asymptomatic HIV seropositive homosexual men. In *Abstracts of the Eighth International Conference on AIDS, July 19–24.* Amsterdam, The Netherlands. Abstract PoB3809.

Munjack, D. J., Brown, R. A., McDowell, D., et al. 1989. Actual medication versus therapist guesses: In a blind study, how blind is blind [letter to the editor]. *Journal of Clinical Psychopharmacology* 9:148–49.

Murphy, W. F. 1951. Problems in evaluating the results of psychotherapy. *Archives of Neurology and Psychiatry* 66:643.

Nagel, E. 1959. Methodological issues in psychoanalytic theory. In S. Hook, ed., *Psychoanalysis, Scientific Method, and Philosophy.* New York: Grove Press.

Nash, H. 1959. The design and conduct of experiments on the psychological effects of drugs. *Journal of Nervous and Mental Disease* 128:129.

———. 1962. The double-blind procedure: Rationale and empirical evaluation. *Journal of Nervous and Mental Disease* 134:34–47.

Nassif, E. G., Weinberger, M., Thompson, R., et al. 1981. The value of maintenance theophylline in steroid-dependent asthma. *New England Journal of Medicine* 304:71–75.

New English Dictionary on Historical Principles. 1933. Edited by J.A.H. Murray. Oxford: Clarendon Press.

New York Hospital Archives. 1992. Reports on and reprints of H. Gold, W. Riker, and H. Stewart. New York City.

New York State Journal of Medicine. 1993. 93:85–141.

Ney, P. G., Collins, C., and Spensor, C. 1986. Double blind: Double talk or are there ways to do better research. *Medical Hypotheses* 21:119–26.

Nowak, R. 1994. Problems in clinical trials go far beyond misconduct. *Science* 264:1538–41.

Nowlis, V., and Nowlis, H. H. 1956. The description and analysis of mood. *Annals of the New York Academy of Sciences* 65:345–55.

Noyes, A. P. 1948. *Modern Clinical Psychiatry,* 3d ed. Philadelphia: W. B. Saunders.

Ohashi, K. 1995. Memorandum on the origin of Rx, the symbol employed to the heading in the prescription. *Japanese Society for History of Pharmacy* 30:91–95.

O'Neill, M. 1993. A healer for the age of Aquarius. *New York Times,* September 3, Metro Report, p. 45.

Orne, M. T. 1962. On the social psychology of the psychological experiment: With particular reference to demand characteristics and other implications. *American Psychologist* 17:776–83.

Osler, W. 1892. *The Principles and Practice of Medicine.* New York: D. Appleton.

———. 1932. *Medicine in the Nineteenth Century.* In *Aequanimitas,* 3d ed. Philadelphia: P. Blakeston's Son.

Osmond, H. 1970. Letter to A. K. Shapiro, August 4.

Ostling, G. 1970. Letter to A. K. Shapiro, August 24.

Ottenbacher, K. 1992. Impact of random assignment on study outcome: An empirical examination. *Controlled Clinical Trials* 13:50–61.

The Oxford English Dictionary. 1989. 2d ed. Oxford: Clarendon Press.

Oxford English Dictionary: Compact Edition. See *Compact Edition of the Oxford English Dictionary.* 1971.

Pachter, H. M. 1951. *Magic into Science: The Story of Paracelsus.* New York: Henry Schuman.

Palmer, R. S. 1955. The hypotensive action of Rauwolfia serpentina and reserpine: A double hidden placebo study of ambulatory patients with hypertension. *American Practitioner and Digest of Treatment* 6:1323–37.

Park, L. C., and Covi, L. 1965. Nonblind placebo trial: An exploration of neurotic patients' responses to placebo when its inert content is disclosed. *Archives of General Psychiatry* 12:336–45.

Parker, W. B. 1908–9. *Psychotherapy: A Course of Readings in Sound Psychology, Sound Medicine, and Sound Religion.* Vols. 1–3. New York: Centre Publishing.

Parloff, M. B. 1980. Psychotherapy research: An anaclitic depression. *Psychiatry* 43:279–93.

———. 1982. Psychotherapy research evidence and reimbursement decisions: Bambi meets Godzilla. *American Journal of Psychiatry* 139:718–27.

———. 1986. Placebo controls in psychotherapy research: A sine qua non or a placebo for research problems? *Journal of Consulting and Clinical Psychology* 54:79–87.

Parr, B. 1809. *London Medical Dictionary.* London: J. Johnson.

———. 1820. *London Medical Dictionary.* Vols. 1 and 2. Philadelphia: Mitchell Ames and White.

Paulshock, B. Z. 1982. William Heberden, M.D., and the end of theriac. *New York State Journal of Medicine* 82:1612–14.

Penick, S. B., and Fisher, S. 1965. Drug set interaction: Psychological and physiological effects of epinephrine under differential expectations. *Psychosomatic Medicine* 27:177–82.

Pepper, O.H.P. 1945. A note on the placebo. *American Journal of Pharmacology* 117:409.

Perry, S. 1994. In reply [letter to the editor]. *Archives of General Psychiatry* 51:247–48.

Perry, S., and Fishman, B. 1993. Depression and HIV: How does one affect the other. *JAMA* 270:2609–10.

Perry, S., Fishman, B., Jacobsberg, I., et al. 1992. Relationships over one year between lymphocyte subsets and psychosocial variables among adults with infection by human immunodeficiency virus. *Archives of General Psychiatry* 49:396–401.

Pfeiffer, C. C. 1957. Critical discussion of research designs for determining the effect of therapy which may increase or decrease the schizophrenic state. *Modern Hospital* 88:104–10.

Phillips, E. D. 1987. *Aspects of Greek Medicine.* Philadelphia: Charles Press.

Pichot, P. 1970. Interview by A. K. Shapiro, Paris, France, September 2.

Pichot, P., and Oliver-Martin, R. 1974. *Psychological Measurements in Psychopharmacology.* Vol. 7. Basel: S. Karger.

Pierce, C. S., and Jastrow, J. 1885. On small differences of sensation. *Memoirs of the National Academy of Sciences* 3:75–83.

Plotkin, W. B. 1985. A psychological approach to placebo: The role of faith in therapy and treatment. In L. White, B. Tursky, and G. E. Schwartz, eds., *Placebo: Theory, Research, and Mechanisms.* New York: Guilford Press. Pp. 237–54.

Podmore, F. 1963. *From Mesmer to Christian Science.* New Hyde Park, N.Y.: University Books.

Pogge, R. 1963. The toxic placebo. *Medical Times* 91:773–78.

Prien, R. F. 1988. Methods and models for placebo use in psychopharmacotherapeutic trials. *Psychopharmacology Bulletin* 24:4–8.

Prioleau, L., Murdoch, M., and Brody, N. 1983. An analysis of psychotherapy v. placebo studies. *Behavioral and Brain Sciences* 6:275–310.

Propst, L. R., Ostrom, R., Watkins, P., et al. 1992. Comparative efficacy of religious and nonreligious cognitive-behavioral therapy for the treatment of clinical depression in religious individuals. *Journal of Consulting and Clinical Psychology* 60:94–103.

Quen, J. M. 1963. Elisha Perkins, physician, nostrum-vendor, or charlatan? *Bulletin of the History of Medicine* 37:159–66.

Quincy, J. 1787. *Lexicon Physico-Medicum* . . . , 10th ed. London: A. Bell.

———. 1794. *Lexicon Physico-Medicum* . . . , 11th ed. London: A. Bell.

Rabkin, J. G., Markowitz, J. S., Stewart, J., et al. 1986. How blind is blind? Assessment of patient and doctor medication guesses in a placebo-controlled trial of imipramine and phenelzine. *Psychiatric Research* 19:75–86.

Rachman, S., and Wilson, G. T. 1980. *The Effects of Psychological Therapy,* 2d ed. New York: Pergamon Press.

Randell, T. 1993. Morphine receptor cloned: Improved analgesics, addiction therapy expected. *JAMA* 270:1165–66.

Rapport, S., and Wright, H. 1952. *Great Adventures in Medicine*. New York: Dial Press.

Rawlinson, M. C. 1985. Truth-telling and paternalism in the clinic: Philosophical reflections on the use of placebos in medical practice. In L. White, B. Tursky, and G. E. Schwartz, eds., *Placebo: Theory, Research, and Mechanisms*. New York: Guilford Press. Pp. 403–18.

Reinharez, D. 1978. Errors in the placebo test. *Phlebologie* 31:313–20.

Remmen, E., Cohen, S., Ditman, K. S., et al. 1962. *Psychochemotherapy: The Physicians's Manual*. Los Angeles: Western Medical Publications.

Reyburn, R. 1990. Curiosities of homeopathic pharmacy: One hundred years ago. *JAMA* 264:1724.

Reznikoff, M., and Toomey, L. C. 1959. *Evaluation of Changes Associated with Psychiatric Treatment*. Springfield, Ill.: Charles C Thomas.

Rickels, K. 1968. *Non-Specific Factors in Drug Therapy*. Springfield, Ill.: Charles C Thomas.

———. 1986. Use of placebo in clinical trials. *Psychopharmacology Bulletin* 22:19–24.

Rickels, K., Raab, E., and Carranza, J. 1965. Doctor medication guesses: An indicator of clinical improvement in double-blind studies. *Journal of New Drugs* 5:67–71.

Rickels, K., Hesbacher, P. T., Weise, C. C., et al. 1970a. Pills and improvement: A study of placebo response in psychoneurotic outpatients. *Psychopharmacologia* (Berlin) 16:318–28.

Rickels, K., Lipman, R. S., Fisher, S., et al. 1970b. Is a double-blind clinical trial really double-blind? A report of doctors' medication guesses. *Psychopharmacologia* (Berlin) 16:329–36.

Riker, W. 1992. Telephone interview with A. K. Shapiro, New Jersey.

Rinkel, M. 1963. *Specific and Non-Specific Factors in Psychopharmacology*. New York: Philosophic Library.

Rinzler, S. H., Bakst, H., Benjamin, Z. H., et al. 1950. Failure of alpha tocopherol to influence chest pain in patients with heart disease. *Circulation* 1:288–93.

Rivers, W.H.R. 1908. *The Influence of Alcohol and Other Drugs on Fatigue*. London: Arnold.

———. 1927. *Medicine, Magic, and Religion*. London: Macmillan.

Robbins, F. C. 1993. Eradication of polio in the Americas. *JAMA* 270:1857–59.

Roberts, A. H., Kewman, D. G., Mercier, L., et al. 1993. The power of nonspecific effects in healing: Implications for psychosocial and biological treatment. *Clinical Psychology Review* 13:375–91.

Roccatagliata, G. 1986. *A History of Ancient Psychiatry*. New York: Greenwood Press.

Rose, G. 1982. Bias. *British Journal of Clinical Pharmacology* 13:157–62.

Rose, L. 1971. *Faith Healing*. Harmondsworth, Middlesex, England: Penguin Books.

Rosen, G. 1968. *Madness in Society*. Chicago: University of Chicago Press.

Rosenthal, D., and Frank, J. D. 1956. Psychotherapy and the placebo effect. *Psychological Bulletin* 55:294.

Rosenthal, R. 1966. *Experimenter Effects in Behavioral Research*. New York: Appleton-Century-Crofts.

———. 1970. Letter to A. K. Shapiro, August 10, 1970.

———. 1985. Designing, analyzing, interpreting, and summarizing placebo studies. In L. White, B. Tursky, and G. E. Schwartz, eds., *Placebo: Theory, Research, and Mechanisms.* New York: Guilford Press. Pp. 110–36.

Rosenthal, R., and Rosnow, R. L. 1975. *The Volunteer Subject.* New York: John Wiley and Sons.

Ross, O.B.J. 1951. Use of controls in medical research. *JAMA* 145:72–75.

Ross, S., and Buckalew, L. W. 1985. Placebo agentry: Assessment of drug and placebo effects. In L. White, B. Tursky, and G. E. Schwartz, eds., *Placebo: Theory, Research, and Mechanisms.* New York: Guilford Press. Pp. 67–82.

Rothman, D. J. 1991. *Strangers at the Bedside.* New York: Basic Books.

Roueché, B. 1960. Annals of medicine: Placebo. *New Yorker,* October 15, p. 85.

Rubin, S. 1974. *Medieval English Medicine.* New York: Barnes and Noble.

Sainz, A., Biegelow, N., and Barwise, C. 1957. On a methodology for the clinical evaluation of phrenopraxic drugs. *Psychiatric Quarterly* 31:10.

Salter, A. 1952. *The Case against Psychoanalysis.* New York: Henry Holt.

Sandifer, M. G., and Hawkings, D. R. 1958. A double-blind study of the effects of drugs on mood, mentation, and sedation. Paper presented at the convention of the American Psychiatric Association, San Francisco, May 15.

Sargant, W., and Slater, E. 1956. *An Introduction to Physical Methods of Treatment in Psychiatry,* 3d ed. Edinburgh: E. and S. Livingstone.

Schafer, A. 1982. The ethics of the randomized clinical trial. *New England Journal of Medicine* 307:719–21.

Scheff, T. J. 1979. *Catharsis in Healing, Ritual, and Drama.* Berkeley: University of California Press.

Schmideberg, M. 1958. Values and goals in psychotherapy. *Psychiatric Quarterly* 32:234.

Schmidt, F. L. 1992. What do data really mean? Research findings, meta-analysis, and cumulative knowledge in psychology. *American Psychologist* 47:1173–81.

Schulz, K. F., Chalmers, I., Hayes, R. J., et al. 1995. Empirical evidence of bias. *JAMA* 273:408–12.

Scriven, M. 1959. The experimental investigation of psychoanalysis. In S. Hook, ed., *Psychoanalysis, Scientific Method, and Philosophy.* New York: Grove Press.

Seigworth, G. R. 1980. Bloodletting over the centuries. *New York State Journal of Medicine* December:2022–28.

Shadish, W. R., Montgomery, L. M., Wilson, P., et al. 1993. Effects of family and marital psychotherapies: A meta-analysis. *Journal of Consulting and Clinical Psychology* 61:992–1002.

Shapiro, A. K. 1956. An attempt to demonstrate a catatonigenic agent in cerebro-spinal fluid of catatonic patients. *Journal of Nervous and Mental Disease* 123:65–71.

———. 1959. The placebo effect in the history of medical treatment. *American Journal of Psychiatry* 116:298–304.

――――. 1960a. Attitudes toward the use of placebos in treatment. *Journal of Nervous and Mental Disease* 130:200–211.

――――. 1960b. A contribution to a history of the placebo effect. *Behavioral Science* 5:109–35.

――――. 1963. The psychological use of medication. In H. I. Lief, V. F. Lief, and N. R. Lief, eds., *The Psychological Basis of Medical Practice*. New York: Harper Brothers.

――――. 1964a. Etiological factors in placebo effect. *JAMA* 187:712–14.

――――. 1964b. Factors contributing to the placebo effect and their implications for psychotherapy. *American Journal of Psychotherapy* 18:73–88.

――――. 1964c. A historic and heuristic definition of the placebo. *Psychiatry* 27:52–58.

――――. 1964d. Placebogenics and iatroplacebogenics. *Medical Times* 92:1037–43.

――――. 1964e. Rational use of psychopharmaceuticals. *New York State Journal of Medicine* 64:1084–95.

――――. 1964f. Rejoinder. *Psychiatry* 27:178–81.

――――. 1964g. Review: *Specific and Non-Specific Factors in Psychopharmacology*, edited by M. Rinkel. *Psychosomatic Medicine* 26:193–94.

――――. 1968. Semantics of the placebo. *Psychiatric Quarterly* 42:653–95.

――――. 1969. Iatroplacebogenics. *International Pharmacopsychiatry* 2:215–48.

――――. 1971. Placebo effects in psychotherapy and psychoanalysis. In A. E. Bergin and S. L. Garfield, eds., *Handbook of Psychotherapy and Behavior Change*. New York: Aldine Publishing. Pp. 439–73.

――――. 1976. Psychochemotherapy. In R. G. Grenell and S. Gabay, eds., *Biological Foundations of Psychiatry*. New York: Raven Press. Pp. 793–836.

――――. 1978. The placebo effect. In W. G. Clark and J. Del Guidice, eds., *Principles of Psychopharmacology*. New York: Academic Press.

――――. 1984. Opening comments. In J.B.W. Williams and R. L. Spitzer, eds., *Psychotherapy Research: Where Are We and Where Should We Go?* New York: Guilford Press. Pp. 106–7.

Shapiro, A. K., and Morris, L. 1978. The placebo effect in healing. In S. L. Garfield and A. E. Bergin, eds., *Handbook of Psychotherapy and Behavior Change*. New York: Aldine Publishing. Pp. 477–536.

Shapiro, A. K., and Shapiro, E. 1984a. Controlled study of pimozide vs. placebo in Tourette syndrome. *Journal of the American Academy of Child Psychiatry* 23:161–73.

――――. 1984b. Patient-provider relationships and the placebo effect. In J. D. Matarazzo, S. M. Weiss, J. A. Herd, et al., eds., *Behavioral Health: A Handbook of Health Enhancement and Disease Prevention*. New York: John Wiley and Sons. Pp. 371–83.

Shapiro, A. K., and Struening, E. L. 1973a. Defensiveness in the definition of placebo. *Comprehensive Psychiatry* 14:107–20.

――――. 1973b. The use of placebos: A study of ethics and physicians' attitudes. *Psychiatric Medicine* 4:17–29.

————. 1974. A comparison of the attitudes of a sample of physicians about the effectiveness of their treatment and the treatment of other physicians. *Journal of Psychiatric Research* 10:217–29.

Shapiro, A. K., Dussik, C. T., and Tolentino, J. C., et al. 1960. A "browsing" double blind study of iponiazid in geriatric patients. *Diseases of the Nervous System* 21:223.

Shapiro, A. K., Frick, R., Morris, L., et al. 1974. Placebo induced side effects. *Journal of Operational Psychiatry* 6:43–46.

Shapiro, A. K., Shapiro, E., Young, J. G., et al. 1988. *Gilles de la Tourette Syndrome*, 2d ed. New York: Raven Press.

Shapiro, A. K., Struening, E. L., Barten, H., et al. 1975. Correlates of placebo reaction in an outpatient population. *Psychological Medicine* 5:389–96.

Shapiro, A. K., Struening, E. L., and Shapiro, E. 1980. Reliability and validity of a placebo test. *Journal of Psychiatric Research* 15:253–90.

Shapiro, A. K., Struening, E. L., Shapiro, E., et al. 1983. Diazepam: How much better than placebo? *Journal of Psychiatric Research* 17:51–73.

Shapiro, A. K., Wilensky, H., and Struening, E. 1968. Study of the placebo effect with a placebo test. *Comprehensive Psychiatry* 9:118–37.

Shapiro, D. A., and Shapiro, D. 1982. Meta-analysis of comparative therapy outcome studies: A replication and refinement. *Psychological Bulletin* 92:581–604.

Shapiro, D. A., Barkham, M., Rees, A., et al. 1994. Effects of treatment duration and severity of depression on the effectiveness of cognitive-behavioral and psychodynamic-interpersonal psychotherapy. *Journal of Consulting and Clinical Psychology* 62:522–34.

Shapiro, E., Shapiro, A. K., Fulop, G., et al. 1989. Controlled study of haloperidol, pimozide, and placebo for the treatment of Gilles de la Tourette's syndrome. *Archives of General Psychiatry* 46:722–30.

Shear, M. K., Pilkonis, P. A., Cloitre, M., et al. 1994. Cognitive behavioral treatment compared with nonprescriptive treatment of panic disorder. *Archives of General Psychiatry* 51:395–401.

Shepard, O. 1930. *The Lore of the Unicorn.* Boston: Houghton Mifflin.

Shepherd, M. 1979. Psychoanalysis, psychotherapy, and health services. *British Medical Journal* 2:1557–59.

Shlien, J. M., Mosak, H. H., and Dreikurs, R. 1962. Effect on time limits: A comparison of two psychotherapies. *Journal of Counseling Psychology* 9:31–34.

Sifneos, P. 1972. *Short-time Psychotherapy and Emotional Crisis.* Cambridge: Harvard University Press.

Sigerist, H. E. 1958. *The Great Doctors.* New York: Doubleday.

Silverman, W. A. 1979. Controlled trials and medical ethics. *Lancet* 1:160–61.

————. 1989. The myth of informed consent: In daily practice and in clinical trials. *Journal of Medical Ethics* 15:6–11.

Silverman, W. A., and Chalmers, I. 1992. Sir Austin Bradford Hill: An appreciation. *Controlled Clinical Trials* 13:100–105.

Simmons, B. 1978. Problems in deceptive medical procedures: An ethical and legal analysis of the administration of placebos. *Journal of Medical Ethics* 4:176.

Sixty Plus Reinfarction Study Research Group. 1980. A double-blind trial to assess long-term oral anticoagulant therapy in elderly patients after myocardial infarction. *Lancet* 2:989–93.

Sledge, W. H. 1994. Psychotherapy in the United States: Challenges and opportunities. *American Journal of Psychiatry* 151:1267–70.

Sleisenger, M. H. 1958. Reply to Dr. Tomenius. *American Journal of Digestive Diseases* 3:415–16.

Sloane, R. B., and Staples, F. R. 1984. Psychotherapy versus behavior therapy: Implications for future psychotherapy research. In J.B.W. Williams and R. L. Spitzer, eds., *Psychotherapy Research: Where Are We and Where Should We Go?* New York: Guilford Press. Pp. 203–14.

Sloane, R. B., Staples, F. R., Cristol, A. H., et al. 1975. *Psychotherapy versus Behavior Therapy.* Cambridge: Harvard University Press.

Smith, J. A., and Wittson, L. L. 1957. Evaluation of treatment procedures in psychiatry. *Diseases of the Nervous System* 18:1.

Smith, M. L., and Glass, C. V. 1977. Meta-analysis of psychotherapy outcome studies. *American Psychologist* 32:752–60.

Smith, M. L., Glass, G. V., and Miller, T. J. 1980. *The Benefits of Psychotherapy.* Baltimore: Johns Hopkins University Press.

Smith Kline and French. 1962. "Do-nothing" drugs: Placebos in pharmaceutical research. *Psychiatric Reporter* 3:3.

Smyrnios, K. X., and Kirkby, R. J. 1993. Long-term comparison of brief versus unlimited psychodynamic treatments with children and their parents. *Journal of Consulting and Clinical Psychology* 61:1020–27.

Sollmann, T. 1912. Experimental therapeutics. *JAMA* 58:242–44.

———. 1916. The Therapeutic Research Committee. *JAMA* 67:1439–42.

———. 1917. The crucial test of therapeutic evidence. *JAMA* 69:198–99.

———. 1930. The evaluation of therapeutic remedies in the hospital. *JAMA* 94:1279–81.

Solomon, R. L. 1949. An extension of control group design. *Psychological Bulletin* 46:137–50.

Spiegel, D. 1993. Psychosocial intervention in cancer. *Journal of the National Cancer Institute* 85:1198–1205.

Sprott, D. A. 1968. A theoretical examination of double-blind design [letter to the editor]. *Canadian Medical Association Journal* 98:124.

Stallone, F., Mendlewicz, J., and Fieve, R. R. 1974. How blind is the double-blind? An assessment in a lithium-prophylaxis study [letter to the editor]. *Lancet* 1:619–20.

————. 1975. Double-blind procedure: An assessment in a study of lithium prophylaxis. *Psychological Medicine* 5:78–82.

Standards Reporting Trials Group. 1994. A proposal for structured reporting of randomized controlled trials. *JAMA* 272:1926–31.

Stanley, B. 1988. An integration of ethical and clinical considerations in the use of placebos. *Psychopharmacology Bulletin* 24:18–20.

Stein, M. 1992. Future directions for brain, behavior, and the immune system. *Bulletin of the New York Academy of Medicine* 68:390–410.

Stein, M., Miller, A. H., and Trestman, R. L. 1991. Depression, the immune system, and health and illness: Findings in search of meaning. *Archives of General Psychiatry* 48:171–78.

Stein, S., Hermanson, K., and Spiegel, D. 1993. New directions in psycho-oncology. *Current Opinion in Psychiatry* 6:838–46.

Steinmark, S. W., and Borkovec, T. D. 1974. Active and placebo treatment effects on moderate insomnia under counterdemand and positive demand instructions. *Journal of Abnormal Psychology* 83:157–63.

Stevens, W. K. 1993. Want a room with a view: Idea may be in the genes. *New York Times,* November 30, C1, C13.

Strupp, H. H. 1994. Retrospective review: *Psychoanalytic Therapy,* by F. Alexander and T. M. French (New York: Ronald Press, 1946). *Contemporary Psychology* 39:355–57.

Strupp, H. H., and Binder, J. L. 1982. *Time Limited Dynamic Psychotherapy (TKDP): A Treatment Manual.* Nashville, Tenn.: Vanderbilt University, Center for Psychotherapy Research, Department of Psychology.

Strupp, H. H., and Hadley, S. W. 1979. Specific vs. nonspecific factors in psychotherapy. *Archives of General Psychiatry* 36:1125–36.

Sutton, H. G., 1865. Cases of rheumatic fever treated for the most part by mint water. *Guy's Hospital Report* 2:392.

Taber, C. W. 1905. *Taber's Medical Dictionary for Nurses.* N.p.: C. W. Taber.

Temoshok, L., Heller, B. W., and Sageviel, R. W. 1985. The relationship of psychological factors of prognostic indicators in cutaneous malignant melanoma. *Journal of Psychosomatic Research* 28:139–53.

Terry, C. E., and Pellens, M. 1928. *The Opium Problem.* New York: Bureau of Social Hygiene.

Tetreault, L., and Bordeleau, J. M. 1971. On the usefulness of the placebo and of the double-blind technique in the evaluation of psychotropic drugs. *Psychopharmacology Bulletin* 7:44–54.

Thompson, L. W., Gallagher, D., and Breckenridge, J. S. 1987. Comparative effectiveness of psychotherapies for depressed elders. *Journal of Consulting and Clinical Psychology* 55:385–90.

Thomson, R. 1982. Side effects and placebo amplification. *British Journal of Psychiatry* 140:64–68.

Thorndike, E. L., and Woodworth, R. S. 1901. The influence of improvement in one mental function upon the efficiency of other functions. *Psychological Review* 8:553–64.

Thorner, M. W. 1935. The psycho-pharmacology of sodium amytal. *Journal of Nervous and Mental Disease* 81:161–67.

Tibbets, R. W., and Hawkings, J. R. 1956. The placebo response. *Journal of Mental Science* 102:60–66.

Tomenius, J. 1958. The double-blind test in the evaluation of the therapeutic effect of drugs. *American Journal of Digestive Diseases* 3:411–15.

Torrey, E. F. 1972. What western psychotherapists can learn from witchdoctors. *American Journal of Orthopsychiatry* 42:69–76.

———. 1992. *Freudian Fraud.* New York: Harper Collins.

Travell, J. 1953. Assessment of drugs for therapeutic efficacy. *American Journal of Physical Medicine* 34:129–40.

Trohler, U. 1978. Quantification in British medicine and surgery, 1750–1830, with special reference to its introduction into therapeutics. Ph.D. diss. London: University College.

Trousseau, A. 1833. *Dictionnaire de médecine* Paris: Libraire de la Faculté de Médecine. Translated in H. Bernheim, *Suggestive Therapeutics.* New York: G. A. Putnam's Sons, 1889.

Trouton, D. S. 1957. Placebos and their psychological effects. *Journal of Mental Science* 103:344–54.

Tuke, H. 1886. *Le corps et l'esprit: Action du moral et de l'imagination sur le physique.* Paris. Translated in H. Bernheim, *Suggestive Therapeutics.* New York: G. A. Putnam's Sons, 1989.

Turner, J. L., Gallimore, R., and Fox-Hemming, C. 1980. An annotated bibliography of placebo research. Manuscript 2063, pts. 1 and 2. Abstracted in *Journal Supplement Abstract Service Catalog of Selected Documents in Psychology* 10:1–296.

Turner, R. M., and Ascher, L. M. 1979. Controlled comparison of progressive relaxation, stimulus control, and paradoxical intention therapies for insomnia. *Journal of Consulting and Clinical Psychology* 47:500–508.

Twain, M. 1899. *Christian Science.* New York: Harper.

Tyler, V. E., Brady, L. R., and Robbers, J. E. 1976. *Pharmacology,* 7th ed. Philadelphia: Lea and Febiger.

Ubell, E. 1959. Why useless drugs often cure patients. *New York Herald Tribune,* October 10.

Uhr, L., and Miller, J. G. 1960. *Drugs and Behavior.* New York: John Wiley and Sons.

Usdin, M. E., and Efron, D. H. 1967. *Psychotropic Drugs and Related Compounds.* Washington, D.C.: U.S. Department of Health, Education, and Welfare, Health Services and Mental Health Administration.

———. 1972. *Psychotropic Drugs and Related Compounds,* 2d ed. Washington, D.C.: U.S.

Department of Health, Education, and Welfare, Health Services and Mental Health Administration.

U.S. Department of Health, Education, and Welfare. 1966. *Report on Current and Emerging Problems of the Food and Drug Administration.* Washington, D.C.: U.S. Department of Health, Education, and Welfare.

U.S. Food and Drug Administration (FDA). 1970. Adequate and well-controlled clinical evaluations. *Federal Register* 35:7250.

————. 1974. Guidelines for psychotropic drugs. *Psychopharmacology Bulletin* 10:184.

————. 1978. Guidelines for the clinical evaluation of psychotropic drugs: Antidepressants and antianxiety drugs. *Psychopharmacology Bulletin* 14:45–63.

U.S. Office of the Adjutant General. 1947. *Trials of War Criminals.* Vol. 2. Washington, D.C.: Government Printing Office.

U.S. Public Health Service. 1966. *Policy and Procedure Order No. 129, July 1.* Washington, D.C.: U.S. Government Printing Office.

Van Dyke, H. B. 1947. The weapons of panacea. *Science Monthly* 64:322.

Veith, I. 1972. *The Yellow Emperor's Classic of Internal Medicine,* new ed. Berkeley: University of California Press.

Volgyesi, F. A. 1954. "School for patients" hypnosis-therapy and psychoprophylaxis. *British Journal of Medical Hypnotism* 5:8.

Von Felsinger, J. M., Lasagna, L., and Beecher, H. K. 1955. Drug-induced mood changes in man: Personality and reaction to drugs. *JAMA* 157:1113–19.

Von Sholly, A. L., and Park, W. H. 1921. Report of the prophylactic vaccination of 1536 persons against acute respiratory diseases, 1919–1920. *Journal of Immunology* 6:103–15.

Waife, S. O., and Shapiro, A. P., eds. 1959. *The Clinical Evaluation of New Drugs.* New York: Paul B. Hoeber.

Walker, K. 1959. *The Story of Medicine.* Tiptree, Essex: Anchor Press.

Walton, A. H. 1958. *Aphrodisiacs: From Legend to Prescription.* Westport, Conn.: Associated Booksellers.

Watson, G. 1966. *Theriac and Mithridatium: A Study in Therapeutics.* Vol. 9. London: Wellcome Historical Medical Library.

Waxler-Morrison, N., Hislop, T. G., and Mears, B. 1992. Effects of social relationships on survival for women with breast cancer: A prospective study. *Social Science and Medicine* 33:177–83.

Wayne, E. J. 1956. Placeboes. *British Medical Journal* 11:157.

Webster's An American Dictionary of the English Language. 1838. New York: N.N.J. White.

Webster's New International Dictionary of the English Language. 1934. 2d ed. Springfield, Mass.: G. and C. Merriam.

Webster's Third New International Dictionary. 1961. Springfield, Mass.: G. and C. Merriam.

Webster-Stratton, C., Hollinsworth, T., and Kolpacoff, M. 1989. The long-term effectiveness and clinical significance of three cost-effective training programs for families with conduct-problem children. *Journal of Consulting and Clinical Psychology* 57:550–53.

Weinberger, M. A. 1973. The blind technique. *Science* 282:219–20.

Weintraub, W., and Aronson, H. 1963. Clinical judgment in psychopharmacological research. *Journal of Neuropsychiatry* 5:65–70.

Weisz, J. R., Weiss, B., and Donenberg, G. R. 1992. The lab versus the clinic: Effects of child and adolescent psychotherapy. *American Psychologist* 47:1578–85.

Welsh, A. L. 1958. *Psychotherapeutic Drugs.* Springfield, Ill.: Charles C Thomas.

White, L., Tursky, B., and Schwartz, G. E., eds. 1985. *Placebo: Theory, Research, and Mechanisms.* New York: Guilford Press.

White, L., Kando, J., Park, T., et al. 1992. Side effects and the "blindability" of clinical drug trials. *American Journal of Psychiatry* 149:1730–31.

White, S. 1985. Medicine's humble humbug: Four periods in the understanding of the placebo. *Pharmacy History* 27:51–60.

Whitehorn, J. C. 1958. Psychiatric implications of the "placebo effect." *American Journal of Psychiatry* 114:662–64.

Wickramasekera, I. 1985. A conditioned response model of the placebo effect: Predictions from the model. In L. White, B. Tursky, and G. E. Schwartz, eds., *Placebo: Theory, Research, and Mechanisms.* New York: Guilford Press. Pp. 255–87.

Wilkins, W. 1985. Placebo controls and concepts in chemotherapy and psychotherapy research. In L. White, B. Tursky, and G. E. Schwartz, eds., *Placebo: Theory, Research, and Mechanisms.* New York: Guilford Press. Pp. 83–109.

Williams, J.B.W., and Spitzer, R. L. 1984. *Psychotherapy Research: Where Are We and Where Should We Go?* New York: Guilford Press.

Williams, J.B.W., Rabkin, J. G., Remien, R. H., et al. 1991. Multidisciplinary baseline assessment of homosexual men with and without human immunodeficiency virus infection. *Archives of General Psychiatry* 48:124–30.

Wilson, C.W.M. 1962. An analysis of factors contributing to placebo responses. *Proceedings of the Royal Society of Medicine* 55:780–85.

Wilson, E. O. 1978. *On Human Nature.* Cambridge: Harvard University Press.

———. 1984. *The Biophilia Hypothesis.* Cambridge: Harvard University Press.

Wilson, J. R. 1960. *The Double Blind.* New York: Doubleday.

Witts, L. J. 1960. Controlled clinical trials. Papers presented at the conference of the Council for International Organization of Medical Scientists. Oxford: Blackwell Scientific Publications.

Wolberg, L. 1977. *The Technique of Psychotherapy,* 3d ed. New York: Grune and Stratton.

Wolf, S. 1950. Effects of suggestion and conditioning on the action of chemical agents in human subjects: The pharmacology of placebos. *Journal of Clinical Investigation* 29:100–109.

———. 1955. The evaluation of therapy in disease. *Transactions of the American Clinical and Climatological Association* 66:61–75.

————. 1959a. Placebos. In D. R. Lawrence, ed., *Quantitative Methods in Human Pharmacology and Therapeutics.* New York: Pergamon Press.

————. 1959b. The pharmacology of placebos. *Pharmacological Reviews* 2:689–704.

————. 1968. Telephone interview by A. K. Shapiro, Tulsa, Okla., May 17.

————. 1992. Telephone interview by A. K. Shapiro, Tulsa, Okla., August 20.

Wolf, S., and Pinsky, R. H. 1954. Effects of placebo administration and occurrence of toxic reactions. *JAMA* 155:339–41.

Wolf, S., and Wolff, H. G. 1947. *Human Gastric Function: An Experimental Study of a Man and His Stomach,* 2d ed. New York: Oxford University Press.

Wolf, S., Doering, C. R., Clark, M. L., et al. 1957. Chance distribution and the placebo reactor. *Journal of Laboratory and Clinical Medicine* 49:37.

World Health Assembly. 1976. Declaration of Tokyo. *Bulletin of the American College of Physicians* 17:15.

World Medical Association. 1964. Declaration of Helsinki. Pamphlet of the Eighteenth World Medical Assembly. New York: World Medical Association. Pp. 4–7.

World Psychiatric Association. 1977. Declaration of Hawaii. *British Medical Journal* 2:1204–5.

Wyckoff, J., Du Bois, E. F., and Woodruff, I. O. 1930. The therapeutic value of digitalis in pneumonia. *JAMA* 95:1243–49.

Young, J. H. 1961. *Toadstool Millionaires.* Princeton, N.J.: Princeton University Press.

————. 1967. *The Medical Messiahs.* Princeton, N.J.: Princeton University Press.

————. 1992. *American Health Quackery.* Princeton, N.J.: Princeton University Press.

Yusuf, S., Wittes, J., Probstfield, J., et al. 1991. Analysis and interpretation of treatment effects in subgroups of patients in randomized clinical trials. *JAMA* 266:93–96.

Zifferblatt, S. M., and Wilbur, C. S. 1978. A psychological perspective for double-blind trials. *Clinical Pharmacology and Therapeutics* 23:1–10.

Zilboorg G., and Henry, G. W. 1941. *A History of Medical Psychology.* New York: W. W. Norton.

Zorc, J. J., Larson, D. B., Lyons, J. S., et al. 1991. Expenditures for psychotropic medications in the United States in 1985. *Journal de Psychologie Normale et Pathologique* 148:644–67.

Zweig, S. 1932. *Mental Healers: Franz Anton Mesmer, Mary Baker Eddy, Sigmund Freud.* Translated by E. C. Paul. New York: Viking Press.

Index

Library of Congress Cataloging-in-Publication Data

Shapiro, Arthur K., 1923–1995.

    The powerful placebo : from ancient priest to modern physician /
Arthur K. Shapiro and Elaine Shapiro.

      p.   cm.

    Includes bibliographical references and index.

    ISBN 0-8018-5569-1 (alk. paper)

    1. Placebo (Medicine)   2. Clinical trials.   I. Shapiro, Elaine.
II. Title.

    [DNLM: 1. Placebo Effect.   2. Placebos—history.   WB 330 S529p
1997]

RM331.S53   1997

615.5'8'072—dc21

DNLM/DLC

for Library of Congress   97-6754
                                                      CIP